The natural way to
BETTER
BABIES

PRECONCEPTION HEALTH CARE
for PROSPECTIVE PARENTS

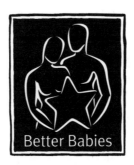

Better Babies

For our children and our children's children

FRANCESCA NAISH &
JANETTE ROBERTS

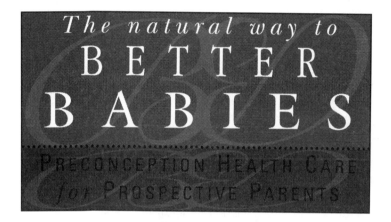

The natural way to
BETTER
BABIES

PRECONCEPTION HEALTH CARE
for PROSPECTIVE PARENTS

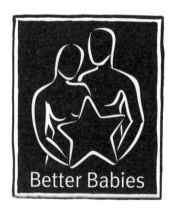

Better Babies

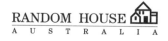

RANDOM HOUSE
AUSTRALIA

Random House Australia Pty Ltd
20 Alfred Street, Milsons Point, NSW 2061

Sydney New York Toronto
London Auckland Johannesburg
and agencies throughout the world

First published in 1996

National Library of Australia
Cataloguing-in-Publication Data

Naish, Francesca.
    The natural way to better babies.

    Includes index.
    ISBN 0 09 183 135 0

    1. Preconception care. 2. Prenatal care. 3. Pregnant women–
    Health and hygiene. 4. Parenthood. I. Roberts, Janette.
    II. Title

618.24

Design by Yolande Gray
Illustrations by Jacqueline Bateman
Text diagrams and illustrations by Anna Warren

Typeset by DOCUPRO, Sydney
Printed by Griffin Press Pty Ltd, Adelaide
A Division of PMP Communications

10 9 8 7

ABOUT THE AUTHORS

ABOUT FRANCESCA

Francesca Naish was born in England in 1946. She studied mathematics at Sussex University, but after arrival in Australia, when in her late twenties, established a Natural Birth Control practice in Paddington, Sydney. This grew into The Village Healing and Growth Centre, one of the first holistic health-care practices in Australia. Since 1994 she has trained health professionals in the use of her unique Natural Fertility Management techniques. In 1995, after 20 years in clinical practice, she established the Jocelyn Centre in Woollahra, Sydney. This is the first clinic in Australia to specialise in natural methods for fertility management, reproductive health and preconception care. Francesca is a qualified naturopath, herbalist and hypnotherapist. She writes extensively for the press, appears regularly on radio and television and is sought after as a public speaker and lecturer. She also pioneered the teaching in Australia of natural vision improvement. She has written two previous books *The Lunar Cycle* (1989) and *Natural Fertility* (1991). Francesca lives in Bondi with her family.

ABOUT JANETTE

Janette Roberts was born in Sydney in 1947. She graduated with an Honours Degree in Pharmacy from Sydney University in 1968.

During the next 20 years she worked in London and then in Sydney as a community pharmacist. She received a postgraduate diploma in clinical nutrition in 1983. Janette retired from her full-time pharmacy career before the birth of her first child in 1985 and since then she has been a stay-at-home mother. In 1987 she became the Australian secretary of Foresight—the Association for the Promotion of Preconception Care. To further the work of the Association she has distributed regular newsletters, appeared on radio and television, lectured to health professionals and written numerous articles on the benefits of preconception care. *Better Babies* is her first book. Janette lives in Birchgrove with her partner and their two sons.

ACKNOWLEDGMENTS

FRANCESCA'S ACKNOWLEDGMENTS

Acknowledging the sources of the seeds of inspiration, their germination into ideas, and then the (sometimes almost uncontrollable) growth of these ideas into a book, is an almost impossible task. For me, this book is the outcome of 20 years in clinical practice and all that this involves. Those who have been influential over this time and helped my understanding of, and ability to treat, the numerous facets of reproductive health are innumerable, so before I begin, my heartfelt thanks to all those who have ever worked with, and contributed to, the areas that we cover in this book. No author, or therapist, can start from scratch. We all build on each other's work and hopefully our book is just another step on the way, for others to take further.

There are, however, some particular thanks due—firstly to all those at the Village Healing and Growth Centre, one of Sydney's first holistic health centres, which grew around my practice and which helped my practice grow. My second home and family for 20 years, this has now evolved into the Jocelyn Centre for Natural Fertility Management and Holistic Medicine. My team of colleagues has given me enormous support, without which I could never have stretched my working days to meet the needs of this book. Special thanks go to Jane Bennett for her contributions on yoga and in many other areas, to Vicki Turner for her expertise and many suggestions, to Miriam Camara and Sally Charles for advice on acupressure points, to Jane Zabrana for her medical knowledge, to Sarah Parsons and Karina Quinlan for typing my incomprehensible scrawl (being a Luddite my first draft is always handwritten) and to Anna Brennan, Veronica Sumegi and Pamela Williams for their 'holiday homes' to work in (some day I'll be back for a holiday).

If it weren't for my clients, of course, I would not have been spurred ever onwards to learn what they, and I, needed to know, and if they (the majority of them anyway) had not been such delightful people, I might not have done it with such enthusiasm.

Many of those whose work I have drawn on were acknowledged in my previous book, *Natural Fertility*, but there has been one particularly important influence since then. This is the work of Foresight, the British Medical Association for the Promotion of Preconception Care. Their findings have brought a new dimension and legitimacy to my work which, funded as it is only by my own earnings in practice, has of necessity been focused more towards clinical practice than research and evaluation. To my co-author, Jan Roberts, the Australian secretary of this association, I owe a huge debt. Her skills and knowledge, through her newsletters, were invaluable to me well before we met, and our working relationship while writing *Better Babies* has been a delight. With a life already full to overflowing, without her I could never have taken on this project. She has done much more than her share of the 'legwork' for which I am eternally grateful.

Further thanks go to Margaret Sullivan of Random House, for persuading me to write the book in the first place, and for her patience in being handed a manuscript which was twice as long as she wanted. Thanks also to Julia Cain, our editor, for helping us to reduce it in ways which still left it intact, and for her meticulous care with the text. My dear friend Jacqueline Bateman has once again contributed beautiful illustrations to add to the great work done by Yolande Gray our designer, and Anna Warren who produced the text diagrams and illustrations. Thanks also to our proofreader, Ella Martin, and our indexer, Barbara Crighton.

My previous publisher, Sally Milner, deserves great thanks for allowing me to build on the information in *Natural Fertility*, making *Better Babies* a wonderful complement for my previously published work, and for her support through the growth of Natural Fertility Management.

Lastly, my love and thanks to my family, past and present. To my mother, Jocelyn, the first environmentalist I ever met, who passed on to me her gift with words and her belief in individual integrity, and on her recent death made it financially possible for me to start my new centre. To my present family, for their forbearance when my attention and time are absorbed by work. To Malcolm, my partner, for helping plan and raise our two 'better babies' who prove that it has all been worthwhile!

JANETTE'S ACKNOWLEDGMENTS

This list would be incomplete if I did not first acknowledge the (unwitting) contribution of my grandmother, Elizabeth Henderson. It was her chronic asthma, treated most successfully in the 1930s with healthy diet and herbal medicine, which led directly to my interest in all that follows. My mother, Margaret Roberts, who fed me salads when all around were eating chocolate spread on white bread, also has a lot to answer for. She alone must accept responsibility for my lifetime of excellent health, and for my unshakeable belief in myself and my actions.

My training in clinical nutrition was made a reality by Dr Robert Buist who also planted the seeds which led to this book. My initial interest in the work of the Foresight Association I owe to Dr Stephen Davies (UK) and special thanks must go to Belinda Barnes, the founder of Foresight, an endlessly supportive and enthusiastic voice on the end of a long-distance telephone line. Anna Priest was a storehouse of information on the toxic effects of mercury and was exceptionally generous in sharing her knowledge. Morris Karam of Balmain Life Fitness not only checked the accuracy of the text on exercise, but together with Bill Moore and Ian Riley provided the best equipped gym and finest training program in Sydney, where this author not only kept her level of endorphins high, but while cycling, stepping, running and pushing weights, mentally wrote a great deal of the manuscript. My confidante, Jennifer Macdiarmid, contributed in ways which are difficult to specify, but which are in part attributable to a keen intellect and a great ability to listen. To all those couples who have contacted me to share their disappointments and their subsequent successes thanks to preconception care, I also owe a great debt, for they have reinforced my belief in the importance of the information in this book.

My co-author Francesca Naish deserves a very special mention, for when we embarked on this venture we were barely acquainted. However, no author could have wished for a more harmonious working relationship and Francesca's vast knowledge, her writing skills and her sense of humour have made this whole undertaking an enormously rewarding and enjoyable experience. Our publisher Margaret Sullivan and editor Julia Cain should not remain anonymous, for they have worked tirelessly to ensure that Francesca and I feel that this is still very much our book.

The contribution of Alexander Nemeth, my partner of 25 years, is significant in a whole host of ways, for it was he who first goaded me to learn more about nutrition. Despite initial scepticism he gave up smoking and drinking Coca-Cola and took to eating lentils, soya beans and supplements. Now, as a community pharmacist, he preaches what we practised. But to David and Michael our two sons, who have had 'better beginnings' and are undoubtedly 'better boys' because of this, must go the greatest thanks of all, for without them this book most certainly would never have been written!

Sydney, June 1996

CONTENTS

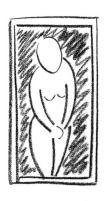

PART ONE
What you can do in your everyday life

PART TWO
How your health practitioner can help

PART THREE
Time to conceive

INTRODUCTION

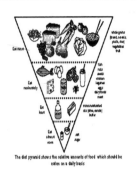

The diet pyramid shows the relative amounts of food which should be
eaten on a daily basis

'BETTER BABIES' IS NOT just an idle boast nor simply a catchy
title to our book. You can make a positive difference to the health
of your child and the rewards of following the recommendations you
will find on the following pages will extend far beyond that. Your
own physical and mental health will improve, your environment will
benefit too, and we would also like to think that, as preconception
care becomes more widely practised, the health of future generations
will be vastly improved. The natural way to having 'better babies'
also avoids the many problems associated with reproductive technology and genetic engineering, and all of their 'brave new world' type
implications.

We say this to you with the confidence of our own experience
with preconception care. One of us, Francesca, has not only had two
'better babies' herself, but for the past 20 years has run a clinic where
she has helped thousands of couples to overcome fertility and other
reproductive problems, and has seen the vast majority of them go on
to have beautiful, bright, healthy children. Francesca's clinic is now
the first in Australia to deal exclusively with healthy preparation for
pregnancy.

Like many women, Janette decided quite late in life that she
wanted a family. She knew about the importance of preconception
care, but she had no luck in finding a practitioner who knew any
more about it than she did. The gynaecologist she originally con-
sulted simply declared that she was a healthy woman and she should

go away and have a healthy baby. That was when Janette was already 37 years old, so she and her partner decided to work their way through the information they had from Foresight—the British Association for the Promotion of Preconception Care. They were rewarded for their efforts with a very quick conception, a healthy 40-week pregnancy, a three-hour labour and a birth at home of an absolutely beautiful, bright and exceptionally healthy baby boy who nursed until he was four and a half years old. That baby boy and his brother, who was born five years later, were catalysts for Janette's work on behalf of the Foresight Association in Australia and her contribution to this book.

Despite the fact that both of us have been involved in promoting preconception care for some considerable time, we have always known that information on the subject was not widely available and that, for the most part, health practitioners were completely unaware of the very significant benefits of such care and of all the factors requiring attention. This book is an attempt to address both of those problems. To do this, we have written many more words than we originally intended—but they are all important. We have been as comprehensive as possible, although some specialist areas will require further help. We have not always given cross references, but you will find that everything we refer to is mentioned elsewhere in the book, and you can easily find it by referring to the Contents or the Index.

We have dealt with self-help and practitioner-guided treatments, as both are necessary. Because of the huge diversity of health practitioners and the differences in the understanding of the needs during the preconception period, it is sometimes difficult to separate what you should do on your own from what requires professional help. If you are in any doubt, always seek help. If you are treating any condition which may have serious health repercussions with natural remedies, make sure that diagnostic checks are regularly performed by your medical practitioner.

Sometimes you may find that the advice you receive conflicts with what we have said here. In these instances there are two things that you need to bear in mind. Firstly, each individual has different health concerns and requires different changes in their lifestyle. As far as your health is concerned, there may be sound medical reasons why you cannot follow some of the advice in this book. However, it may also be worth your while to be sure that the medical advice you receive is from a practitioner who has a commitment to using as natural and non-interventionist an approach as possible.

Secondly, not all practitioners are aware of the needs during the preconception period (if they were, there would be no need for this book). Many medical practitioners are not trained in nutritional medicine and have little understanding of natural medicines. Some natural health practitioners have no access to expert medical, diagnostic or pathology procedures. Even a practitioner trained in, for example, nutrition, may not be aware of the level of nutrients required to ensure an optimally healthy pregnancy and baby.

Therefore, we suggest that the best way to use the information presented here, and still follow the advice of your health practitioner, is to take this book with you when you consult him or her, and refer to it together. Most health practitioners have to deal with a huge diversity of health concerns and cannot be expected to be up-to-date on all new research findings. If they truly have your concerns at heart (which nearly all of them will) then they should be only too pleased to use the information we present as a reference. Perhaps you will be able to inspire them to further study in the area. (We run training programs for professionals and will be delighted to help increase the numbers of informed practitioners.)

We know that some of you might find all that needs attention a little daunting and, unfortunately, we cannot change that. What we do hope we have done, however, is provide *all* the information that you need, whatever your state of health, to have a truly 'better baby'. We strongly believe that if you start early, work through one aspect of your diet or lifestyle modification at a time, stay positive and focused on the things that you can do and which are relevant to you, rather than on those which still remain to be tackled, then things do fall naturally into place. As you make the changes you will feel healthier and you will find that your confidence and motivation to continue will increase, and you will also find that it's not really as complex as it looks. It is also particularly important that you do as much as you possibly can without creating blame, resentment or guilt about any aspects of the program that are not fully attended to.

We know that raising absolutely healthy children is hard work. Raising children with allergies, learning problems, not to mention a more severe disability, is much harder work still, so much so, in fact, that what you have done to prepare yourselves for pregnancy actually pales into insignificance. As our cover shows, the health of your children rests entirely in your hands. We hope that you will take this opportunity to give them something priceless—their sound physical and mental health.

PROLOGUE

Why preconception care?

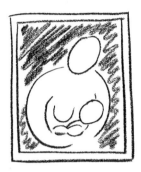

IN THE FOLLOWING PAGES you will find the most up-to-date information on the many dietary, lifestyle and environmental factors which are known to affect fertility, general reproductive health and the health of your child. Recent research has clearly shown that every aspect of our reproduction is adversely affected in some way by our twentieth-century lifestyle and living conditions. While this might seem a very negative statement for an introduction to this book, the good news is that studies have also clearly shown that if both prospective parents improve their general health, and if they avoid many common lifestyle factors and environmental hazards in the months preceding conception, they can greatly improve reproductive outcomes. The most important improvement being seen is in the physical, mental and emotional health of their child.

Preconception care for both partners is the key ingredient in ensuring optimal reproductive health, and the various aspects of this care are consequently the major focus of this book. The steps outlined here are those which will ensure that your child gets off to the very best possible start. By taking all the necessary steps to ensure a beautiful, bright, healthy baby, you will also improve your fertility, be much more likely to have a healthy, full-term pregnancy, a short and straightforward labour without medical intervention and have no difficulty breastfeeding your child.

We believe that all couples who plan to have a child should read this book. Whether your plans are for a first or a further child, whether your plans are for now or for later, this information has the potential to significantly improve the outcome of any future pregnancy. Our hope is that all potentially child-bearing couples, and those involved in caring for those couples, will read these words. They also hold a particularly important message for those who have experienced a previous reproductive problem. The reasons for much infertility, for many miscarriages, premature births, congenital defects and for much infant and child ill health are frequently dismissed as 'nobody really knows' or 'just one of those things', but the most recent research clearly shows otherwise. What follows is a clear summary of just what that current research has shown, and what this means in practical terms, if you are a couple planning to have a child.

We both have a strong commitment to making this information generally available in a form which is easily understood and readily applied, although the backgrounds from which we come are diverse. One of us has spent almost 20 years in the delivery of orthodox health care, the latter half of those years involved in nutritional and lifestyle counselling. The other has spent a similar length of time in a clinical practice using natural and traditional therapies. In the following pages we have combined our knowledge to present to you a step-by-step guide for the preconception period. This tells you everything that you should do, as well as what you should avoid. In the case of any unavoidable risk factors, we try to give you ways to compensate for such exposure.

Ideally, the preconception preparation is best implemented over the longest possible period of time. But because many of you will have left your child-bearing till late in life, or may feel impatient for various reasons, we have tried to give alternatives which may be effective in a short period of time. We both firmly believe that natural or complementary treatments are to be preferred, but we have also made reference to those which are more orthodox.

Preconception care will be a new idea to many of you, but thousands of couples in Australia, the United Kingdom and the United States have already discovered the benefits of this approach in improving their reproductive health and the health of their children. It is a simple, non-invasive, low technology approach, and basic preventive medicine, which is the best medicine of all. Preconception care is also an alternative which, we believe, is far preferable to genetic engineering and all its ramifications. It is certainly a far healthier and less stressful treatment for infertility than drugs and assisted-conception technologies. Preconception care is cheaper, has a much higher success rate and is free of any ethical, religious, legal or social dilemmas.

WHAT YOU CAN DO

There are certain things that can be done to ensure that you are in the best health, that your pregnancy, labour and postnatal experience are as successful as they can be, and that your baby is beautiful, bright and healthy. All these topics are covered in later chapters.

Fertility enhancement

Females

Regulate ovulation.
Balance hormone levels.
Improve health of ovaries and ova.
Reduce endometriosis and improve uterine health.
Clear blocked Fallopian tubes and improve tubal function.
Discover and treat hidden infections in the reproductive tract.
Treat Pelvic Inflammatory Disease (PID).
Soften scar tissue and adhesions.
Lessen cervical damage from erosion/infection/surgery.
Enhance quality and quantity of fertile mucus.

Males

Improve sperm count.
Improve sperm motility.
Improve health and quality of sperm.

Mutual problems

Help with:
Antibodies.
Hostile mucus.

Conscious conception
Timing—avoid old egg and sperm—conceive at the optimum time in your cycle.
Welcome the child—be aware of its existence from the earliest days.

Normal, healthy, full-term pregnancy
Suffer much less (or hopefully not at all) from minor discomforts such as morning sickness, varicose veins, haemorrhoids, constipation, heartburn, stretch marks, poor memory/mood swings, increased skin pigmentation, hair loss, bleeding gums, increased susceptibility to infection e.g. thrush, breakthrough bleeding, fatigue.

Greatly reduce incidence of more severe complications such as hyperemesis, ectopic pregnancy, miscarriage, toxaemia, preterm birth, stillbirth.

Short and straightforward labour
Strong and effective contractions.
Perineum more inclined to stretch than tear.
Quick recovery from any grazes or tears.
Enhanced bonding.
Reduced need for induction, drugs, surgery, other interventions.
Reduced likelihood of breech birth, postpartum haemorrhage, postnatal depression.

Beautiful, bright, health baby
Completely sound physical and mental development.
Greatly reduce incidence of severe conditions such as congenital defects, even for older parents.
Also reduce incidence of excessive crying, colic, nappy rash, thrush, eczema, cradle cap, teething problems, allergies such as asthma, learning and behaviour problems.

Successful breastfeeding
Improve quantity and nutrient quality of breast milk.
Improve physical and mental health of child.
Avoid artificial contraception.
Greatly reduce incidence of conditions such as cracked nipples, mastitis, inadequate supply of milk, tiredness/exhaustion.

TWO STORIES—WITH AND WITHOUT PRECONCEPTION CARE

Just in case you still have a few doubts about what you have just read, we would like to tell you two short stories which better illustrate what can be achieved with preconception care and, on the other hand, what you might experience without it.

The first couple, who are in their late 30s, conceive at their first attempt after attending to all of the recommendations in *Better Babies*. This mother-to-be suffers a little tiredness during the early weeks of her pregnancy, but by the end of the first three months, she feels like her usual self again. Her pregnancy progresses without a problem, she gains a modest amount of weight, feels well and looks wonderful. The only discomfort she suffers is some indigestion as the size of her baby increases, and her usually sound sleep pattern changes to a more fragmented one.

She goes into labour shortly after her expected date. Her contractions are strong and effective, and throughout her very short labour she moves and groans instinctively. After her baby is delivered, she has a tiny labial graze, but an intact perineum. Her newborn's health is rated at the top of the scale. The placenta is delivered, with minimal loss of blood. Breastfeeding is quickly and easily established.

In the days that follow the new mother is euphoric. She is confident and at ease in the handling of her new baby. He is particularly handsome, and he has a large perfectly shaped head, with broad, and evenly spaced facial features. His skin glows with good health. He is alert, but content. He knows night from day and even as a newborn he spends long periods of the daylight hours awake and observing all around him. He wakes at fairly regular intervals throughout the night when he nurses, but goes straight back to sleep. He never cries for longer than it takes for his mother to attend to his needs. She seems to know instinctively what he wants and when he wants it.

As he grows he reaches all his developmental milestones well ahead of his peers. He suffers from none of the usual ills of infancy. His mother has an abundant milk supply and he continues to breastfeed. He is strong, well-coordinated, exceptionally healthy and very bright, he suffers from no learning or behaviour problems. He is quite simply a wonderful child to have around!

We could go on, for this is *not* really the end of the story, but we will leave this mother and her baby here, and we now hear of another couple, who also decide that they want to start a family.

After trying unsuccessfully for three years to conceive (and after suffering two early miscarriages), they are referred to a GIFT program. After four unsuccessful attempts they decide not to try again, but twelve months later the woman discovers to her delight that she is pregnant.

During the early weeks of her pregnancy, this mother-to-be suffers badly from nausea and vomiting. Eventually this stage passes, but in the following months she develops haemorrhoids, varicose veins and stretch marks, though she wears these and her increased skin pigmentation and weird food cravings as a badge of her impending motherhood.

She gains a great deal of weight and towards the end of her pregnancy she is unable to eat a meal or to sleep with any degree of comfort. She also develops pre-eclampsia and is threatened with an induction. Fortunately, her labour begins spontaneously, although it progresses slowly. After 24 hours with very little progress, she is exhausted, demoralised, and agreeable to some help. This speeds things up, but it also makes her contractions quite unbearable. She has an epidural, an episiotomy and a forceps delivery in quick succession.

Her baby, at birth, is limp and a poor colour and is taken to the neonatal ward for observation. When he is returned to her she puts him to the breast, but he has an abnormally shaped palate and does not suckle well. He cries in frustration. She cries in frustration too, but perseveres and, with the help of a lactation consultant, breastfeeding is eventually established. However, her nipples are badly cracked, and she has an infection in her episiotomy wound. With the help of a nipple shield and a rubber cushion she survives the next few weeks, but she cries a lot. Finally, her nipples and her episiotomy heal, but she remains weepy and depressed. Her baby cries a lot too, sometimes for hours on end and these sessions always leave her feeling totally useless and rejected.

Finally, she decides to wean the baby, and things improve a bit, but he is still a sickly child. His skin is rough and blotchy, his head is rather small, his features are pinched, he has a pot belly. After a short time on the cow's milk formula, he develops eczema, so the mother changes to a soya formula and for a while she notices some improvement, but he still has nappy rash, which frequently becomes infected, has cradle cap and is miserable when he is teething. He is a fussy eater, and as well there are numerous foods which disagree with him. He is clumsy and accident-prone.

When he starts school he finds it difficult to sit still, his attention span is short, he is disruptive and is diagnosed as having a learning problem. He has constant colds and develops glue ear. He continues to wet the bed.

We could go on, but let us leave the stories here, for it is now probably clear that the first story is about a new family who have a 'better baby', and the second about a family who do not.

SOME HISTORICAL FACTS AND SOME RECENT STUDIES

You may be surprised to learn that your diet prior to conception, your lifestyle and environment all have a direct and profound bearing on your reproductive health and on the health of your baby. Certainly many prospective fathers are unaware that they have a very significant role to play in achieving sound physical and mental development in their child. So, if preparing for pregnancy means no more to you than deciding that you want a baby, and if preconception care simply sounds like the latest buzz word, it might interest you to know that the idea, and in fact the practice, of *care before conception*, is very, very old.

In the early days of the Roman Empire young women of child-bearing age were banned from drinking alcohol, and in Ancient Greece, the city fathers of Sparta and Carthage did not allow newly-weds to drink. In other words, both the Greeks and Romans were aware that alcohol taken before and around the time of conception had adverse effects on the development of the foetus. In the Bible, the following words were used to caution the mother-to-be of Samson: 'Thou shalt conceive and bear a son. Now therefore beware, I pray thee, and drink no wine or strong drink, and eat not any unclean thing.'

More recently, but still as long ago as the early 1930s, Dr Weston Price, a dentist, studied the effects of different dietary habits on teeth, general health and reproduction in numerous traditional societies throughout the world. He linked a change from a wholefood to a refined diet to a number of health and reproductive problems. In his classic work *Nutrition and Physical Degeneration*, he clearly demonstrated an increase in the incidence of dental decay, crooked teeth and bite, physical deformity and allergies, as well as a loss of mental acuity and a decrease in the efficiency of the birthing process, with a change from a society's traditional diet to one containing products made from white flour and sugar.

Weston Price has been called the 'Darwin of Nutrition'. Further work by his contemporaries Francis Pottenger and Robert McCarrison showed that optimal reproductive and foetal health depended on the consumption of whole and largely raw food grown on healthy soil. They also demonstrated the importance of the health of the male in achieving the best reproductive outcome. It is worthwhile remembering that these pioneering studies were carried out almost 60 years ago.

Large numbers of studies with animals show that when either parent is deficient in one, or a number of, essential nutrients, the offspring will be spontaneously aborted, or they will suffer from a variety of malformations. These malformations, which in the past were believed to be genetic, can be manipulated at will by inducing a deficiency or deficiencies in one or more of the essential vitamins and minerals. Furthermore, the nutrient-deficient mother will have a difficult and lengthy labour, and the way in which she nurtures her offspring will also be affected.

Finally, research carried out in the United Kingdom over the last eighteen years by Foresight—the Association for the Promotion of Preconception Care, which was established in 1978, has shown conclusively that if, in the months preceding conception, both prospective parents eat a nutritious diet, follow a healthy lifestyle, avoid exposure to environmental pollutants and if infections or allergies are treated, they will not only improve their fertility, but will also significantly reduce their chance of suffering a miscarriage, premature or stillbirth, or of giving birth to a baby with a congenital defect.

A recent study conducted by Foresight in conjunction with Surrey University followed the progress of 367 couples over a period of eighteen months (results were published in *The Journal of Nutritional and Environmental Medicine*, 1995).

The women participating in the study ranged in age from 22 to 45 years, the men from 25 to 59 years. Upon coming to Foresight, 41 per cent of the couples had no previous adverse reproductive history, but older couples were included among these. The remainder had suffered infertility (37 per cent), previous miscarriage (38 per cent), therapeutic abortion (11 per cent), stillbirth (3 per cent), 'small for dates' or low birth weight babies (15 per cent) or babies with a malformation (2 per cent).

By the end of the study, *89 per cent of all the couples had given birth, including 81 per cent of those who were previously infertile.* The average age at birth was 38.5 weeks, and no baby was born before 36 weeks. The average weight of males was 7 lb 4½ oz (3,305 g), average weight of females was 7 lb 2 oz (3,232 g) and no baby was lighter than 5 lb 3 oz (2,353 g). There were no miscarriages, no perinatal deaths and no malformations! No baby was admitted to Intensive Care! In a similar population sample of people who have practised no preconception care, you would expect about 70 women to experience a miscarriage and about twelve children to be born with a malformation.

The study's very significant results are borne out by the clinical experience of one of us, Francesca, who, over the last 20 years has treated well over 5,000 women and couples to improve their general reproductive health. Many of these people had experienced fertility problems, difficult pregnancies and births, or had previous children with health disorders. Some couples came simply to ensure that they experienced none of these things.

Although there are, as yet, no exact statistics, work is currently underway to assess the overall effectiveness of these treatments. However, what we are sure of is that holistic treatment of the type espoused in this book, has proven itself to be remarkably effective in improving reproductive outcomes and infant health.

WHY PRECONCEPTION CARE NOW?

You will probably agree that the human population has generally chosen to ignore historical facts and earlier scientific findings and, as far as having babies is concerned, has just left it to Nature to 'get it right'. You might therefore be forgiven for asking 'why change now?' Well, the truth of the matter is, Nature is finding it increasingly difficult to 'get it right'.

If you are wondering why this is so, you might take a minute to reflect on how our diet, lifestyle and the environment in which we live, differ from that of our ancestors. The many changes which have been wrought in the environment and the further changes which have occurred in the way we live over the last 200 years, far outweigh all those which have occurred during preceding millenia. What we eat and drink today is probably dramatically different from what previous populations consumed for hundreds of thousands of years. What was once an active lifestyle, is now, for the majority of us, a sedentary one, and possibly a stressful one at that. The environment in which we live has been flooded with chemicals, our food and water supply has been tampered with, and many of us use tobacco, alcohol and drugs (prescribed or otherwise) on a regular basis. The availability of oral contraceptives has led to an increased degree of sexual activity, with the increased risk of sexually transmitted disease, and has also given us the option of bearing children at a much later age.

Risk factors
Poor nutrition
Tobacco/alcohol/drugs
Environmental pollution
Lack of exercise
Stress
Oral contraceptives
Genito-urinary infections
Other infections e.g. Candida
Allergies
Child-bearing at older age

Research has now shown that each one of these factors alone may have adverse effects on fertility, reproductive and general health. When these factors are present in combination, the adverse effects are likely to be much more pronounced, and to occur with increasing frequency. Indeed, the full extent of compromised reproductive outcomes becomes apparent if you consider the following statistics.

In Australia at present one couple in *six* is infertile, one woman in *five* will miscarry, one woman in *ten* suffers from toxaemia or the high blood pressure of pregnancy, almost one woman in every *five* undergoes a Caesarean section, one baby in *ten* is born prematurely or 'small for dates', and one baby in *thirty* is born with a congenital defect. Some degree of postnatal depression affects more than one woman in every *three*, and only one woman in *ten* breastfeeds her child for more than twelve months. More than one child in every *ten* is affected by a learning or behaviour problem, and one child in *five* suffers from asthma.

These facts and figures are not given here to discourage you from having a child, nor are they meant to make you apprehensive about what a future pregnancy might hold. What we hope they will do is convince you that it is no longer good enough to leave the bearing of healthy children to chance. Rather, we hope these figures will encourage you to take the necessary steps to prevent problems with the pregnancy, birth and baby. Assuming that you now recognise that a healthy body is a fertile body, and that it is important to actively prepare for your child's conception, you also need to know exactly what this preparation involves.

WHAT DOES PRECONCEPTION CARE INVOLVE?

Put very simply, preconception care involves making sure that there is an adequate supply of all those factors which are essential to the health of your sperm and ova and to foetal development, and an absence of all those things which have been shown to be harmful. The formation of sperm may take up to 116 days, and ova are susceptible to damage during their period of maturation, which is approximately 100 days before ovulation.

Ideally, you both need to enjoy a period of optimum health which spans a period of *at least four months* immediately preceding any attempt to conceive. Some of the following recommendations may take some time to implement, as may the appropriate treatment of a pre-existing condition, so the more time you can give yourselves for your preparation, the more effective it is likely to be.

There are a number of areas which require attention. There are some issues which you can address for yourselves, and there are others which will require help from a professional. We have tried to make it very clear which is which.

We know that for some of you, the following recommendations will mean major diet and lifestyle adjustments. Consequently, we have tried to make each section of the book as user-friendly as possible. We also know that if the biological clock is ticking, then to faithfully follow all of the recommendations might take more time than you feel you have. For those of you who fall into this category, we have tried to give alternatives, which may save time without overly compromising the outcome. We are also aware that frequently the 'spirit is willing, but the flesh is weak,' so if exposure to a known harmful substance or substances is unavoidable, we have tried to give some compensatory action. We also know that occasionally one partner may be reluctant to accept any responsibility for creating a healthy baby. In answer to that we should say that perhaps the reluctant partner's commitment to becoming a parent must be questioned, but at the same time, some preconception care (or care by one partner) is obviously better than none at all.

However, we want to emphasise again that it takes two very healthy partners to make a very healthy baby. Ideally, therefore, every aspect of the preconception preparation should involve both of you equally, for nothing will be quite as effective as both prospective parents attending faithfully to all that follows in this book.

PART ONE

- - - - - - - - - - - - - - - - -

What you can do in
your everyday life

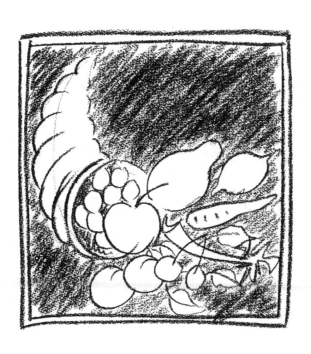

NUTRIENTS FOR 'BETTER BABIES'

AT LEAST FOUR MONTHS before you plan to conceive, both of you must eat an excellent diet. This means that you should:

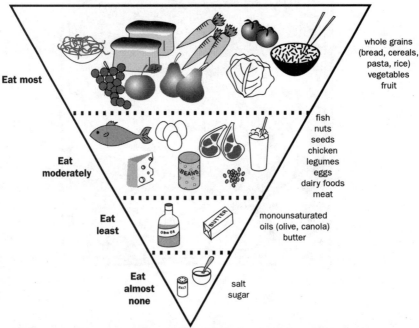

The diet pyramid shows the relative amounts of food which should be eaten on a daily basis

AS WELL, WE RECOMMEND that you *buy
organically grown (or fed) produce, buy in season,
buy unprocessed.*
THEN WE RECOMMEND THAT you *eat it whole,
eat it raw if possible, eat it freshly prepared.*

SOME OF YOU WILL find that these dietary guidelines mean major changes to your eating habits. If this is the case, we have listed below the different food categories and given you some more specific information. At the end of the chapter we have enlarged on our recommendations for buying organically grown or fed, unprocessed, and so on, and we have also given you a few useful tips for getting started.

FOODS TO EAT

Grains

Try to use only organically grown grains. Grains may be eaten in the form of wholegrain bread, wholemeal pasta, brown rice or corn. You might like to try others such as oats, rye, millet, or barley. Grains can be eaten alone as bread, muesli, pasta or porridge, or you can combine them with vegetables, or with protein dishes of animal or vegetable origin.

Vegetables

Try to use only organically grown vegetables. You should eat lots of them every day—in fact vegetables should make up *at least 40 per cent* of your total food intake. All vegetables (except potatoes) can be eaten *raw*, although if you have relied heavily on cooked vegetables in the past, introduce raw vegies gradually so that your digestive system has time to adjust. Root vegetables such as carrots can be shredded, grated, juiced or lightly cooked to allow for maximum absorption of nutrients. Potatoes should always be cooked and any green ones discarded. Juicing or shredding (which increases the surface area of the food which is available to your digestive enzymes) are good ways to accustom your body to a diet which is high in raw vegetables. Make sure that juicing or shredding is done immediately before you eat, to minimise nutrient loss.

Be adventurous, try vegetables you haven't eaten before! Eat the widest possible variety, especially dark green leafy and red and orange ones. Avocados are particularly nutritious. You can add chopped fresh herbs such as parsley and watercress, and all sprouts (especially alfalfa) to your salads. If you are using juices, celery, beetroot and carrot make a good base—add others for a vegetable cocktail.

If you do cook your vegies, methods such as stir-frying, steaming or dry-baking, which keep nutrient losses to a minimum, are better than roasting and boiling. Scrubbing rather than peeling also reduces nutrient loss. When making soups, use a blender rather than boiling the foods to death. Since there are studies which show that food which has been cooked in a microwave oven suffers molecular damage, and when eaten, causes abnormal changes in human blood and immune systems, we recommend that you use other cooking methods, such as a wok or a steamer.

Fruit

Try to use only organically grown fruit. You should eat two or three (apple-sized) pieces of fruit every day, but no more since the sugar content is high. This amount of fruit includes any pieces which are juiced, and these should be diluted 50/50 with purified water. Dried fruit is very high in sugar, so try to avoid it altogether or eat it very sparingly.

Protein

You need an average-sized serving of protein-providing food at least twice a day. This should be a food which gives you either an animal protein which is a complete (or primary) protein, or the appropriate combination of plant (or secondary) proteins. Primary proteins contain all the essential amino acids which are needed to build and repair tissue, muscles, organs and hair. They are also necessary for the formation of semen, for the optimum functioning of the testes and for the manufacture of digestive enzymes. Protein also buffers against excessive acidity, which is important because an environment which is too acidic is hostile to sperm. We recommend that you increase your protein intake by approximately 20 per cent, once you know you are pregnant. To ensure optimal birth weight, you need good quality protein and plenty of it.

There are studies showing a strong link between low birth weight, infant mortality and congenital defects, and low protein intake. It's too late to change to a higher protein intake during pregnancy—you need it before conception, since adequate protein is vital for both quantity and quality of eggs produced, for healthy sperm, for the fertilisation process, and the early development of the embryo.

Because excessively high protein diets seem to create problems in much the same way as those that are protein deficient, there's no need to go overboard. However, the implications are serious for the vegetarian or vegan who gets little, if any, primary protein.

Since plant proteins are incomplete proteins, you need to combine them so that you get your full complement of essential amino acids. To do this, you should combine at one meal foods from *two* of the following groups:

(1) Nuts,   (2) Grains/Seeds, and   (3) Legumes/Pulses.

For example, you could choose to have rice and beans, nuts and lentils, or nuts and seeds, and so on.

We recommend that you buy animal produce which has been fed on organically grown grain and raised without the use of antibiotics and hormones. You should be aware that the words 'free range' refer to the manner in which the livestock is allowed to graze, rather than to what it is fed, although produce which has been organically fed may also be grazed in a free-range manner. You should ask your butcher very specific questions if you are in doubt, although you will generally find that the produce which you seek will be carefully packed and labelled accordingly.

If you are unable to find a supplier of organically fed meat products, you can minimise your exposure to chemical contamination by alternating your sources of protein. Some protein-providing foods are more suitable than others. We have marked them with an appropriate number of stars to show their suitability (more stars mean they are more suitable).

*** *Fish* is low in saturated fats and high in essential fatty acids (see the later section on Essential Nutrients). Deep-sea/ocean/cold-water fish (such as salmon, trout, cod and herring) are particularly beneficial, and they are also less likely to be polluted. Your diet can include small quantities of tinned salmon and sardines, though not too much since the metal can leach into the oil. It is wise to limit your intake of tuna, whether fresh or tinned. Tuna is high in the food chain, and may be contaminated with mercury, as may swordfish and shark.

*** *Nuts/seeds* are the best plant or secondary proteins. Eat them raw, unsalted and fresh. Use them in salads, stir-fries and pasta dishes, or as a snack. Combine them as described above for a complete protein source. Avoid the combinations of nuts with dried fruit because of the high sugar content.

** *Chicken* should only be eaten if you are able to get chooks of the organically fed variety. Battery fed chickens (and even some free-range) may be fed large amounts of hormones (though these are officially illegal in Australia) and antobiotics. Trim the skin to avoid fats.

** *Legumes/pulses/grains* legumes and pulses include soya, tofu, tempeh, lentils and all the many varieties of bean, and the grains include those we have already listed (see Grains). These are good secondary proteins, but you need to combine them as we have shown.

* *Eggs* should be from organically fed chooks. Eat no more than two or three eggs per week, and only if you are not allergic to them.

* *Dairy produce* should be eaten very sparingly. It is a common allergen and creates mucus in the Fallopian tubes in most women, sets up a malabsorption syndrome in the gut and studies have linked its consumption with reduced fertility—it is preferable to use soya or goat's milk (and cheese) as an alternative. Yoghurt is good. This means Acidophilus yoghurt *with no added sugar*. If you know for certain that you are allergic to cow's milk, avoid it completely and get your dietary calcium from other sources. Further suggestions will be found in Chapter 12.

* *Red meat* with the fat trimmed can be eaten in moderation. The fat should be avoided since it is the storage site for pollutants such as pesticides, and animal fats can also upset your hormonal balance. Unless you can get organically fed meat, avoid offal, mince and sausage. If you need mince, ask your butcher to mince a chosen piece of lean meat on site. Offal may contain high levels of pesticides and chemical hormones.

Fats

Use olive oil (or canola oil) for cooking and stir-frying. Both olive and canola are monounsaturated oils and will not saturate on heating, unlike polyunsaturates. In other words, they are least susceptible to the chemical changes caused by high temperatures. Always discard used oil and keep the unused portion in the refrigerator.

Use lots of cold-pressed olive oil on salads. This oil contains essential fatty acids if it has never been heated (that is, if it is cold-pressed). You can add lemon, pepper, garlic or herbs to the dressing.

Use butter very sparingly. For a change, try using avocado, banana, hummus or nut spreads on your bread, instead of butter.

Water

Try to drink 10 to 12 glasses of filtered, purified or bottled water daily. Use only this type of water in your saucepans and kettle as well. This recommendation is important if you are to avoid ingesting toxins such as heavy metals and chemicals which may be present in tap-water. Even rainwater collected in tanks should be filtered since the roof it is collected from, and the tank itself, may be sources of toxic substances.

FOODS TO AVOID

Products containing white flour or sugar

A large proportion of essential vitamins and minerals is removed in the refining processes which lead to the production of white flour and sugar. Consequently, when you consume refined products, these nutrients will be leached from your body's stores, since they are still required for the metabolism of the carbohydrate (flour and sugar). Since *chromium* is one of these nutrients, and a chromium deficiency increases sugar cravings, you can be caught in an endless cycle of consuming nutrient-depleted foods. *Zinc* and *folic acid* (which is part of the B-complex group of vitamins) are the other most affected nutrients. As you will see, zinc and folate are two of the most important preconception nutrients.

Just remember that despite the catchy slogan of the sugar industry, 'it's a natural part of life', your body does not require refined sugar of any sort for its energy requirements. All your sugar needs are met when your body metabolises or breaks down complex carbohydrate-containing foods such as whole grains, legumes, fruit and vegetables.

If you are going to avoid these nutrient-depleted products, you must become a careful label reader—for example, coloured pastas and some brown breads may contain refined white flour with dye added. Sugar may be listed as any one of the following—sugar, dextrose, glucose, glucose syrup, fructose, corn syrup, honey or sorbitol. Some very popular muesli bars, which have the outward appearance of being a healthy snack, actually contain four different types of sugar.

Remember too that honey, although it does contain some nutrients, is still sugar. Fruit juices contain large amounts of fructose, which although preferable to refined sugar, may still be a problem in large quantities. This is why we recommend that you limit your fruit intake (including any pieces juiced) to three pieces daily. If you suffer from Candida, it is important that you recognise the sugar content of foods since these must be avoided on the anti-Candida diet.

A diet which is high in products containing sugar also has a depressant effect on the immune system. Sugar competes with Vitamin C for uptake into immune cells. Too much sugar is also responsible for increasing cholesterol levels, and is also implicated in much gastrointestinal disease, gallstones, kidney stones, diabetes, obesity and a variety of skin conditions including acne.

Green potatoes
Avoid potatoes which have gone green—they are toxic.

Fats and fried foods
You need to avoid saturated fats which means animal fats and fats (or oils) which have been heated. Saturated fats upset the metabolism of essential fatty acids, and consequently disturb your hormonal balance. *Avoid margarine.* Although butter and margarine are both saturated fats, butter, unlike margarine, has not been heated. Margarine is also full of added chemicals.

Foods that contain additives
Almost everything which comes in a can, packet or bottle has some sort of chemical added to stabilise it, preserve it, or help it keep its colour, smell or texture. Apart from the fact that you may be sensitive to additives, your body will also use a number of essential nutrients to detoxify these chemicals. Read the labels on food carefully.

You should avoid all delicatessen or processed meats, for example salami. These are high in salt as well as fat, and the nitrites (which are used as preservatives in these products) are particularly toxic. Processed meats also contain offal which is high in herbicides, pesticides and chemical hormones.

Food which has been reheated or left standing

Food of this nature has lost most of its nutrients and may contain moulds. It is particularly important that you avoid moulds if you suffer from Candida.

Salt

Avoid salting your food, unless your diet contains absolutely no pre-prepared food at all. Remember that bread is a pre-prepared food and you will get all your salt requirements (and more) from this.

Coffee and tea

We will deal further with the many reasons for avoiding drinks containing caffeine in Chapter 2. Replace coffee and tea with herbal teas—there are lots of different varieties to choose from. Alternatively, drink filtered water or juice a piece of fruit. If you find that complete abstinence from tea and coffee is difficult initially, then allow yourself two cups of tea (not coffee) per day—*but no more*!

Junk foods

This goes without saying since junk foods invariably fall into one (sometimes all) of the above 'do not eat' categories.

Allergens

Do not eat a particular food if you suspect you are allergic to it, even if it is an excellent source of a nutrient you need.

SOME OTHER THINGS TO CONSIDER

Acid/alkali balance

The acid/alkali balance of your diet is important, because if your cervical mucus is too acidic it will destroy sperm. A post-coital test can easily determine if this is occurring—see Chapters 7 and 14). Acidity also predisposes to heavy metals and radiation toxicity.

Acid-forming foods include meat and other animal products, fish, eggs, grains, seeds, sugar, coffee, tea and alcohol. Prunes, plums and cranberries are also acid forming. Do not confuse foods which *contain* acids, such as tomatoes, pineapple and oranges, with those that are *acid forming*.

Alkali-forming foods are the ones which you need to eat in abundance. They include all the vegetables (especially alfalfa and red clover sprouts), all fruit (except prunes, plums and cranberries) and nuts (especially almonds and hazelnuts). Milk, although an animal food, may buffer against acidity, but it should be used with caution as it is a very common allergen.

Food combining

The foregoing dietary changes will give many of you quite enough to do and to think about. Others will be quite comfortable with our recommendations and will be prepared to go one extra step. For those of you who fall into this category, we suggest that food combining can greatly assist your body to absorb nutrients. In short, there are certain categories of foods which need to be kept separate from one another. If you think that you could take another dietary recommendation on board, we recommend that you consult *The Food Combining Diet* by Katherine Marsden.

Your correct weight

If you are either too thin or too fat, your fertility may be affected. Women need about 25 per cent of their body weight as fat if they are to menstruate and ovulate normally. When fat levels fall too low, the body does not produce enough oestrogen. Consequently, if you are much leaner than this, your periods may be irregular or scanty or they may cease altogether (this is merely Nature's way of making sure you don't conceive until you have sufficient body fat to sustain a pregnancy). If you do conceive while you are very thin you have a much higher chance of giving birth to a low birth weight infant. These tiny babies are, of course, much more likely to suffer from a variety of health problems.

If you are significantly heavier than the ideal, your higher fat content may also disrupt your hormonal balance and contribute to the risk of fertility problems. If you do conceive while you are overweight you have a greater risk of suffering from gestational diabetes and toxaemia of pregnancy. Both these conditions carry a very serious risk to your baby.

What then is your ideal weight? We know that your weight will usually, given ample time, approach an appropriate level if you attend faithfully to all that we recommend here. However, you may feel happier if you know approximately what you should be aiming for!

As a guide to your ideal weight you can calculate your Quetelet index (Q index).

To do this: $\text{Q index} = \dfrac{\text{Weight in Kilograms}}{\text{Height in Metres}^2}$

For example, if you weigh 65 kg and are 167 cm tall your calculation looks like this:

$$\text{Q index} = \frac{65}{1.67 \times 1.67} = \frac{65}{2.8} = 23.2$$

An index of between 20 and 25 puts you in the desirable weight range. If your Q index is significantly lower than 20, then we recommend that you gain an appropriate amount of weight before you try to conceive and if your index is significantly higher than 25 then you need to lose some weight before your pregnancy. It is probably a good idea to try to reach your ideal weight before that all important four month period which immediately precedes conception.

And remember:

- No fad diets
- No fasting—an exception may be made for a one day fast of vegetable juices. This is best done under supervision, and only if you are definitely not pregnant.

TIPS TO IMPROVE YOUR DIET

Don't try to do it all at once

If your eating habits are really in need of a major overhaul, then the prospect of implementing big changes can be daunting. If you try to do it all at once, the failure rate is likely to be high. Work on one aspect at a time, bearing in mind that a really healthy diet for both of you should be in place for at least four months before conception. Give yourself plenty of time to implement the necessary changes.

Set some realistic goals

For example, if you salt your food heavily, you might consider stopping this as a first step. Once your tastebuds are accustomed to food without salt, they will appreciate more subtle flavours such as fruit and vegetables, and other changes may then be a little easier to make.

Perhaps you're zinc deficient?

If you constantly crave very salty (or sweet or spicy) food in preference to everything else, you may be suffering from a zinc deficiency. Adequate zinc status is necessary for proper taste sensation—in other words, if you are zinc deficient, food which is not very salty, sweet or spicy, simply tastes like cardboard. To test for zinc status, buy Zinc Challenge or Zinc Tally from your local pharmacy and follow the instructions (see also Chapter 9). Once you respond positively to this test, you can take zinc supplements in tablet form.

One sugar hit leads to another

Perhaps you need to give up all those soft drinks (very high in sugar) in favour of filtered water, as a first step to improving your eating habits. Maybe all those chocolate bars should be the first to go. Perhaps you ought to stop all those sugared cups of coffee. If you seem to need an endless succession of sugary snacks or drinks to get you through your day you may be suffering from a sugar metabolism problem. This will be made worse by having a sugar hit every time you feel your energy levels drop. Refined sugar, since it enters the bloodstream rapidly, can cause wild fluctuations in blood sugar levels in sensitive individuals. Since the brain depends entirely on a constant supply of glucose for its proper function, these fluctuating levels can leave you feeling angry, moody, depressed, sleepy, lethargic, faint, headachy or restless.

If this sounds like you, try the following recommendation—*eat a good breakfast* and follow it with a wholesome lunch and evening meal. If your energy levels really sag between meals you may do better if you *eat little and often*. Include *lots of complex carbohydrate-containing foods* in your diet. Remember these are vegetables, fruit, legumes and whole grains. The body metabolises these to glucose, but at a rate which gives you a constant and steady supply of the substance, rather than the brief highs and subsequent lows which you get from sugary snacks and drinks. Snacks such as almonds can also help to keep your blood sugar levels steady. Many of the supplements which we look at later in this chapter will help to reduce sugar cravings.

Eat a good breakfast

Even if sugar metabolism is not a problem for you, a substantial, wholesome breakfast is still important. With this under your belt you will be much less likely to crave unsuitable snacks or drinks during the day. Be careful of commercial breakfast cereals, because some of them contain large amounts of sugar. Prepare your own muesli or look for one which is sugar free and without too much dried fruit. Wholegrain toast, with a suitable spread, is a possible alternative. Try getting up a little earlier each day so that you have enough time to follow this recommendation.

Take a packed lunch from home

This is much more likely to be an appropriate lunch than something which you pick up from the local fast food shop. Even ready prepared salads or other foods, which on the surface appear healthy, may have been standing for a considerable time, they may have been reheated, and may have had preservatives added to extend their fresh appearance. There are notable exceptions, however, and you may be fortunate to have, near your workplace, a simply wonderful health food bar which offers a range of freshly prepared, wholefood meals.

Shop when you are well fed

This is the only wise way to shop—you are far less likely to pick up inappropriate snacks.

Keep healthy snacks on hand

Once you have eaten all the unsuitable processed foods and snacks which you have stockpiled in your cupboard, do not replace them. Better still, throw them out or give them away right now. If they are not in the house, you can't be tempted. Make sure you have only healthy, tasty, and easily prepared food available for the times when you are hungry.

Find a good recipe book

Whole, healthy food does not have to be boring. In fact, nothing looks more appetising than freshly prepared wholefood which is attractively presented. In Contacts and Resources we have listed some books which give good examples of easily prepared food which is not only healthy, but appetising and interesting. These books contain recipes which we think are well suited to the Australian climate.

Say an affirmation

'*I am making a conscious choice to eat a healthy diet for my sake and for the sake of my children,*' or '*healthy food, healthy body, healthy children*' and repeat whenever your resolve weakens.

The odd transgression is OK

If for some reason you do stray from the straight and narrow, don't burden yourself with guilt. Guilt is destructive. Enjoy the chocolate mud cake or whatever your particular poison is—occasionally—if you must. The odd unhealthy meal or snack is unlikely to matter greatly. It is what you eat *most of the time* that's important.

On the other hand, don't plan to break your diet. This can turn into an ever more frequently used excuse.

WHY EACH MOUTHFUL MUST COUNT

The food and drink that you put into your mouth is the source of all fluid, fat, protein, carbohydrate and essential vitamins and minerals. All the enzyme systems which keep your various organ systems functioning, the formation of hormones and chemical transmitters, the repair and formation of new cells and the energy to fuel all these processes depend on a supply of basic building blocks which are found in what you eat or drink, and digest and absorb. These basic building blocks, which are called *nutrients*, include essential amino acids, essential fatty acids and trace minerals and vitamins.

More specifically, the formation of healthy, vigorous sperm and the maturation of one ovum per month are both processes which require an adequate supply of many essential nutrients. As well, these processes are controlled by hormones, which in turn depend on the availability of numerous nutrients for their formation. Having a healthy vagina and cervix which will, at the time of ovulation, nurture the sperm as they make their long journey towards the ripe ovum, depends on an adequate supply of nutritional factors. A fertilised ovum is nourished by secretions as it makes its journey through the Fallopian tube and the formation of these also depends on a plentiful supply of a variety of building blocks. Once a fertilised egg implants itself in the uterus and development of the embryo begins in earnest, nutritional requirements increase dramatically.

From conception to the end of the first three months, the mass of the embryo increases over $2\frac{1}{2}$ million times. This is the period during which cells differentiate and organs are formed. This rapid phase of growth requires levels of nutrients which are many times higher than those required by your body in its pre-pregnant state. There is little doubt that a diet with deficiencies which may go unnoticed in day-to-day life may fail to support a pregnancy. The development during this critical and rapid phase of growth and cell division also occurs to a very strict timetable. For example, if the nutrients needed for the satisfactory closure of the neural tube are absent, on day 28 or 29 of the pregnancy, or present in insufficient quantities, development will proceed regardless, but a neural tube defect such as spina bifida will result.

The requirements for all nutrients remain high throughout your pregnancy. Increased amounts are necessary not only to meet the demands of the developing foetus, but to manufacture the hormones which maintain the pregnancy, prepare the breasts for lactation and the muscles of the uterus for labour. They are needed in order to manufacture the greater volume of circulating blood and to prevent stretch marks on your belly and breasts as they increase in size. Inevitably, still further nutrients are required to initiate the birthing process; adequate amounts must be present if the ligaments and muscles of the pelvic girdle are to relax sufficiently, the cervix is to soften and ripen and the muscles of the uterus are to contract strongly and effectively, and if the tissue of the perineum is to stretch adequately to allow your baby to be born easily.

Still more nutrients are required for the manufacture of hormones controlling the delivery of the placenta. Following birth, others are needed to help the blood clot, and so that any necessary healing can take place. The maternal hormones associated with bonding, and oxytocin, which ensures that the uterus clamps down on itself and returns to its normal size, are only manufactured successfully in the presence of good nutrition.

The manufacture of the hormones associated with successful lactation, and the formation of the hundreds of complex substances contained in breast milk, are once again totally dependent on the nutrients which you absorb from your food, and the optimal growth and development of your baby is dependent on the presence of an adequate supply of all nutritional factors.

In other words, your diet, is of the utmost importance. Put quite simply, it means that there must be a sufficient supply of *all* the essential nutritional factors present *at all times*, if the many marvellously complex and interdependent processes which constitute the full reproductive cycle are to proceed without a hiccup. These processes of course begin well before conception, continue throughout the pregnancy and the birth of your baby and finish after the baby is weaned.

As well, an excellent diet and the resulting adequate nutritional status means that your body has a plentiful supply of essential nutrients from which to draw for its work of detoxifying chemical or heavy metal pollutants. It means that there will be a sufficient supply of anti-oxidants to counteract the damage caused by these contaminants and by various types of radiation. Adequate nutritional status also means a competent immune system, with the likelihood of fewer or much milder infections and less likelihood of allergies or sensitivity reactions.

It also means that you will be emotionally stable, have plenty of energy, be more resistant to the effects of stress, will have faster wound healing and much, much more. While these factors may not seem to be as important as the health of sperm and ova, or the health of the placenta, there is no doubt that they have a significant role to play in ensuring a healthy pregnancy, birth and baby.

A CLOSER LOOK AT SOME INDIVIDUAL NUTRIENTS

At the risk of belabouring the importance of an excellent diet, we have listed below each individual nutrient and looked a little more closely at the many functions of each, with particular emphasis on those actions which are essential for good reproductive outcomes. We have chosen to do this so that you will be aware of the importance of ensuring that every mouthful is a nutritious one. To help you make every mouthful count, we have also included a list of the foods in which you will find each of the various nutrients. You will also see that we have included a recommended dose range for the supplementation of each. The need for supplementation may be surprising to some, but if you read on, the reasons for this recommendation will become clear.

Zinc

Last in the alphabetical scheme of things might seem an odd place to start our list of nutrients, but since zinc is intimately involved in so many aspects of reproductive function, we will deal with it first and in detail. Zinc has antibacterial, antiviral, antifungal, anticancer and antiradiation properties. It is involved at many levels of reproductive function, and in the formation of the brain and the immune system. It is, in fact, a part of over 300 enzyme systems in the body. Of the elemental micro-nutrients or trace elements, zinc has the widest range of essential functions, and is *the most important nutrient for the pregnant woman.*

A recent quote from Professor Derek Bryce-Smith, Professor of Organic Chemistry at the University of Reading in the United Kingdom, will leave you in no doubt about the importance of zinc: 'If a new drug had been found with this broad range of properties it would have been hailed as the discovery of the century.'

However, zinc is lost during the refining of grains, uptake from the soil is reduced by non-sustainable (or non-organic) farming methods, its excretion is increased by alcohol, sugar, refined grains and diuretics (caffeine is a diuretic), smokers have an increased requirement for zinc, and zinc status is seriously disrupted by oral contraceptives, by copper IUDs, by the copper present in many water supplies, and also by the use of inorganic iron supplements, which are frequently prescribed for anaemic women, and very commonly prescribed during pregnancy. Calcium (high in dairy produce) also inhibits the absorption of zinc, and vegetarians are frequently found to be zinc deficient. Zinc is also utilised by your body as it excretes toxic metals, such as cadmium and lead, and your requirements for zinc are increased in times of growth, and during stress, illness, or periods of inflammation and infection.

Does it occur to you that your zinc status might, perhaps, be inadequate? Many researchers have shown, in fact, that zinc deficiency is widespread among the general population. A study by the CSIRO found that the levels of zinc (and magnesium) were marginal in the diets of 67 per cent of Australian men and 85 per cent of women! Look around you at the many individuals with white spots on their fingernails, who are exhibiting just one of the signs of a zinc deficiency. Consider also the following statistics, which give further indication of the frequency with which marginal or inadequate zinc status now occurs.

Zinc is necessary for proper fertility in both the male and female. Adequate zinc is needed for a viable sperm count, and a high percentage of live, well-formed sperm in semen. Zinc is present in fairly large amounts in semen, and excessive ejaculation (intercourse or masturbation), may cause a loss of 2 to 5 mg of zinc a day. Zinc is the most important mineral for male reproductive health, and a deficiency can cause chromosomal aberrations and lowered testosterone levels.

Infertility rates have increased several fold in recent years, with the incidence of male responsibility for infertility rising from 10 per cent to 25 per cent in less than a decade. Recent Belgian studies show that as many as 40 per cent of young men have below normal sperm concentration and poor sperm movement and shape, whereas seventeen years ago only 4.9 per cent showed such abnormalities. Figures from the United States show that the number of infertile women aged between 20 and 25 has tripled in 30 years, and as many as one-quarter of women between the ages of 35 and 39 are involuntarily infertile. Present estimates give one couple in six considered to be infertile at some time, or unable to conceive after two and a half years.

Zinc is one of the nutrients necessary for proper formation of elastin chains in connective tissue. Zinc deficient women develop stretch marks, they have perineums which do not stretch but tear, (or need cutting), and they have nipples which crack readily. There are no exact statistics for the frequency of stretch marks or cracked nipples but you will certainly be aware that they are common; and in many hospitals, episiotomies (the cutting of the perineum to allow the baby to be born) are performed routinely.

Maternal tissue zinc depletion has been found to be associated with foetal growth retardation. One baby in ten is born prematurely or 'small for dates'. Some very recent studies from the University of Liverpool (United Kingdom) have linked SIDS (Sudden Infant Death Syndrome) with foetal growth retardation.

Zinc deficiency causes women to have prolonged labours. In zinc deficient women there are gaps in the uterine membrane which compromise its ability to contract. At present in Australia, in some hospitals, fewer than half of the births occur spontaneously, and in the last 20 years there has been a 300 per cent increase in the number of Caesarean sections performed. This rate now approaches 17 per cent. It seems entirely probable that not all interventions are due to the increasing medicalisation of the birthing process.

Adequate zinc status is essential to maintain the *correct ratio of copper to zinc* in the body. Copper and zinc are called antagonistic minerals. Research has linked high copper levels (which occur when zinc is deficient) to spontaneous abortions and premature births. High copper levels have also been linked to toxaemia, or the high blood pressure of pregnancy, which may affect as many as one woman in ten.

Copper levels normally rise during the third trimester of pregnancy and zinc packs into the placenta. In fact, the placenta is the richest source of zinc known and contains from 300 to 650 mg of elemental zinc depending on its size, which is why it is traditionally eaten. The high copper levels are thought to act as a trigger on the central nervous system initiating the phenomena of birth. Many researchers have linked postnatal depression to these high copper levels which fail to return to normal after the birth, because of lack of zinc.

Zinc is also intimately involved in the correct formation and functioning of the immune system. Statistics show that, in Australia, one child in five and one adult in ten suffers from asthma. These figures also show the high percentage of the population which has compromised immune function. Recent statistics also show that the number of childhood asthma sufferers has doubled in the last ten years.

Zinc is essential for the correct formation and functioning of the brain. Learning and behaviour problems affect increasing numbers of children. Figures from the United States show that as many as 4.5 million American children bear the official designation ADD or ADHD (Attention Deficit Disorder with or without hyperactivity). Boys are ten times more likely to be affected than girls. It is an interesting fact that boys (because of testicular tissue), require *five times more zinc* for their development than girls!

Because of its involvement in such a wide range of enzyme systems, zinc deficiency has been implicated in many types of congenital defects. Figures from the United Kingdom show a rise in the incidence of congenital abnormalities, especially among baby boys. Congenital malformation rates per 10,000 births rose from 159 in 1965 to 221 in 1983, with a peak of 245 for boys compared to 190 for girls. Undescended testes is now such a common condition (seven times as common as in 1969) that it is no longer recorded as a malformation.

Zinc is also needed for adequate infant growth. It is in fact a critical factor in the development of skeletal muscle and bones both before and after birth. A recent study from France showed a significant increase in weight and length when breastfed babies were given a modest zinc supplement. The results were particularly evident in baby boys.

Zinc deficient babies have been shown to cry excessively and are frequently also inconsolable and jittery. Babies like this are at much greater risk of being abused—statistics for infant abuse of course also show a trend which is not only alarming but on the increase.

You might perhaps find it interesting to observe how the incidence of many of the conditions which we have listed above has increased dramatically with the widespread use of *oral contraceptives*, which cause profound, and in some long-term users, irreversible changes in zinc status.

A final word on zinc. The RDA (Recommended Daily Allowance) for mature adults is given as 12 to 15 mg (elemental zinc) but this rises to 20 mg during pregnancy. The demand for zinc during breastfeeding is even greater than during pregnancy.

Zinc supplements are best taken on an empty stomach, or last thing at night. This improves absorption since there is no interference from, or competition with, other nutrients.

Blood plasma levels are not a good measure of your zinc status. White blood cell zinc (or sweat zinc, although this test may not be readily available) is the best clinical marker. There is also a simple test which you can do at home to assess zinc status, and we give full details in Chapter 9. We recommend that you both take this test as soon as possible and implement appropriate measures if you are found to be zinc deficient—the effects on your fertility, on any pregnancy and on the health of your infant will be significant!

Selenium

This mineral is an important anti-oxidant, but levels of selenium in Australian soil are very low. A deficiency of selenium has been linked to cot death, Down Syndrome and asthma, and too little selenium (or Vitamin E) can increase the risk of cystic fibrosis. It is an important nutrient in the treatment of breast disease, and for older parents, since it can reduce their risk of having a child with a congenital abnormality. A lack of selenium decreases sperm production and motility. It is lost through frequent ejaculation since it is present in semen. If you want to obtain a selenium supplement you will need a prescription from your doctor. It occurs naturally in garlic and onions (although not in large amounts). Higher doses are required if there is much toxicity or radiation in your environment.

Potassium

This mineral is involved in maintaining the correct fluid balance in the body and if your diet contains too much salt (sodium), this balance will be disturbed. Potassium is also needed for glandular health, sperm motility and correct nerve and muscle function. Diuretics, which are commonly used to treat fluid retention, will lead to an excessive loss of potassium.

Manganese

Manganese is an essential mineral which has some important functions during reproduction. It is involved in the building and breakdown cycles of protein and nucleic acids which are the carriers of genetic information. Through certain enzymes, manganese affects the glandular secretions underlying maternal instinct. It contributes to a mother's love and the instinctive desire to protect her child. The body also utilises manganese to rid itself of lead, and low manganese levels have been linked to learning and behaviour problems in small children, to poor blood sugar control and ligamentous pain. A deficiency of manganese can be a cause of infertility, can lead to a total lack of sperm, spontaneous abortion and bone, heart and nervous system defects.

It is not always easy for you to get adequate amounts of this mineral in your diet, since uptake of manganese from the soil is blocked by the use of the commonly used organophosphate pesticides, which are used routinely in non-sustainable (non-organic) farming operations.

Magnesium

This mineral is essential for correct function of both nerve and muscle. It is necessary for the production of oestrogen and progesterone and is involved in the metabolism of carbohydrates. A deficiency can lead to nervousness, irritability and fluid retention, and to the toxaemia of pregnancy, compromised immune function and can also adversely affect the muscular contractions of the Fallopian tubes which are essential for transport of egg and sperm. A deficiency can also lead to low levels of endorphins (the body's natural pain-killers) and therefore to increased period and labour pain. In the foetus a magnesium deficiency can lead to miscarriage, and retarded development including low birth weight. Even a mild magnesium deficiency can cause free radical damage to sperm and testes.

Magnesium can relieve cravings for sugar, and particularly for chocolate (which is actually very high in magnesium). An adequate supply of this nutrient can therefore help you to avoid eating inappropriate snacks.

The non-pregnant requirement for magnesium is 300 mg daily. This requirement rises to 450 mg daily during pregnancy. Magnesium supplements given throughout pregnancy have been shown to prevent thrombosis, improve vasodilation (preventing toxaemia) and also prevent premature uterine contractions. The supplement which provides optimal absorption of this mineral is magnesium glycinate.

A survey of 568 women showed that a dose of 1 g of magnesium sulphate caused a decrease in hospitalisation time, transfer rates to neonatal units and premature labour, and an increase in the size of the baby.

Iron

During pregnancy the volume of circulating blood increases by approximately one-third. Adequate iron stores are necessary for the increased production of haemoglobin, the oxygen-carrying component of the blood. Iron is also needed to ensure the integrity of the mother's mucous membranes, and for proper thyroid and immune function. Adequate amounts are needed for the correct formation of foetal blood, brain, eye and bone, and for a healthy growth rate. A deficiency can cause infertility and inhibit menstrual flow.

The best source of iron is haem-iron, or iron which is contained in red meat. Iron is also found in green leafy vegetables (non-haem iron), from which it is quite poorly absorbed. Iron requires the presence of Vitamin C to be properly absorbed. The homoeopathic cell salt, ferrum phos, also aids absorption, which is inhibited if tea, coffee or soft drinks are drunk with the meal.

An iron supplement should never be given alone, and should only be given if there is a *proven need* (see Chapter 9). This need should be established well before pregnancy and appropriate supplementation given to ensure that serum ferritin levels are in the range of 55 to 65 micrograms (mcg) per litre well before conception occurs. If supplementation is shown to be necessary, the chosen product should be both organic and chelated. Inorganic iron (which is the type usually prescribed for anaemic women, especially during pregnancy) should not be used, since it destroys Vitamin E, competes with zinc for uptake and metabolism, can cause constipation, and if taken while breastfeeding, may cause colic in the baby.

Iron taken in excess can be toxic. Your body has elaborate mechanisms for ensuring that dietary iron is absorbed and utilised, but has no such mechanisms (apart from menstrual losses) for excreting excess iron.

Iron deficiency may be indicated if you suffer from shortness of breath, palpitations, dull headaches, fatigue, if your nails have ridges or if they separate, if you are very pale, or if you crave non-food items such as ice, starch, clay, dirt or paper. Be aware that unusual cravings in a child may indicate mineral deficiencies.

Iodine

Iodine is essential for the correct functioning of the thyroid gland which controls hormone balance. An under active thyroid may lead to anovulatory cycles (in which no ovulation takes place). Iodine deficiency during pregnancy can lead to damage to the thyroid and causes impairment of brain development in the baby. Iodine is toxic in excess, but it can be useful in cases of excessive bleeding.

Copper

Both a deficiency and an excess of copper can lead to fertility problems. Since water which has run through copper piping contains high levels of this mineral, a deficiency is not often considered to be a problem in Australia. However, an excess of copper can lead to low levels of zinc, and zinc deficiency is implicated in many reproductive problems as we have already discussed. Hair trace mineral analysis combined with a blood test will show if you are suffering from an excessive burden of copper (see Chapter 9).

Chromium

This mineral is a part of GTF (Glucose Tolerance Factor) and is intimately involved in the metabolism of glucose. As you have already learned, your brain depends entirely on a steady supply of glucose to fuel all its processes. Glucose is also necessary for every movement of nerve and muscle. As well, the foetus is dependent on a constant and stable supply of blood glucose for its energy. In other words, since no energy for foetal growth is generated from protein or fat, a maternal chromium deficiency will affect this steady supply of glucose and will consequently affect foetal development. A lack of chromium may also predispose to arteriosclerosis, hypertension and diabetes in later life.

Chromium is found in whole grains, since it is necessary for their metabolic breakdown, but is almost completely removed during the refining process. When you eat refined grains, chromium is leached from your body's stores. To compound this problem, chromium is not easily absorbed but is readily removed from the body. Chromium can be used to stabilise blood sugar levels and thereby help control the nausea of pregnancy and sugar cravings.

Calcium

There are dietary and lifestyle habits which lead to calcium deficiency. These include a diet which is high in phosphorus. Phosphorus is a buffering agent and is present in all processed foods. It is present in particularly high concentrations in soft drinks, where it is necessary to stop the otherwise acidic fluid from dissolving your teeth. As well, a diet which is high in red meat (which is also high in phosphorus), a high protein diet, a high intake of salt or sugar, smoking, drinking alchohol, consumption of caffeine and lack of exercise all contribute to calcium loss. Calcium is also used by the body as it endeavours to rid itself of lead. Calcium absorption may also be compromised if magnesium and Vitamin D (as well as oestrogen) are deficient.

Calcium is essential for proper dental and skeletal development in the embryo and for the formation of muscle and nerve tissue. Dental decay and a need for orthodontic treatment, the latter increasingly common, are just two signs of a calcium deficiency.

Calcium is also necessary for the formation of fertile or 'stretchy' mucus and can also improve the ability of the sperm to swim through it. Calcium counteracts the negative effect of too much manganese, which causes the mucus to become 'sticky' or infertile.

A calcium deficiency can lead to nervous tension and fluid retention, and has also been linked to the toxaemia of pregnancy. Since calcium is essential for proper muscle contraction, and is also necessary for controlling blood clotting mechanisms, there are further implications for the birthing woman.

The recommended daily allowance for calcium during pregnancy is 1,200 mg daily. Calcium supplements must be balanced with magnesium (calcium:magnesium in the ratio 2:1). Calcium levels which are too high compared with those of magnesium can lead to the formation of kidney stones. It is important to know that if you take calcium carbonate as a supplement, only 10 per cent is absorbed. Calcitite (if available) is a supplement made from bone and also contains the hormonal factors which aid absorption.

Boron

Boron is found in most plant foods, but is unlikely to be found in supplements (because it is now only available on prescription). If you eat plenty of fresh fruit and vegetables you should receive sufficient of this mineral. A diet which is high in boron can double the levels of oestrogen in the blood.

Vitamin A

Vitamin A is an anti-oxidant and therefore has an important role to play in detoxification. It enhances the metabolic efficiency of essential fatty acids. It is necessary for the maintenance of the gastrointestinal tract, lungs and mucous membranes, and it keeps the cilia (tiny hair-like projections) inside the Fallopian tubes healthy. It is also necessary for the health of the testes, for sperm production, and is needed for the conversion of cholesterol to the male hormone, testosterone. It can prevent heavy periods and premenstrual depression.

Vitamin A is an oil-soluble vitamin and is stored by the body. It is usually recommended that doses of this supplement are carefully monitored before and during pregnancy, since an excessive intake has been linked to birth defects. However, the doses of Vitamin A found to cause foetal abnormalities were in the range of 25,000 to 500,000 iu (international units) per day.

On the other hand, Vitamin A deficiency has been linked to infertility, miscarriage and to a number of abnormalities such as cleft palate and absence of eyes. Therefore, do not avoid supplementation with this nutrient completely. Worldwide studies which showed a lowering of the incidence of birth defects, gave supplements which contained levels of Vitamin A up to 6,000 iu per day. Alternatively, you may prefer to supplement with beta-carotene which your body will convert to Vitamin A as required.

Beta-carotene

Beta-carotene is a precursor of Vitamin A and occurs naturally in all red and orange vegetables. It is an anti-oxidant and improves your immune response.

B-complex vitamins

These vitamins include the Vitamins B1 (thiamine), B2 (riboflavin), B3 (niacin), B5 (pantothenic acid), B6 (pyridoxine), B12 (cobalamin), PABA (para-aminobenzoic acid), inositol, choline and folic acid. These nutrients always occur together and are needed for a large number of bodily functions including the metabolism of carbohydrates, the utilisation of energy, correct digestive function, manufacture of the sex hormones and maintenance of healthy tissue. The metabolism of essential fatty acids and the subsequent production of the correct balance of oestrogen and progesterone is also dependent on the presence of adequate levels of the B-complex vitamins. Male fertility is particularly dependent on B5 (healthy testes), B12 (to increase sperm count and motility) and Inositol (healthy prostate).

B-complex vitamins are found in a variety of foods including organ meats and whole grains, and they may also be manufactured by the healthy gastrointestinal tract. However, together with many of the trace minerals, the B vitamins are removed during the manufacturing processes which give us white flour, white rice and refined sugar. Their synthesis in the gut is inhibited by commonly used antibiotics and further loss may be caused by other drugs, including oral contraceptives, by smoking, or by the consumption of alcohol and coffee. During periods of stress there is a greatly increased need for all the B vitamins. This stress may be emotional but can also include periods of rapid growth, pregnancy, birth, lactation and injury or infection.

In the animal foetus, problems which occur due to a deficiency of one or more of the B vitamins may include miscarriage or stillbirth, low birth weight and increased incidence of neonatal or perinatal death. Since the roles of these nutrients are so varied, defects in all organ systems including the heart, genito-urinary system, blood vessels, spinal cord, skeleton, eye, lung, kidney and brain have been observed.

The B vitamins occur together in nature and although pyridoxine (Vitamin B6) and folic acid may sometimes be recommended as single supplements, we want to emphasise that the full complement of B vitamins should always be given together. If one of the B vitamins is given alone, a deficiency in another may arise.

Vitamin B2 (riboflavin)

This vitamin affects the level of oestrogen which is needed to develop the follicle. If you are on a dairy-free diet or exercise intensively you may be deficient in this nutrient. There have been suggestions that the mutagenic effect of thalidomide was due to its interference in the absorption of this vitamin.

Vitamin B6 (pyridoxine)

Conditions which may benefit from supplementation with Vitamin B6 include fluid retention, breast tenderness, premenstrual tension and the nausea of pregnancy. This vitamin can increase progesterone levels (necessary for preparation of the endometrium to receive the fertilised ovum), and inhibit the excessive production of prolactin which is caused by a dysfunctional pituitary gland. Vitamin B6 also promotes the absorption of zinc.

Vitamin B12 (cobalamin)

This vitamin has been shown to enhance fertility and a deficiency can cause spinal cord damage in the infant. Vegetarians beware—the main source of B12 is animal products.

Folic acid

Folic acid is essential for the formation of DNA and RNA. These compounds are essentially the genetic material, so an adequate supply of this vitamin is especially important during the first three months of pregnancy when cells are dividing and organs are forming. A deficiency can lead to infertility (by reducing production of eggs and sperm). Studies have now shown conclusively that giving a supplement of folic acid before and around the time of conception can prevent neural tube defects such as spina bifida, and anencephaly by 70 to 75 per cent. Spina bifida is a split or divided spine and is usually associated with hydrocephalus (fluid on the brain). One in every 700 to 800 babies born in Australia has spina bifida. Anencephaly means the complete absence of a brain (these babies do not survive).

Many doctors now recommend that all women of child-bearing age should receive a supplement of this nutrient, but once again, we want to emphasis that folic acid should always be taken in conjunction with the other vitamins of the B group. Folic acid is found in all green leafy vegetables (foliage), hence its name. Since oral contraceptives deplete folic acid stores, special care must be taken after stopping their use before conceiving.

Vitamin C (ascorbic acid) and bioflavonoids

Vitamin C is a powerful anti-oxidant which protects against the toxicity of lead, pesticides and other environmental pollutants, and against mutagenic activity. Good levels can protect against genetic abnormalities (more often resulting from faulty paternal DNA than maternal). The ovaries are very rich in Vitamin C which indicates a strong need for the presence of this nutrient, which has been shown to promote ovulation in women whose cycles are anovular. Vitamin C has also been shown to prevent the agglutination (clumping together) of sperm. It is necessary for hormone production, for the metabolism of essential fatty acids and must be present for the proper absorption of iron. It is important for appropriate immune function— the level of Vitamin C in immune cells may be up to 100 times higher than that found in other tissues.

Vitamin C is needed for the production of collagen and it therefore promotes the integrity of skin, tissue and bone, and protects them from invasion by viruses, bacteria or other foreign organisms. It is obviously an extremely important nutrient during pregnancy when foetal skin and bones are developing, but also because your needs for sound collagen must be satisfied as the size of your breasts and belly increase. Lack of Vitamin C during pregnancy has been linked to an increased risk of miscarriage, spontaneous rupture of the membranes, and brain tumours in the offspring.

Vitamin C deficiency in children may cause them to be listless and lethargic, they may bruise easily and their bones may be brittle. Lack of Vitamin C in adults may mean that they have poor resistance to infection, poor wound healing, bleeding gums and dandruff and small haemorrhages due to capillary fragility. Vitamin C levels in the body are reduced by stress, smoking and infections. Vitamin C and the bioflavonoids occur together naturally in all fresh fruits and vegetables.

Vitamin D

Vitamin D is sometimes considered to be a hormone rather than a nutrient. It is involved in the uptake and utilisation of calcium and phosphorus and is manufactured in the skin in the presence of sunlight. In Australia, Vitamin D deficiency is not generally considered to be a problem, although in colder climates where sunlight is limited, people with dark skin are at risk of rickets, a Vitamin D deficiency. A deficiency has been shown to be a factor in many congenital abnormalities.

Vitamin E

Vitamin E is an anti-oxidant and therefore protects against mutagenic activity. Although there is no known acute deficiency disease for this nutrient (such as scurvy for Vitamin C), Vitamin E is important for proper fertility in both the male and female. Adequate levels of Vitamin E are necessary to ensure a conception, a healthy pregnancy and an easy delivery. It is required for the metabolism of essential fatty acids and selenium. It regulates oestrogen levels, and has an important role to play in the treatment of premenstrual syndrome (PMS). It is especially useful for symptoms such as lumpy breasts (fibrocystic breast disease), headache, sweet cravings, increased appetite, fatigue, dizziness and palpitations.

Vitamin E reduces the body's requirements for oxygen, it improves circulation and can protect against varicose veins and haemorrhoids. A deficiency can lead to spontaneous abortion, and if severe, to a total lack of sperm and, together with selenium deficiency, can increase the risk of having a child with cystic fibrosis. Once again this nutrient is lost during the refining of grains. Supplements of Vitamin E should be used with caution in patients with high blood pressure.

Essential fatty acids (EFAs)

The essential fatty acids are necessary for the formation of the prostaglandins. Those substances have a wide variety of biological functions, including responsibility for correct hormonal balance, and for the fine-tuning of the baby's bodily functions. EFAs are needed for fully functioning sex glands, and for the formation of the pros-taglandins which are present in semen. Males need more EFAs than females. EFAs help to reduce the 'bad' prostaglandins (those that cause pain, cramping, PMS, hypertension and benign breast disease) and increase the 'good' prostaglandins. They are essential for the correct formation of all cell walls and for the development of the foetal brain and nervous system. They have beneficial effects on uterine blood flow and may protect against cot death (SIDS). Defi-ciencies can lead to chromosomal defects, subtle brain disorders such as dyslexia, spontaneous abortion and may delay labour.

EFAs are found in high concentrations in deep dwelling and cold-water fish. They are especially high in Evening primrose oil and are also found in cold-pressed oils such as olive and sunflower, but they are readily destroyed by excessive heat and their metabolism is blocked by saturated fats. The two main essential fatty acid supplements are *Evening primrose oil* (which contains gamma-linolenic acid or GLA) and *fish oil* (which contains docosahexaenoic and eicosapentaenoic acids) and is widely available as MaxEPA.

Special note: Supplements of Evening primrose oil are contraindicated for anyone suffering from epilepsy. An alternative source of EFAs is as follows:

3 parts linseeds
1 part sunflower seeds
1 part almonds
Combine all and grind to a paste.

Amino acids

Amino acids are essential for the formation and repair of tissue, muscle, organs and hair, and for the formation of semen and digestive enzymes. All the essential amino acids occur together in primary proteins (proteins from an animal source) but if secondary proteins (vegetable origin) are eaten, they must be combined as you have already seen to give the full complement of these essential building blocks.

An adequate intake of protein is particularly important *before conception* since it is necessary for healthy sperm and eggs (both quantity as well as quality), for proper fertilisation and the healthy early development of the embryo.

Complex carbohydrates

As we have already discussed, complex carbohydrate containing foods are necessary for energy.

NUTRIENT FOOD SOURCES

Now that you have read through this long list, the implications should be fairly obvious. The roles of the essential nutrients are many and varied, and adequate nutritional status is unquestionably of enormous importance not only in ensuring good health in both prospective parents, but in all phases of the reproductive cycle, and for sound physical and mental foetal development as well.

You can see why an excellent diet is important if you want to receive an adequate supply of all essential nutrients, and in the table following we have listed the best food sources of each. You may find that, in some instances, we have not listed what is traditionally the richest source of a nutrient (for example, liver is the richest source of Vitamin A). However, the richest source may perhaps be a food that we recommend you avoid—liver (and other organ meats or offal) are the detoxification routes for the animal, and may therefore contain high concentrations of chemicals, pesticides and heavy metals. Likewise, dairy foods, because they are a common allergen, may not be a useful source of nutrients for many people. (See also pages 57–8 for supplements and suggested daily dosages.)

Nutrient	Good food source
Vitamin A	Red, orange and green vegetables, particularly red capsicums, dandelion greens, carrots, sweet potatoes, parsley, spinach, butternut pumpkin, watercress, mangoes.
Vitamin E	Whole grains, oatmeal, brown rice, wheat germ and oil, sunflower seeds and oil, safflower oil, almonds, sesame oil, olive oil, soya bean oil, spinach, salmon.
Vitamin D	sardines, salmon, prawns, sunflower seeds, eggs, mushrooms.
B-complex vitamins	Whole grains, wheat germ, sunflower seeds, soya beans and other legumes, nuts, poultry, seafoods (including deep-sea fish and shellfish), eggs.
Folic Acid	Beans (soy, kidney, mung, lima, navy), blackeye and split peas, lentils, whole wheat, barley, broccoli, spinach, kale, asparagus, berries.
Vitamin C and Bioflavonoids	Red and green capsicums, kale, spinach, parsley, broccoli, brussel sprouts, watercress, cauliflower, red cabbage, berries, cherries, papaya, citrus fruits, grapes, rose hips.

Calcium	Swiss and cheddar cheese, whole milk, yoghurt, goat's milk, seaweed, collard leaves, beet, dandelion and turnip greens, parsley, watercress, broccoli, spinach, sesame seeds (hulled), almonds, brazil nuts, tofu, ripe olives, cooked soya beans, salmon and sardines (with bones).
Magnesium	Seaweed, wheat grain, wheat bran, wheat germ, buckwheat, millet, brown rice, cooked soya beans, almonds, cashews, brazil nuts, sunflower seeds, hazelnuts, spinach, Swiss chard, parsley, beet greens, avocado, tofu.
Potassium	Seaweed, sunflower seeds, wheat germ, millet, almonds, pecans, brazil nuts, raisins, dates, dried figs, spinach, Swiss chard, parsley, broccoli, beans and soya beans (cooked), yams, avocado, garlic, lean beef, whole wheat, rye, corn, snapper, chicken.
Iron	Lean beef, seaweed, wheat bran, wheat germ, millet, pumpkin seeds, sunflower seeds, almonds, cashews, brazil nuts, sesame seeds (hulled), cooked dry beans, parsley, dandelion and beet greens, Swiss chard, Jerusalem artichoke, clams, egg yolk.
Manganese	Barley, rye, buckwheat, whole wheat, oatmeal, oats, cornmeal, millet, walnuts, brazil nuts, almonds, split peas (dry), spinach, turnip and beet greens, rhubarb, brussel sprouts.
Zinc	Fresh oysters, ground round steak, lamb chops (meat is best source of absorbable zinc), chicken, pecans, brazil nuts, hazel nuts, walnuts, almonds, whole wheat, rye, oats, split peas (dry), lima beans, sardines, anchovies.
Chromium	Wholewheat bread, wheat bran, rye bread, wheat germ, beef (round), fresh chilli, green capsicum, potatoes, apple, parsnips, hen's eggs, chicken, oysters.
Selenium	Wheat germ, wholewheat bread, brown rice, oats, bran, barley, brazil nuts, scallops, lobster, prawns, crab, oysters, apple cider vinegar, garlic.

| Iodine | Seaweed, prawns, haddock, halibut, oysters, salmon, sardines (canned), wholewheat bread, eggs, lettuce, spinach, pineapple. |
| Essential Fatty Acids (EFAs) | Deep-sea/ocean/coldwater fish e.g. salmon, trout, cod, herring; monounsaturated cold pressed oils e.g. olive, canola, sunflower, linseed; flax and blackcurrant seeds; walnuts. |

WHY A GOOD DIET IS NOT GOOD ENOUGH

For at *least four months prior to conception*, both prospective parents should take a combination of supplements which will provide an adequate supply of all the essential nutrients. The mother should continue this *supplementation throughout her pregnancy and during the full period of breastfeeding*. But, don't ignore this advice: don't take single nutrients in isolation unless it appears certain from hair trace mineral analysis or another clinical marker that you have a greater than normal need for a particular mineral or vitamin; and do not take nutrients in megadoses, unless instructed to do so by a practitioner who is fully trained in the use of nutritional therapies.

Nutrients from diet alone?

In our many discussions with couples on the topic of supplements we frequently hear the retort, 'Oh, I try to get my vitamins and minerals from my diet!' Of course this is an absolutely sensible and worthy sentiment, and we want to emphasise at the outset that nothing can take the place of a truly excellent diet. However, we would now like to give you some of the reasons why optimal nutritional intake may not, for many of you, be possible from diet alone, or why a good diet may simply not be good enough. On closer examination of the many reasons why your diet may not provide all that you need in terms of nutrients, the logical place to start is down on the farm.

How nutritious is your food?

What happens on the farm?

Much of the soil in Australia is nutrient poor due to its great age. The farming techniques which are practised on this soil are still, almost universally, non-sustainable, and will therefore exacerbate the problem of nutrient poor soil. Continual farming of land and the use of inorganic fertilisers means that the many nutrients such as manganese, zinc, iron, chromium, cobalt, magnesium, molybdenum and calcium to name a few, which the growing plant takes from the soil, are never fully replaced. Subsequent crops therefore have increasingly low levels of essential nutrients from which to draw, making them more susceptible to disease and requiring more frequent applications of fertilisers. These fertilisers boost growth but fail to give the plant time to take up what nutrients are there. The disease-susceptible crops must then be sprayed many times with a variety of pesticides. Some of these are known to destroy choline and inhibit the uptake of manganese.

The result is produce which is large, but which may be so only by virtue of its high water content. It may be tasteless and have a vitamin and mineral content significantly lower than produce which has been grown by sustainable or organic methods. It is probably not too surprising that animals and birds which have been intensively farmed or battery bred have a fatty acid composition which differs markedly from livestock which has been fed organically and grazed in a free-range manner.

Sustainable farming techniques such as green manuring, composting, companion planting and crop rotation will ensure that the soil is healthy and has an adequate supply of nutrients for the plant to draw from. By contrast, the produce from sustainable farms is not generally distinguished by its large size, or by its unblemished appearance. It is, however, distinguished by its superior taste and by its freedom from pesticide and other chemical residues. Most importantly it is distinguished by its superior vitamin and mineral content.

From the farm to your table

You can clearly see that before conventionally grown crops have even been picked, they may be of extremely variable nutritional quality. Once they are picked, the loss of essential nutrients continues. Once they are off the tree, or out of the ground, fruit and vegetables may have a long journey before they reach your table. Initially, they may be put into cold storage. They will then be transported and perhaps stored again. The trip from greengrocers' shelves to your dinner plates means further loss of essential nutrients as produce is refrigerated, then cooked by a variety of methods. Some of these preserve nutrients, while others destroy them. The cooked food may then be frozen and reheated, which contributes even further to nutrient loss.

Some fresh produce will go to canning or packaging plants. Many of the processes used here will also destroy nutrients. For example, the chemical chelating agent which is used to ensure that frozen peas retain their bright green colour when cooked, also removes all traces of zinc from the vegetable. Canned tomatoes have lost 80 per cent of their zinc content, and storing cans for prolonged periods results in even further nutrient loss.

What happens during refining?

Grains such as wheat and rice are milled or crushed in refining processes which give us our widely consumed white flour and white rice or other refined grains. These processes separate the outer coating (bran), and the growing point (germ), which contain the greatest proportion of vitamins and trace minerals, and leave the white endosperm which is largely complex carbohydrate (starch) with very few vitamins and minerals. Unfortunately, the remaining complex carbohydrate requires all of the nutrients with which it occurs naturally, but from which it has now been separated, for its metabolism. Consequently, when you consume any of the refined grains such as white flour or white rice, those vitamins and minerals which are required for the breakdown of carbohydrates, will be leached or stolen from your body stores.

Sugar-cane refining is a similar story, with the loss of a great proportion of essential trace minerals and vitamins in the production of raw or brown sugar, and all nutrients completely removed to give the highly refined white product. Your body has no need at all for refined sugar. The body's metabolic processes break down the molecules of complex carbohydrates which are found in fruit, vegetables, whole grains and legumes, to give the simple sugars which your body requires for its energy. The essential nutrients required for these metabolic processes always occur naturally in conjunction with the *complex* carbohydrates, but these same nutrients will be leached from your body's reserves when you consume *refined* carbohydrates.

However, refining of flour and production of refined sugar is only the beginning of the road to many finished food products. Bread, for example, has an extraordinary number and variety of chemicals added during its manufacture. These are used to ensure that the flour is easy for the baker to work with, that the texture of the loaf is acceptable, that it has good keeping qualities and much more. The label may say 'no additives' but if your loaf is made from breadmaking flour it actually contains a number of added chemicals. As well, today's food technologists are able to produce an amazing array of edible goods from starting products which have more in common with the stuff of petrochemical plants than food as we know it.

What happens during processing?

In America it has been estimated that as many as 20,000 chemicals are presently used in food production with 3,000 of those added directly to the food supply. Most of these will be added to processed food. As your consumption of processed and fast food increases, so the use of chemical additives continues to increase and in the United States has doubled in the last fifteen years from 181 million kg to 363 million kg. Chemicals can be used to enhance flavour or colour, they are used to buffer, extend, stabilise and preserve. Apart from the fact that a great deal of processed food is already of extremely poor nutrient quality due to the large proportion of refined flour and sugar used in its manufacture, your body must use many essential vitamins and minerals to rid itself of chemical additives.

Furthermore, a significant number of you may be adversely affected in a much more direct manner, by many of these chemicals. The most common offenders are preservatives and food colourings; infants and children, partly because of their small body size, partly because their enzyme detoxification systems are immature and partly because their brains are still developing, are particularly susceptible to the adverse effects of these chemicals.

The sensitivity reactions or allergies as they are sometimes called may occur in any of your body's organ systems. The symptoms may be neurological, with hyperactivity or learning and behaviour problems particularly prominent, there may be skin reactions, gastrointestinal disturbances, hay fever or asthma type symptoms. Whatever the reaction, your body must then use many of its precious nutrients to try to repair the damage or to restore itself to good health.

An ever increasing number of meals, perhaps as many as one in four, are now prepared outside the home. Many of these meals would have been standing for long periods, and have had a variety of chemicals added to extend their life, and to help them retain their appearance.

Hopefully, the reasons for our dietary recommendations are now clearer to you. The reasons for supplementation should be a little clearer too. For many people, the typical twentieth-century diet has probably been, at least until you picked up this book, the diet which sustained you (and possibly your parents and maybe your grandparents too). Put simply this diet is one of oversupply/undernutrition. If you are the third or fourth generation who has lived largely on a diet of this nature, your body's nutrient stores may be severely depleted, and even if you now undergo a religious conversion to improving your eating habits, those depleted nutrient stores will almost certainly stay depleted without the help of supplementation to put them right.

Further reasons for supplementing
Medical conditions
Many of you may have suffered throughout your life from undiagnosed allergies, sensitivities or other conditions which have affected your body's ability to absorb nutrients. You may have had recurring or long-term low grade infections (see Chapters 10 and 11). We know that all of these conditions create further demand for nutrients.

Lifestyle and environmental factors
The use of tobacco, alcohol, caffeine, oral contraceptives and other drugs may have robbed your body of vitamins and minerals. Your body also uses a variety of nutrients to detoxify and protect itself from the damage of polluting factors such as chemicals, radiation and heavy metals such as lead. Stress, in all its guises, causes an increased demand for a variety of essential nutritional factors. We will talk more about all of these in the following chapters.

Increasing age of child-bearing couples

You are probably aware that, on average, first time parents are considerably older than they once were. The mean age for a couple having a first child is now late 20s, where just two decades ago it was early 20s. Many couples are putting off starting a family until late 30s and frequently beyond. While the optimal age for a woman having a first child is suggested as late teens, we firmly believe that many of the complications which are said to arise with older mothers (and with older fathers) can be completely avoided with good pre-conception care. Many problems arise because nutrient stores in the older population are depleted. This is because they have spent more years eating processed and refined food, older couples have used nutrient-depleting lifestyle factors such as alcohol, tobacco, tea, coffee and other drugs, including oral contraceptives, for longer, and have had more sustained exposure to environmental pollution.

Biochemical individuality

As well, everyone is biochemically different and it may be quite impossible for you to achieve adequate nutritional status from a wholefood diet alone. Unfortunately, it is not yet possible to completely and accurately assess each individual's specific needs and the popular recommended daily allowance (RDA) is a mean or average amount and makes no allowance for those whose needs for a nutrient are much greater than average. Furthermore, the RDA may only be of use in calculating the dose required to prevent a frank deficiency state, such as scurvy, from occurring. This measure may be of little use in assessing the amount of a nutrient required to achieve or maintain optimal health.

Increased nutritional needs during gestation

Finally, as we have already outlined, the needs for all essential nutrients during every phase of reproduction are critical. In fact, while food requirements during pregnancy increase by 15 to 20 per cent, the requirements for a particular nutrient may double. It seems to be universally true that nutrition that is merely good enough to keep adults alive, may fail to support reproduction. Deficiencies which may go completely unnoticed in adult life can severely compromise the development of the foetus.

Therefore, because of non-sustainable farming techniques, because nutrients may be lost or destroyed due to a variety of environmental and lifestyle factors, because the nutritional needs of individuals are extremely variable, because many of you have left your child-bearing till late in life, and because the needs during reproduction are so critical, we recommend that you take a combination of supplements which will provide you with a complete and well balanced supply of all essential vitamins, minerals, amino and fatty acids. Think of these supplements as an insurance policy and in no way assume that they will take the place of an improved diet or a healthier lifestyle. Both of you should take these supplements for *at least four months* prior to conception and the mother should continue their use through-out her pregnancy and during the full period of breastfeeding.

Popular misconceptions about supplements

A significant proportion of the general population and some medical practitioners are still firmly of the opinion that if you eat a reasonably varied diet you will be assured of an adequate supply of all the essential vitamins and minerals. Unfortunately, orthodox medical training in Australia does not include adequate information on nutri-tion. Even those practitioners trained in nutrition may not be aware of the unique needs of the preconception period.

From the huge advances made in nutritional research we now know that in between optimal health and frank deficiency states there exists a vast grey area of sub-clinical deficiencies of many kinds.

What about the old stand-bys?

Traditionally, many gynaecologists and obstetricians have recognised the vastly increased need for nutrients during gestation. They have also recognised the fact that these needs may not be met from dietary sources alone, and have prescribed supplements of *iron, folic acid* and *calcium* for pregnant women.

The volume of circulating blood increases by approximately one-third during pregnancy. Extra iron is needed for the increased production of haemoglobin which carries oxygen in the blood to the tissues. Folic acid is involved in the formation of red blood cells, but is of particular importance during pregnancy since it is necessary for the division and formation of all new cells. Calcium is essential to ensure strong bones and teeth and to ensure proper nerve and muscle function in the developing foetus.

However, the practice of giving these three nutrients in isolation does not reflect their relative importance. It indicates, instead, rather outdated knowledge of nutrition and gestational requirements. By this we do not mean that iron, folate and calcium are unimportant nutrients. In fact, a recent eight-year study from 33 international centres has shown that folic acid given before and around the time of conception will prevent neural tube defects such as spina bifida.

But what we do mean to say is that these nutrients are no more important than a host of others, and that our present state of knowledge indicates that single nutrients should not be given in isolation. All nutritional factors work in unison, one nutrient may on occasion be able to substitute for another—indeed the interactions and the balances and checks are extraordinarily complex. It is rare for a deficiency of one single nutrient to occur in Nature. Consequently, if one vitamin or mineral is given alone or in megadoses, a deficiency of another nutrient may arise, such as the example of inorganic iron supplements competing with zinc for uptake.

To sum up

The recognition that supplements may be necessary to meet nutritional needs during reproduction is nothing new. However, in light of what has recently been learned about nutritional requirements and nutrient/nutrient interactions you must ensure that the combination of supplements which you take is complete and well balanced. When using supplements, also remember that they should not be used in place of an improved diet and a healthier lifestyle, nor should they be used in megadoses. Remember too that individual nutrients should be added to a basic general formula only under the supervision of a practitioner who is fully trained in the use of nutritional therapies.

Nutrient	Supplement and suggested daily dosage
Vitamin A	10,000 iu or 6 mg beta-carotene
Vitamin E	500 iu
Vitamin D	200 iu
B-complex vitamins	B1, B2, B3, B5—up to 50 mg each; B12—400 micrograms (mcg); B6—up to 250

Nutrient	Supplement and suggested daily dosage
	milligrams (mg); biotin—200 mcg; choline, inositol and PABA—25 mg
Folic acid	500–1000 mcg (0.5 to 1.0 mg) daily (1000 mcg (1.0 mg) daily if you have had a previous miscarriage or if there is a history of neural tube defects in your family)
Vitamin C and Bioflavonoids	2000–3000 mg (2 to 3 g) Vitamin C (up to 5 g if you are suffering from infection) and 300 mg bioflavonoids
Calcium	800 mg (twice the amount of magnesium). Avoid dolomite and bone meal supplements which may be contaminated with lead
Magnesium	400 mg (half the amount of calcium)
Potassium	15 mg or as potassium chloride cell salt
Iron	15 mg taken with iron phosphate (usually called ferrum phos). Iron should be organic and chelated, but should only be taken if need is proven. Dairy foods decrease availability of iron from diet
Manganese	10 mg
Zinc	20–60 mg elemental (depending on results of Zinc Tally. Take separately, on an empty stomach, last thing at night)
Chromium	100–200 mcg (upper levels for those with sugar cravings)
Selenium	100–200 mcg (upper levels for those exposed to heavy pollution) (You need a prescription for selenium supplements as they are restricted, Schedule 4 in Australia)
Iodine	75 mcg (or as kelp—150 mg)
Evening primrose oil	500–1000 mg three times daily
MaxEPA	500–1000 mg three times daily, especially if diet contains little deep-sea fish
Acidophilus and Bifidus	½–1 teaspoon of each, one to two times daily (upper level for those with Candida problems)

A *few hints about supplements*

- Obviously, it is impossible to take all these supplements separately. Look around for a good multivitamin and mineral formula which contains approximately the dosages recommended. There are several 'women's' formulae or 'PMS' products on the market which will contain similar doses to those listed above, and will reduce the number of extra tablets required.
- Digestive enzymes will help you to absorb nutrients.
- Take vitamins and minerals just before, during or after meals—this aids absorption since there are co-factors present in food which are absent from supplements.
- Take your supplements every day.
- If you cannot swallow tablets, the micellised form of a supplement can be added to water or juice. Micelles are very well absorbed.
- If supplements are made from oils, they should be refrigerated and their expiry date adhered to. Rancid oils will increase serum levels of free radicals which are very damaging.

A *few cautions about supplements*

- Avoid mega-vitamins. Some vitamins taken in large quantities can have adverse effects. For example:
- High levels of folic acid can mask a B12 deficiency.
- Too much B6 can be toxic and lead to numbness in hands and feet (up to 250 mg daily is very safe, and up to 400 mg should present no problems, even during pregnancy. However, levels above 250 mg should be supervised).
- Too much copper can decrease zinc levels (and fertility).
- Too much iron affects zinc absorption.
- Too much phosphorus increases the need for calcium.
- Too much manganese can make your mucus 'sticky'.
- Too much Vitamin A can lead to foetal abnormalities, but up to 10,000 iu daily is very safe (see also page 42).
- All of these nutrients are essential—if you are in any doubt about what constitutes too much, consult a health professional who is trained in nutrition.

Digestion/Absorption

We have just given you guidelines for making sure that you receive all the nutrients necessary for optimum health, but we also want to say that if your digestion and/or absorption are below par, then the best diet and the most comprehensive supplementation program may be largely in vain. There are some symptoms which may indicate if your digestion and/or absorption is inadequate:

- Bad breath/coated tongue.
- Indigestion/heartburn.
- Constipation/diverticulitis.
- Flatulence/bloating.
- Belching.
- Low minerals levels revealed by hair trace mineral analysis.

There are several factors which may contribute to poor digestion and absorption:

- Lack of hydrochloric acid in the stomach—supplementation can correct.
- Lack of pancreatic enzymes—supplementation can correct.
- Generally poor nutritional status—ironically you need good nutrition for good digestion and absorption, as well as vice versa!
- Candida.
- Allergies.
- Coeliac or other genetic condition.
- Alcohol/other drug use.

If you suffer from any of the above symptoms, or if your hair trace mineral analysis indicates the possibility of malabsorption, it is essential that you (ideally with the help of a practitioner) track down the cause of the problem and implement appropriate treatment. Without attention to the underlying condition, all your efforts to eat well and all your supplementing may not do you a great deal of good, and the effects on the foetus of poor digestion/absorption can of course be severe.

2

IMPROVING YOUR
LIFESTYLE

AT LEAST FOUR MONTHS (preferably longer) before
you plan to conceive your child, both of you should
stop smoking, *avoid alcohol completely*, *avoid drugs*
and *avoid caffeine*.

WE NOW COME TO a discussion of those lifestyle habits which may
adversely affect your ability to carry a baby and your baby's health.
As you will see, they are all factors over which you can exercise
almost complete personal control. However, they are such an
entrenched part of our culture, and so well accepted by society, that
many people find it extremely difficult to give them up. As well, many
experts are reluctant to issue more than a mild caution about their use.
In a recent article, which appeared in a leading Australian newspaper,
two obstetricians from prominent teaching hospitals stated that they
could see little evidence for harm in one or two glasses of alcohol,
three cups of tea or coffee and marijuana in small quantities during
pregnancy. Obviously, advice such as this only makes it more difficult
for you to give up habits such as smoking and drinking

Those factors which are capable of adversely affecting the foetus
are also capable of seriously compromising the health of both prospective parents, and consequently the health of sperm and ova, factors on
which, of course, foetal health ultimately depends. They can also
affect fertility, they may be responsible for many complications of

pregnancy, they can affect the ease and duration of labour, the success of lactation and the way in which you nurture your child. An adverse effect on the foetus, is, in fact, only one way in which your reproductive health may be compromised.

Smoking, drinking and drug-taking may exert their adverse effects *directly*, or they may act *indirectly* by compromising that all-important factor—nutritional status. Some of these habits may have both direct and indirect effects and there also exists the possibility that a combination of factors such as smoking and drinking, or drinking and drug taking will have synergistic effects, or effects which are greater than the sum of the individual parts. Therein, of course, lies the danger of experts giving the nod to the consumption of moderate amounts of social drugs.

For this reason we make no apologies whatever for our blanket recommendation that *both prospective parents should completely avoid cigarettes, alcohol, and other drugs including caffeine* (which is found in cola drinks and chocolate, not just in tea and coffee) for *at least four months leading up to conception*. Obviously if you are prepared to give up these habits now, in preparation for a pregnancy at some much later time, the greater the improvement you can expect to see in your general health. Your chances of staying off the cigarettes, the booze and the caffeine will also be significantly better, and the chance of giving birth to a very healthy baby will be greater too! However, if you are already cringing at the thought of nicotine or caffeine withdrawal, it might be appropriate to look at some suggestions for making the withdrawal a little less painful, before we look at the many reasons why we recommend complete avoidance of these ubiquitous substances.

HOW TO GIVE UP AN ADDICTION

- Eat regular, nutritious, wholefood meals.
- Avoid sugary snacks which often exacerbate cravings for tea, coffee, cola drinks, alcohol or cigarettes.
- Always have plenty of nutritious food, or alternative drinks such as herbal teas and dandelion or cereal coffee, ready at hand for the times when you crave something to put in your mouth. Be aware that some instant herbal teas contain sugar and should be avoided.
- Take multivitamin and mineral supplements as directed in the previous chapter. These will redress some of the nutritional

imbalances caused by the addictive substances, and can help to improve your moods, which may be despondent and erratic without your regular fix.

- Avoid situations in which you usually have a drink, a cigarette or a cup of tea or coffee.
- Try to avoid stressful situations, which are also often the times when you reach for your cigarettes, or a drink containing caffeine or alcohol.
- Find another way to resolve or handle stressful situations. This may involve meditation or regular aerobic exercise.
- Keep busy—take up a new hobby or a sport so that the times when you are idle, and likely to be tempted by your addiction, are much reduced.
- Try to find a companion who will keep you company in your efforts to break the addiction. This may well be your partner.
- If you are a smoker as well as a consumer of alcohol, caffeine and other drugs, then give up only one substance at a time. Alternatively, you can cut down very slowly on all substances before stopping completely. If you try to give up all substances totally and all at once, complete success is much less likely.
- Think positively and try to focus particularly on all the excellent reasons for giving up these habits. Positive visualisation is very helpful.
- Say this affirmation—'*I am making a positive choice for my health and the health of my unborn child,*' or '*better choices, better health, better baby!*'
- Be aware that attendance at special clinics, as well as hypnotherapy and acupuncture, may be useful aids to quitting.
- Remember that a minimum period of four months should elapse between complete withdrawal and conception, and that some methods used to ease withdrawal (such as nicotine patches) still deliver significant doses of the drug to your body.

THINGS TO GIVE UP

Alcohol

Alcohol is probably the most widely used social drug after caffeine. It is also a recorded fact that most people seriously understate (or underestimate) the amount of alcohol they consume. Here again you can see why there is a great danger in stating that there appears to be a safe level of one or two drinks during pregnancy. Quite simply, one or two drinks can very easily become three or four (or more).

Alcohol has serious effects on many of the body's organ systems including the liver, the nervous system, the brain and the heart. Alcohol also affects the body's metabolism of essential fatty acids, and seriously affects nutritional status. It has a toxic effect on gut mucosa and decreases the absorption of all B-complex vitamins and also increases the urinary excretion of zinc as well as that of magnesium, calcium, chromium and Vitamin C. Alcohol, because it is a refined carbohydrate, is fermented, and contains yeast, which may also contribute to an overgrowth of Candida in the gut.

These adverse effects have implications for the most fundamental aspect of the reproductive cycle, since the B-complex vitamins are needed for the formation of the sex hormones and zinc is essential for proper fertility. There are direct effects on fertility as well. A binge drinking bout can have severe effects on spermatogenesis, or on the formation of sperm, particularly in the early stages. Alcohol, in fact, has deleterious effects on the *fertility of both partners* and animal studies show a high incidence of foetal deaths and malformations when females are given alcohol preceding ovulation and close to the time of conception. Alcohol appears to have a direct effect on chromosomes, and its ingestion may be a major contributing factor in many miscarriages. Since the formation of sperm may take up to 116 days and since ova are susceptible to damage for about 100 days before ovulation, both prospective parents should abstain from any intake of alcohol for at least four months before an intended pregnancy. If you both allow for a longer alcohol-free period, this will allow for safe and complete withdrawal and will help to ensure that you won't start drinking again.

The term Foetal Alcohol Syndrome (FAS) may be new, but it has long been known that preconceptional and prenatal alcohol consumption has effects on the physical and mental development of the unborn child. The effects of alcohol on the foetus can be wide ranging and include mental retardation of varying degree, retarded growth and Down Syndrome type facial features. There may be heart and dental defects. While the full FAS child is not common, and may appear only twice in every 1,000 births, it is apparent that many children may suffer from a milder form of the syndrome, or from a variety of more subtle effects. Some estimates give as many as 90 children per 1,000 being affected to some degree. If the mother also smoked, had a high intake of caffeine and was a regular user of other drugs the ill-effects may be quite severe.

It seems that there is no threshold level of alcohol consumption below which the development of the foetus is not affected. However, the degree to which adverse effects occur will vary from woman to woman and will depend on a number of other factors including nutritional status. Several studies have linked FAS to zinc deficiency with findings showing that the FAS group had significantly lower plasma zinc levels and increased zinc excretion. Improved nutrition for alcoholics reduces the severity of FAS in their children. It also appears that there are critical times during the development of the foetal brain, when the effects of alcohol may be particularly damaging. In light of our ignorance of these critical times, avoiding alcohol completely during pregnancy and in the preconception period would certainly appear to be the safest course of action.

Alcohol is also passed through the breast milk to your baby. The ill effects on the baby are similar to those in the adult, with the central nervous system at particular risk since the infant brain continues to develop rapidly during the first three years of life. You should therefore continue to avoid alcohol until your child is weaned. Just remember that what may constitute a small drink for you, is in fact a very large drink for the developing foetus and the newborn!

Smoking

The adverse effects of cigarette smoking on the health of adults are well documented, with effects on the immune system equally as deleterious as those on cardiovascular and respiratory systems. The effects on the foetus are similarly well known, but, unfortunately, less publicity is given to the effects on the *fertility* of both partners, and to the effects on the foetus if the father is a smoker.

Smokers have seriously compromised nutritional status. Their serum levels of Vitamin C may be up to 40 per cent lower than the levels of non-smokers, which impairs their body's ability to deal with chemical or heavy metal pollutants. This deficiency may require additional Vitamin C in the dose range of several hundred milligrams per day to redress the balance. Smokers have also been found to have high serum copper levels, with accompanying low zinc levels, that have implications not only for the fertility of both partners, but for other aspects of reproductive health and for both physical and mental foetal development as well.

Male smokers have lower levels of the hormone testosterone, they will also have reduced sperm numbers, and a greater number of deformed sperm. There appear to be direct effects on the hormones of the female as well. In animal studies nicotine intake causes changes in hormone levels which lead to delayed implantation of the ovum and decreased milk production.

There are at least 4,000 compounds in tobacco smoke. At least 30 of these compounds are known mutagens, in other words, compounds which are known to cause genetic damage. At the International Conference on Environmental Mutagens held in Melbourne in 1992, Professor Bruce Ames, a leading cancer researcher, attributed many birth defects and cancers in children to fathers who smoke. He quoted research going back at least 50 years which shows that the majority of congenital defects are from the male line. German research has shown that if the father smokes heavily, the child is two and a half times as likely as the child of a non-smoking father to suffer some malformation. The children of these male smokers may also suffer from a greater number of health problems, particularly respiratory infections, and allergies.

Nicotine, the compound in cigarettes which is addictive, (and which is present in the patches and chewing gums which are often used as aids to quitting), is a vasoconstrictor, and decreases the flow of blood to the placenta, and also reduces placental uptake of amino acids leading to foetal growth retardation. Cadmium, a heavy metal present in cigarette smoke, which displaces trace minerals from essential enzyme systems is also found to concentrate in the placenta. This has further effects on foetal growth. Carbon monoxide reduces the oxygen-carrying capacity of the blood and is the probable reason for smokers' placentas being larger and thinner than those of non-smokers. This makes the placenta more susceptible to haemorrhage and the mother *twice as likely to miscarry.*

These are some of the reasons why women who smoke during pregnancy will have a greater risk of spontaneous abortion, premature birth, and 'small for dates' babies. As well, their babies suffer an increased incidence of congenital abnormalities. Some experts are in fact suggesting the existence of a foetal tobacco syndrome. The children of women smokers are significantly less healthy at birth, are more likely to die in the first year of life and are also much more likely to suffer from later health problems, including impaired intellectual and emotional development. Hyperactivity in the children of smokers is three times more common than in the children of non-smokers.

The foetus also reacts to the stress of the cigarette in well-defined and measurable ways. Part of this is due to the effect of nicotine on the foetal heart rate. What may be more difficult to measure is how this constant level of unresolved stress during a pregnancy affects the later personality and behaviour of the child.

The effects of passive smoking have also been shown to be deleterious. Passive smoke (from the father) inhaled by the pregnant woman has been shown to have almost as large an effect on the foetus as that of direct maternal smoking. Fortunately, passive smoke inhalation in public places is decreasing due to increased awareness of its deleterious effects. However, if you work in a smoke-filled environment you will be at risk, and you must campaign for a smoke-free workplace.

Also at risk are the infants and small children who live in the home of a smoker or smokers. They have a greater than average risk of a large variety of health problems, including cancer, and are more at risk of dying from Sudden Infant Death Syndrome (SIDS). These risks will increase with the number of cigarettes smoked. There is no doubt at all that smoking in either partner has profound effects on all aspects of reproductive health and on foetal and infant health as well.

Caffeine

Caffeine is probably the most ubiquitous social drug of all. However, its consumption is rarely considered as drug ingestion since it is present in tea, coffee, cola drinks, medicines, chocolate and some foods. But caffeine, particularly if its use is excessive and long term, has the ability to cause addiction in just the same way as those substances with which you more usually associate the word 'drugs'.

Caffeine has harmful effects on all aspects of reproductive health. It adversely affects the way in which sperm move forward, and can cause reduced fertility in women as well. The ingestion of caffeine at mealtimes inhibits the absorption of iron and destroys B-complex vitamins. Reports have also linked caffeine consumption to chromosome damage, and in animal experiments it has been shown to have a number of adverse effects on two succeeding generations. Furthermore, its ingestion during pregnancy has been associated with an increased rate of spontaneous abortion and with a number of congenital abnormalities.

Caffeine is excreted through breast milk, and caffeine ingestion by the breastfeeding infant is a significant contributing factor in colic, restlessness and general irritability. Caffeine also has an adverse effect on the production of breast milk.

If possible, you should avoid caffeine-containing drinks or foods altogether. The use of decaffeinated tea or coffee is not recommended. These drinks may avoid the problems associated with caffeine consumption, but they contain other additives and alkaloids which may be harmful. If complete abstinence is impossible for you, then an occasional cup of tea is considered less harmful than an occasional cup of coffee.

Drugs

The word 'drugs' will probably evoke, for many of you, addicts hanging out for their next fix. But this term includes substances such as alcohol, nicotine and caffeine, which we have already discussed, and also includes those substances which may have been prescribed for you. However, because the general population has become such a great consumer of medical services and pharmaceutical products, you may give little thought to the effects that these products have on your general health and on your nutritional status. You may also forget that drugs, while including those which your doctor prescribes, also include those purchased from the pharmacy for the treatment of minor complaints such as hayfever, coughs, colds, pain, indigestion or constipation. Many of these compounds exert strong nutrient interactions which may of course compromise the *nutritional status* of either prospective parent, with repercussions for all aspects of your reproductive health.

Drug/nutrient interactions

Aspirin, for example, which is widely used in many products to relieve pain or to lower a high temperature, increases the urinary excretion of Vitamin C and decreases blood levels of folic acid. Aspirin is also a common cause of sensitivity reactions. Laxatives, because they may speed the passage of food through the gut, can interfere with the correct absorption of all essential nutrients. The use of antacids containing aluminium may contribute to a high body burden of this heavy metal, with implications for foetal development, and can also decrease the absorption of phosphate. Some antacids can lead to a thiamine (Vitamin B1) deficiency.

Penicillin increases the excretion of potassium in the urine. The tetracycline group of antibiotics decreases the absorption of many minerals, as well as amino acids and fat, and increases the excretion of Vitamin C and some B vitamins. All antibiotics have a deleterious effect on the normal body flora which can lead to an inhibition of the synthesis of the B complex vitamins and Vitamin K in the gut. These compounds may also be responsible for an overgrowth of undesirable micro-organisms such as Candida. Diuretics, commonly used in the treatment of hypertension or high blood pressure, premenstrual tension and often inappropriately for weight control, increase the excretion of potassium, magnesium and zinc. Drugs used in the treatment of stomach ulcers act by inhibiting the secretion of hydrochloric acid, but at the same time the uptake of many essential trace minerals such as zinc, manganese and chromium is inhibited, since the absorption of these minerals cannot occur in the absence of hydrochloric acid.

The list of drug–nutrient interactions is as long as the list of drugs themselves. We have chosen just a few examples of the way in which commonly used drugs may affect the uptake, synthesis or excretion of essential nutritional factors, and how they may therefore compromise nutritional status of either prospective parent before conception even takes place.

Drug side-effects

Drugs, may also, by virtue of the fact that they are physiologically powerful substances, exert any number of unwanted side-effects. Ampicillin, some antidepressants and antipsychotics, antihistamines, many cough mixtures, oral contraceptives, and most interestingly clomiphene (commonly known as Clomid—a drug used to treat infertility), affect the production of cervical mucus in a variety of ways. They may cause an increase or decrease in the amount of mucus, and a thickening or thinning of its consistency. Since adequate fertile-type mucus is an essential ingredient if sperm are to reach and fertilise the egg, these drugs have a deleterious effect on the most basic aspect of a woman's reproductive health (see Chapter 8). Prostaglandin inhibitors (such as aspirin and indomethacin), when taken in high doses, may inhibit ovulation. Antihypertensive drugs of the beta-blocker variety may cause impotency, and calcium channel blockers and ACE inhibitors can lead to infertility in the male.

Mutagenic/teratogenic effects

Other drugs may have *mutagenic* effects, which means that they affect the chromosomes in the germ cells (sperm and ova). The numbers of drugs which exert their effect in this manner may be quite unknown just as they way in which they affect inherited characteristics cannot be predicted.

The other adverse effects with which most people are familiar since the thalidomide disaster, are those which are *teratogenic*, or capable of producing birth defects. These effects will be exerted during the first three months or during the period when cells are dividing and organs are forming. While some drugs may have no known teratogenic effects, knowledge of those that do is incomplete. Teratogenic effects may also act through alteration of vitamin and mineral metabolism and consequently these effects may differ depending on your nutritional status. The effects may not always be entirely predictable since they may also depend on the presence of other factors such as smoking, drinking or chemical or heavy metal contamination.

From all that we have said, it should be apparent that you must ask yourself whether in fact your prescriptions are always necessary. You also need to ask yourself whether the medication might be replaced by a natural alternative, or whether in fact you need it at all? This avoidance of drugs is important not only during the first trimester of pregnancy, but should extend to both partners prior to conception and continue throughout your pregnancy, birth, and during the full period of lactation.

Pharmaceutical drugs for chronic conditions

If you are taking prescription medication for asthma, hypertension, epilepsy or any other chronic condition, you would, of course, be most unwise to discontinue its use. However, it may be possible to reduce your need for this medication. It has been found that the treatment of many chronic conditions can often be aided by diet and lifestyle modification, coupled with alternative therapies such as herbs and acupuncture. In these instances, a practitioner who is trained in nutritional and environmental medicine will use dietary measures, coupled with supplementation and avoidance of tobacco, alcohol, oral contraceptives and allergenic compounds to reduce as far as possible your need for pharmaceutical drugs. Such a practitioner will also be able to advise you of appropriate nutritional supplementation to offset those losses caused by any medication still considered necessary to control your condition.

Marijuana, cocaine and other street drugs

It should be apparent by now that the use of any street or recreational drugs such as marijuana, heroin and cocaine should be avoided. Sperm health may be seriously compromised by the use of these compounds and there is evidence of chromosome damage occurring in marijuana users. Animal studies have reported that cocaine is teratogenic even in non-toxic doses.

Apart from the many problems associated with regular drug use or addiction in adults, babies born to addicted mothers will themselves be addicted. As well, these babies are many times more likely to suffer from a range of congenital abnormalities. Therefore, if either of you is a user of any of these, or related substances, on a regular or an occasional basis, it is imperative that you stop their use before any pregnancy is attempted. Professional help will frequently be necessary for this type of addiction.

Now that we have looked at the many reasons for avoiding smoking, drinking alcohol, caffeine and other drugs, we want to say this: breaking the habits of many years and giving up what may, as well, be very strongly addictive substances, is often much easier said than done. If you have a long-standing addiction to any of the substances mentioned, or if you have tried to give up on previous occasions but have failed, you may need to enlist professional help. We know that for many of you, the recommendations in this chapter may be the most difficult of all for you to follow.

For this reason we suggest that you give yourself plenty of time, so that you have at least the minimum period of four months preceding a conception free from all of the things mentioned. Then, if time is not pressing, you will have some breathing space in case you experience an occasional lapse.

3

CLEANING UP YOUR
ENVIRONMENT

IN THE FOUR MONTHS preceding conception both of you must avoid, as far as possible, exposure to the following: *toxic metals* (lead, cadmium, mercury, aluminium), *chemicals* (whether in the home, garden or workplace), *ionising radiation* (X-rays) and *non-ionising radiation* (VDUs, etc.).

YOU PROBABLY DON'T NEED any introduction to the topic of environmental pollution, because widespread publicity has already alerted most of you to the fact that heavy metals, pesticides, herbicides, fungicides, and other agricultural, industrial and household chemicals, as well as radiation in the environment, can be detrimental to your well-being. Of course, if these factors can be detrimental to your general health, then there is little doubt that they have harmful effects on the health of sperm and ova, and on the developing embryo and foetus.

You are also undoubtedly aware that we are living in an environment with a level of pollution unprecedented in history. For this reason you may feel quite helpless in the face of such widespread chemical usage and ever increasing levels of radiation. You might simply be tempted to throw up your hands and say 'but how can anyone have a healthy baby?'

Some heavy metal and chemical ingestion, and some radiation exposure may be unavoidable, but a great deal of it is in fact within your control. In this chapter we look at how you can actually avoid much of this toxicity. You can also, by means of nutritional intervention and modified lifestyle, do a great deal to ensure that your body has the best possible defences against those levels of pollution and radiation which you simply cannot avoid. In fact, everything which we recommend that you do before conception is aimed at achieving exactly this. Finally, in Chapter 4, we will show you ways in which you can rid your body of the toxins which may have accumulated from past exposure.

But first we will look at the reasons for avoiding environmental pollutants wherever possible.

ENVIRONMENTAL POLLUTANTS
Toxic metals

Toxic (or heavy) metals are those which have no role whatever to play in human metabolism. These substances are widespread in the environment and may be ingested or absorbed from a variety of sources. They can accumulate in various cells and organs in your body and will displace essential minerals from enzymes and hormones. The degree to which they do this will depend on how much is ingested, on your individual biochemical make-up (or your genetic inheritance), the acidity of your system, and also to some extent on whether your diet is rich or poor in essential nutrients. Improvement in your nutritional status will increase your body's capacity to remove heavy metals naturally. Degrees of ingestion or absorption will also depend on the presence of other factors such as cigarette smoking, exposure to other toxic substances, and stress. As well, some adverse effects, those of lead, mercury and cadmium for example, may be synergistic, or greater than the sum of the individual parts.

The toxic metals include *lead, cadmium, mercury* and *aluminium*. *Selenium* and *copper*, while in fact needed by the body in small amounts, have also been shown to have adverse effects in high concentrations. Because these substances are capable of affecting all essential enzyme systems, they have the potential to adversely affect every aspect of reproductive and foetal health. Mercury is antagonistic to the all-important mineral zinc, and lead adversely affects iron function. Mercury, cadmium and lead also have the ability to become highly concentrated in the placenta with severe effects on the developing foetus, and the developing foetal and infant brain are exquisitively sensitive to the ill-effects of lead and mercury. As well, all heavy metals have been shown to have strong immuno-suppressive effects.

Lead

The present average body burden of lead is up to 1,000 times higher than that of pre-industrial humans. It is, in fact, impossible to avoid its ingestion. Even when all cars use lead-free petrol, lead will remain in the soil and can be ingested in food and water. All dust in city and roadside areas contains lead, in some instances levels approach those found in lead-bearing ore. Superphosphate fertilisers make further contribution to lead in the soil.

All paint manufactured before the 1960s contained lead. Commercial paints still contain 15 per cent lead. Renovation of old homes which involves scraping or burning of old paint, and disturbing lead-laden dust which has accumulated over many years, can lead to greatly increased ingestion.

Because the renovation of old homes (painted before 1960), especially those in inner-city areas, (where lead-laden dust is an added problem) is a common practice for couples planning to start a family, we have listed below some of the safe renovation practices which are recommended by the appropriate authorities. Make sure that all paint removal and renovations are carried out and completed appropriately well before the important four month preconception period and certainly do not undertake renovation involving paint stripping or dust removal during pregnancy.

You can, of course, have the work carried out professionally, but make sure that all the safety procedures for removal of lead are adhered to. Further information is available from agencies such as the Environmental Protection Authority (see Contacts and Resources).

- Wear a face mask and protective clothing during paint or dust removal.
- Remember that paint removal using a sander or blow torch can create hazardous dust and fumes.

- The poorer the repair of the house, the greater the risk of exposure from dust containing lead.
- Use work practices that minimise dust or fumes. This means wet sanding, or using a chemical stripper, and wet mopping of surfaces, etc.
- Collect and safely remove all paint or dust debris using a wet mop. Do not empty the mop bucket on a children's play area.
- Paint chips and dust should be placed in heavy duty garbage bags and sealed before disposal at an approved waste depot.
- After working, vacuum carpets, window sills and skirting boards thoroughly. A domestic vacuum cleaner is not adequate for filtering the lead in dust.
- Shower after finishing work on renovations, and wash clothing carefully.

There are numerous further guidelines which may be particularly appropriate in your situation, expecially if you already have young children in the house. Since a child's developing brain, nervous system and general metabolism is much more susceptible to the effects of lead than yours, you must pay special attention to preventing lead ingestion by any children present. Even if you are not renovating, small children are still at risk of ingesting lead from soil and dust and we strongly recommend that you familiarise yourself with measures you can take to minimise this.

There are many other sources of lead pollution. Coal burning and printing processes release lead into the environment. Metal polishes and batteries are further sources of lead contamination. Painted glassware and improperly glazed pottery contain lead. Some pesticides contain lead arsenate, and organ meats (especially liver) contain significant amounts. Lead may also be ingested with food (especially if acidic) which is contained in cans with unlined, lead-soldered seams. Lead solder is also used by the plumbing industry. Some wines contain lead. There is lead in tobacco, and cigarette smoking increases lead ingestion by 25 per cent. Some cosmetic preparations such as mascara and hair-darkening products also contain lead.

At present petroleum companies, paint manufacturers and industries which use lead in their manufacturing processes are working closely with government and consumer bodies to ensure that lead levels in the environment are drastically reduced. These are positive and important moves, for the effects of lead on physical, mental and reproductive health are undoubtedly profound. What then are these ill-effects?

The fact that lead can cause abortions has been known since Victorian times. It is also known to deform or kill sperm. Males working in the lead and battery industries are known to have increased rates of malformation and miscarriage in their offspring. Foresight clinics in the United Kingdom have found that some women with 'hostile mucus' or antibodies to their partner's sperm, found the problem resolved when the partner's body burden of lead was reduced (or if previously undiagnosed infections were treated).

This appears to be an attempt by the body to ensure that unacceptable sperm are destroyed, and you might perhaps wonder at the attempts of reproductive technology to bypass this possible fail-safe mechanism. High lead levels in either partner have also been shown to be a factor in many miscarriages, stillbirths, neonatal deaths and congenital abnormalities. Animal studies have shown that lead exposure causes neurological and endocrinological effects on offspring for four consecutive generations.

Most of you will be aware of the overwhelming and incontrovertible evidence of the ability of lead to cause impaired mental function and behaviour and learning problems in small children. It has been estimated that children up to the age of ten years may suffer an IQ deficit of 2 to 3 points for each 10 microgram/decilitre increment in their blood level of lead. These may only be subtle effects for some children, but costly effects for those whose IQ is already in the lower range and also for those children who are more seriously affected. Some estimates put as many as 40 per cent of NSW children (mainly those living in inner-city areas), aged under four years, as being potentially adversely affected by lead. It may not, in fact, be possible to assess whether there is a level below which the immature brain is unaffected.

Of equal concern are recent studies from Surrey University in the United Kingdom which show that by the age of twelve weeks gestation, all foetuses have some lead-induced damage to the brain. A maternal lead burden is a cause of reduced foetal brain size which is irreversible. In light of these findings, present Health Department endeavours to reduce the ingestion of lead by small children in inner-city areas and in the areas surrounding lead smelters, may be like closing the gate after the horse has bolted. A great deal of damage has already been done.

Mercury

Mercury compounds are used in the manufacture of electrical appliances, laboratory measuring equipment, paint and fluorescent lights. Mercury is also a component of batteries which are used to power electronic games, calculators and computers. Compounds of mercury are found in some pesticides, insecticides and fungicides, which are used, for example, to spray seed-wheat before planting, and to inhibit the growth of slime moulds in the paper-making process. Consequently, mercury is found in water which has been contaminated by factory effluent, or if the water receives the run-off from farms using mercury-containing chemicals. Mercury is a heavy metal, and high levels will therefore be found in deep-water or bottom-dwelling fish and crustaceans, and in fish which are high in the food chain, such as tuna, swordfish and shark, since they eat fish which have eaten smaller fish, which have eaten still smaller fish, and so on. Other sources of mercury contamination include soft contact lens solutions and vaccine products which contain thiomersal, some haemorrhoid suppositories, nasal sprays, vaginal gels and some cosmetics such as waterproof mascara.

Those who have worked in the mercury mining and processing industry, photographers, printers, and crematorium workers may be at risk of excessive mercury ingestion. Most commonly, however, ingestion of mercury occurs because of its use in *dental amalgam*, which is a mixture of silver, copper, zinc, tin and mercury (50 per cent). Dentists and dental nurses, who constantly handle amalgam, are particularly at risk of ingesting and accumulating mercury, but a high body burden of mercury may also be a significant problem for many individuals who accumulate this heavy metal in their organs and body tissues from their amalgam fillings.

While the debate rages about whether mercury-containing dental amalgams are safe, it is interesting to note that the product which is used to fill cavities in your teeth, in the United States from 1988, (according to American Occupational Safety and Health Association regulations) became 'hazardous waste' once outside the mouth (that is, scrap amalgam), with special restrictions on its safe and appropriate disposal! It is also interesting to note that Sweden, Austria and Germany have banned the use of mercury-containing dental amalgams in pregnant women. This is the prelude to a total ban being imposed in these countries.

Elemental mercury or non-organic mercury compounds are relatively poorly absorbed and readily excreted, in contrast to the much more toxic organic compounds such as methyl mercury, which incidentally is formed by oral bacteria (*strep. mutans*) in the presence of amalgam. Once again, knowledge of the toxicity of organic compounds of mercury dates back many years. These compounds, once used in the millinery trade, were known to have toxic neurological effects, hence the term 'mad as a hatter'.

As well as behavioural and psychological changes such as short-term memory loss and mood alterations, mercury toxicity may cause neurological disturbances such as loss of coordination, vision and hearing. There may be further disturbances to gastrointestinal, cardiovascular, endocrine, respiratory, collagen and immunological systems, and oral cavity disorders. There are many other signs and symptoms of chronic mercury toxicity, two of the most common being fatigue and depression. A high body burden of mercury has in fact been identified as a major contributing factor in Chronic Fatigue Syndrome, and the evidence points to it being a causative factor in many other diseases.

Mercury accumulates in the pituitary gland, and any effects on the endocrine system will have implications for the fertility of both male and female, since this system is responsible for the production of all the hormones controlling reproduction. Other effects, which may have implications for reproduction, are poor sperm motility and loss of libido, lasting for several years, in men inadvertently exposed to metallic mercury vapour.

Mercury has also been shown to cause birth defects. These defects were highlighted by the incident at Minimata Bay, Japan where children were born suffering from a range of symptoms which resembled cerebral palsy. These varied from mild spasticity to severe mental retardation and even to death. Their mothers exhibited no signs of mercury toxicity but had been exposed to a high level of mercury in their diet, which was high in fish. The fish were heavily contaminated with mercury which had been discharged into Minimata Bay. Mercury is easily passed through the placenta, and foetal blood has been shown to have concentrations of mercury up to 20 per cent higher than the blood of the mother. High maternal levels of mercury have also been linked to poor placental function.

Treatment for chronic mercury toxicity As we have already stated, chronic mercury toxicity may be responsible for much ill health in sensitive individuals, and mercury-containing amalgams are frequently the major source of mercury ingestion. However, we do not recommend that you have your amalgam fillings removed unless you are certain that your symptoms are due to mercury exposure and tissue accumulation. If you suspect that mercury toxicity is a problem for you, or if your hair trace mineral analysis reveals a high body burden of this metal, it is absolutely essential that you seek help from a practitioner who is experienced in diagnosing and dealing with this condition (such as a member of ASOMAT, see Contacts and Resources).

If you are diagnosed as suffering from chronic mercury toxicity and decide to have your dental work redone with an alternative product, then it is essential that you also ensure that your dentist is knowledgeable about the safety procedures and protocols which must be followed for removal of amalgam containing mercury. If amalgam removal and replacement is carried out in an unsafe manner, your health may well deteriorate, rather than improve.

Following the removal of amalgam and replacement with another material, supplementation and dietary measures should be continued, and a follow-up urine challenge test and further hair trace mineral analysis should be carried out. These tests must indicate that you have been free from a high body burden of mercury for a period of at least four months, before you make any attempt to conceive (see Chapter 9).

WARNING: *Do not, under any circumstances*, have amalgams removed and replaced during pregnancy. At this time it is also probably prudent to avoid dental surgeries where amalgam is used, since mercury vapour will be in the air. It should really also go without saying that any dental work which must be done during pregnancy must involve the use of non-amalgam products only!

It is also not recommended to have amalgam replacements as part of preconception care unless they are completed well before conception since mercury levels can easily rise initially.

Cadmium

Cadmium is present in cigarette smoke, and can be ingested by both active and passive smokers. Cadmium is also present in some plumbing alloys and, consequently, water supplies may be contaminated. Cadmium is used in many manufacturing processes including those associated with paint, batteries, electronic equipment and television sets. Other sources of cadmium contamination include photography, burning plastics, electroplating, rustproofing, welding and solders, fungicides, pesticides and ceramics. Shredded rubber tyres found on highways, and the dust accumulating in nearby areas, are a further source of contamination. Many processed foods and evaporated milk contain cadmium. Refined foods also contain a significant amount of this element since levels of zinc and other trace minerals have been substantially lowered by the refining process, leaving a high proportion of cadmium to other essential nutrients. Oysters are high in cadmium (as well as zinc).

Cadmium slowly accumulates in the liver and kidneys. It also becomes concentrated in the placenta with implications for the growth and development of the foetus. High maternal levels of cadmium (as well as lead and mercury) have been linked with stillbirths and neonatal deaths. Animal studies have produced a range of congenital abnormalities which are due to cadmium, and further animal studies link toxaemia of pregnancy to cadmium. The suggestion has been made that toxaemia in humans may be due to lack of the essential nutrients such as zinc, or calcium, which are necessary to counteract the adverse effects of cadmium. Maternal zinc deficiency has been shown to increase the teratogenic effects of cadmium. Because cadmium and zinc are antagonists, if cadmium levels are high, zinc levels will be low. Low zinc levels have been linked to many physical and mental health problems.

It has been shown that both the emotional and mental development of children can be compromised by an excessive burden of any of the toxic metals. What is of greater significance is the fact that levels of lead and cadmium show a close correlation. In other words, if body levels of lead are high, body levels of cadmium are similarly high. Furthermore, there is an inverse relationship between levels of the essential minerals zinc and calcium, and between levels of cadmium and lead. This fact is hardly surprising since you have already learnt that your body needs essential minerals to rid itself of toxic metals.

Aluminium

Aluminium-containing compounds decrease frothing and foaming in food and beverages, and are added to powders such as salt, white flour and baking powder to ensure that they run or flow freely. Aluminium is present in milk substitutes, processed cheese and some food colour additives and preservatives. It is present in anti-perspirants and toothpastes and is also contained in many antacids which are commonly prescribed for heartburn and indigestion during pregnancy. Kaolin for diarrhoea, some aspirin compounds, and vaccine products also contain aluminium. Compounds containing aluminium are also used to treat public water supplies.

However, aluminium cookware is probably the major source of a high body burden of this toxic metal, so stainless steel cookware should be used instead. Some food, such as acid fruits, are particularly liable to leach aluminium from the pan in which they are cooked or stored, and extra amounts will be leached from the container if the water contains fluoride. Tea from aluminium teapots in which the tea has been left to stew are a special problem, since the tea has already been grown on soils which are high in alum. Foods cooked or wrapped in foil, especially those which have a high fat or acid content, will absorb aluminium from the foil. Drinks from aluminium cans and from soft 'poppa' or 'tetra' type packs (which are lined with aluminium), including fruit juices and soya milk, are further sources of contamination.

The ill-effects of a high body burden of aluminium include its interference with fluoride and phosphorus metabolism, leading to mineral loss from bone. Aluminium in fact has a great affinity for other compounds and may exert many of its ill-effects, which can include gastrointestinal disturbances, skin problems and fatigue, by interfering with nutritional status. Infants fed formula containing aluminium have been found to suffer from kidney problems. There is considerable debate about whether aluminium is implicated in Alzheimer's disease. It may also be a factor in lung diseases including pulmonary fibrosis and emphysema.

Copper

Copper levels in the body may be elevated by the use of the oral contraceptive pill (OCP) and by intra-uterine devices (IUDs) containing copper. Copper may also be leached from water pipes, or less commonly from copper pans and kettles. Indian jewellery, or copper bracelets which are sometimes worn by rheumatic sufferers, may also cause a high body burden of this metal. External contamination may come from hair dyes containing henna or from algicides containing copper found in swimming pool water.

Some of the ill-effects of a high body burden of copper have already been discussed. High copper levels occur with low levels of zinc (and iron and manganese) and may cause birth defects (perhaps due to the accompanying low zinc levels). They have been implicated in the toxaemia of pregnancy and in many instances of premature birth, as well as in postnatal depression. High copper levels may cause anaemia since iron levels fall when copper levels rise, and may also cause dermatitis due to depletion of zinc. Copper also destroys histamine, and high copper may therefore lead to food and environmental allergies.

Other toxic metals

Some studies have linked high levels of iron, arsenic, lithium and selenium to birth defects. A high body burden of selenium may result from prolonged use of antidandruff shampoos containing selenium, or from using these shampoos while soaking in the bath. In Australia, low levels of selenium in the body are generally considered to be of greater concern than elevated levels, since there is little of this nutrient in the soil, and you cannot buy a selenium supplement without a doctor's prescription. In vitro studies from America have linked low levels of selenium to Down Syndrome.

What to do about toxic metals

We have just given you some idea of the extent of contamination by toxic metals and a look at how you may ingest them. Hopefully this will make you a little more aware of how you may avoid them. In Chapter 9 we look at the use of hair trace mineral analysis as a diagnostic test to identify whether or not you are already suffering from an excessive burden of any of the toxic metals. Since you now

CLEANING UP YOUR ENVIRONMENT

know that any burden will have adverse effects on your fertility as well as on foetal health, we will also look at what you must do to reduce this toxic burden to acceptable levels before you make any attempt to conceive. To sum up, we recommend that during the four months preceding conception both of you:

- Avoid work which involves the handling of, or exposure to, toxic metals.
- Avoid peeling, scraping and burning off old lead-containing paint (painted before 1960).
- Avoid renovation which involves disturbing lead-laden dust.
- Avoid activity (especially exercising) near heavy traffic congestion.
- Avoid both active and passive smoking.
- Avoid refined and processed foods.
- Limit consumption of tuna and bottom-dwelling fish and crustaceans.
- Get any dental work done well in advance of pregnancy.
- Ask your dentist to use an alternative to amalgam for fillings.
- Avoid aluminium cookware.
- Avoid aluminium-containing antiperspirants, toothpastes, antacids.
- Avoid oral contraceptives (see also Chapter 7).
- Avoid copper IUDs (see also Chapter 7).
- Drink filtered water (for list of types of water filters see Contacts and Resources).
- Increase your consumption of anti-oxidants—these include Vitamins C, E and A, zinc and selenium (see Chapter 4).

Chemicals

Pollution of the chemical type is probably the one with which most people instinctively associate birth defects. It also seems to be the one environmental factor over which you may feel that you have very little control. This is not surprising when you read that residues of the pesticide DDT and other organochlorines are now found in the most remote corners of the globe, as well as in breast milk, and also understandable when you learn that manufacturing industries pump hundreds of millions of kilograms of chemicals into the environment every year.

Nearly 3,000 pesticide products are currently available on the market. A great deal of crop-spraying is done from the air and the pesticide or herbicide drift may land on your homes and gardens.

Further exposure to a variety of toxic substances may occur if your neighbours have their house and surrounding land treated regularly for cockroaches, white ants and spiders. In Sydney, spraying against cockroaches alone, puts 1 million litres of pyrethroids and 7.5 million litres of organophosphates into the environment every year. It is little wonder that you feel that you are being exposed without your consent, and also often without your knowledge to a potent cocktail of substances. While this is certainly true to some extent, you are still in a position to keep your personal chemical exposure to an absolute minimum. You can also improve your body's ability to detoxify, metabolise and excrete chemical pollutants.

Commonly or widely used chemicals may have a variety of undesirable effects. These effects may be mutagenic or teratogenic, carcinogenic or immune-suppressing, to name just a few. Organophosphate pesticides for example are chemically similar to nerve gas and it is hardly surprising that their use has been linked to a number of health problems in adults and children (particularly respiratory problems such as asthma). The problems associated with lead and mercury ingestion have already been discussed. PCBs (polychlorinated biphenyls), vinyl chloride and solvents such as benzene, have all been linked with a variety of general health and reproductive problems.

We have chosen not to list at length the many individual chemicals and their diverse adverse effects, because what is more important is the fact that toxicity studies generally look at one substance in isolation. What is not assessed are the effects that this huge range of pollutants have in combination. The effects on health and reproduction, of what can only be described as an extremely potent chemical cocktail, are truly unknown. Therefore it is essential that you both make whatever efforts you can to reduce your total exposure to these substances.

In the home, garden, toolshed

Oven cleaners, furniture polishes, carpet cleaners, paint thinners, dry cleaning solvents, insecticides, pesticides and herbicides are just a few of the products which are readily available for use by the homemaker, handyman or gardener. Before using any of them, it is vital that you consider carefully whether their use is absolutely necessary or whether there may be alternatives which are less toxic.

For example, flies and mosquitoes can be deterred by the installation of insect screens, or a simple fly swat may be effective. Cockroaches may be unpleasant companions, but they pose little real health threat. If you find it impossible to coexist with these persistent houseguests, there are firms which specialise in ecologically sound methods of pest extermination.

Many of the potent cleaning products you use in your home can be quite simply replaced with substances that are much kinder both to you and to your environment. There are some appropriate commercial products available and we have listed below a few examples of alternatives for use in the kitchen, laundry and bathroom. It is believed that what you use in these three rooms of your home contribute to the highest levels of domestic pollution, so look carefully at all the products in your cupboards and see if you can replace them.

- Sodium bicarbonate (bicarb soda) can be used to clean all sorts of surfaces including stainless steel, chrome and enamel. Use it to clean your refrigerator or freezer.
- Borax is useful for cleaning extra dirty sinks, floors or other tiled surfaces, and two teaspoonsful in a full kettle is a good scale remover (boil for 20 minutes).
- Salt can be used to scour sinks or chopping boards. It has disinfecting as well as cleaning properties. You can use it to clean glass, marble and laminex as well.
- Wipe your oven while still warm and do not allow grease to build up.
- Newspaper can be used as a cloth in many instances since it doesn't absorb the cleaning product as much as a cloth.
- Half a cup of white vinegar in a bucket of hot water can be used on cork, slate, lino or tiled floors.
- One part lemon juice to two parts olive oil can be used as a floor or furniture polish (or use beeswax).
- Use a plunger to clear your drain initially and follow up with boiling water and equal parts baking soda and vinegar (a quarter cup of each should suffice).
- A paste of vinegar and washing soda will remove soap scum from baths and shower recesses.
- Wash your nappies in a hot wash (over 65°C) and dry them in the sun.

- Sunlight soap is a great prewash treatment (add a little elbow grease of course) and the Australian Conservation Foundation suggests this alternative to commercial laundry detergents: grate a third of a cake of pure soap, add a little water and bring to the boil until dissolved (use a potato masher if necessary). In a bucket dissolve a third of a cup of washing soda in a little hot water, add the soap solution, and fill the bucket up with water. This mixture sets into a soft gel. Use 2 cups—or more if necessary— per wash. It is also good for washing dishes, and even hair.
- Use pot-pourri or fresh (scented) flowers to replace your normal air freshener.
- Light a match in the lavatory (after a bowel motion) to burn the methane which is the main component of unpleasant odours.

There are, of course, a great many more alternatives to the very large number of chemical-laden products which you generally find in these three small rooms in your home.

In the garden, you can use companion planting to deter pests (aphids are discouraged by chives, garlic and nasturtiums) and to attract beneficial insects (earthworms like dandelions). Always remember the insects all have a very important role to play and they destroy only weak and unhealthy plants and keep the ecosystem strong and healthy.

If you do need to spray, here are the recipes for a couple of easily made solutions which you can put into a pump pack and use as insecticides. The basic ingredients for both can be purchased from your local pharmacy.

- Dissolve 56 g of soft soap in 4.5 litres of hot water, and allow to cool before you spray.
- Boil 56 g of quassia chips in 2¼ litres of water for 2 hours. Pour off the liquid and dilute one part of the quassia solution with four parts of water. *Label*: Caution—Keep out of reach of children. This spray is for aphids and caterpillars.

You may be involved in hobbies or leisure pursuits which involve contact with chemicals, glues and solvents. Don't forget about these products! Some of them can be quite toxic. If you are a do-it-yourself home handyperson, check out the environmentally friendly chemical alternatives which are appearing on the market. With the realisation that many treatments used on wood and furniture are adversely affecting many aspects of our health, we now have the option to seek out and use those which are less toxic.

If you are presently exposed to chemicals in your home, in the garden, or the toolshed, there are numerous publications which offer environmentally sound alternatives for almost every aspect of chemical use. We have included a list of resource publications in Suggested Reading at the end of this book. There are also numerous 'green' alternatives available. However, when you purchase 'environmentally friendly' products, ensure that the products carry the logo which indicates that the manufacturers' claims have been tested and validated by the appropriate government body.

Buy organically grown

You can easily reduce the amount of chemical residue you ingest on your fresh fruit and vegetables. Although the spraying of crops with organophosphate or other pesticides is fairly universal, many farmers are turning to sustainable agriculture, and increasingly more retail outlets are now selling produce which has been organically grown.

Once again it is important that you check that the fruit and vegetables which are sold as organic are in fact certified and labelled by NASAA (National Association of Sustainable Agriculture Australia), BFA (Biological Farmers of Australia) or Demeter which certifies biodynamic products. This will ensure that you are buying produce which is genuinely free from chemical residues and which has a high content of essential nutrients. NASAA or similar certification will give the produce different grades. These will vary, and will depend on how long the farm has been using sustainable methods, how free the soil is from pesticide residues, and the conditions prevailing in the surrounding areas.

Occupational exposure

Chemicals which are used in the workplace constitute a very serious hazard since exposure to these may be constant and long term and may also be far more difficult to avoid. While general awareness is improving and appropriate regulations are becoming more stringent, it is possible that some of the products you use on a regular basis will be handled carelessly and without knowledge of their effects on health and reproduction. Those at risk include artists and jewellers, workers in the car manufacturing and repair industry, chemical workers, clothing, textile and leather workers, electricians, those working in the fields of electronics and semi-conductors, food workers, workers in general manufacturing, glass and pottery workers, and hospital and health-care staff. The products used in these fields may affect every aspect of reproduction beginning with effects on both male and female fertility.

If you use any sort of chemicals at all in your daily work you must find out exactly what ill-effects these may have. There are numerous agencies that can advise you, and we have listed some helpful names and addresses in the Contacts and Resources section. Once you are armed with the knowledge, you can then make provision for reduced and safer handling of the offending products. You can also take all possible steps to rid yourself of any accumulated toxicity and to ensure that your body has the best possible defence against further exposure.

If necessary, you can arrange for alternative work if you consider the risks to your reproductive health and the health of your future children to be unacceptable. If this is the case, a program of detoxification is still important before you attempt to conceive. This advice is of course equally important for both prospective parents.

Occupational exposure to dust has also been identified as a reproductive risk factor. Male workers who were exposed to dust were found to be more likely to suffer from infertility. Workers in the building, mining and construction industries were just some of those found to be at risk. We have already examined the adverse effects of exposure to lead-laden dust, but as well as lead, dust may contain a number of other substances such as timber, paints, inks, concrete, and rubber from tyres worn on roadways. It seems that if you are exposed regularly to dust during the course of your work, you are probably being exposed to a cocktail of compounds. Working in appropriate protective gear might therefore be a sensible option.

Radiation and other hazards

Radiation is the other great concern if you are planning to have a baby. This concern is understandable after nuclear accidents such as Chernobyl and others which have occurred worldwide, and after the many years (both past and now present) of nuclear weapons testing in the southern Pacific region. But once again, there is a great deal of radiation to which you expose yourself unwittingly, but fairly constantly. It is possible to reduce your radiation exposure to little more than that of background levels, and as well there are nutritional factors which we recommend to strengthen your body's defences against this form of pollution.

First of all you need to be aware that there are two types of radiation. The one which is of greatest concern is the ionising type of radiation. This is the radiation of radioactive material, used to fuel nuclear power stations and nuclear weapons. It is also the type of radiation encountered in X-rays. Ionising radiation has damaging effects on all cells, particularly those which have a high rate of growth and division. It obviously has the potential to damage germ cells (sperm and ova), embryonic and foetal cells and the cells of growing children (as well as those of adults of course, although their rate of cell growth and division is significantly slower). No level of ionising radiation has been proven to be safe.

Very recent findings from Flinders University, South Australia, have linked increased miscarriage rates to either partner undergoing a back or abdominal X-ray at any time in the five years preceding a pregnancy. It would appear sensible in light of these findings, to be very cautious about submitting yourself to this sort of diagnosis unless it is absolutely essential. While it may not be possible to totally avoid X-rays in the years prior to a pregnancy, this is an extremely important recommendation for both prospective parents in the four months preceding conception, and of critical importance for the pregnant woman, particularly during the first three months.

The second type of radiation is much more widespread with effects on reproductive health which are much less clearly defined. This is non-ionising radiation and it comes from lasers, microwaves, electrical appliances in the home, mobile phones, television screens and visual display units. This type of radiation has been shown in animal studies to affect almost every body system. Some of the effects which have been demonstrated in humans are more subjective and include changes in behaviour, irritability and sleeplessness.

There have been numerous studies which have attempted to link the use of computer terminal screens to reproductive problems, but the results have been conflicting. There have been suggestions that the stress of sitting at a VDU for eight hours per day may be the significant factor in compromised reproductive outcomes. Whatever the outcome of the debate, however, management in many countries is now limiting the number of hours which workers can spend in front of a computer terminal. Screens or special clothing to give you some protection from emitted radiation are also sometimes used. The suggestion has been made that women limit their exposure to computer terminals to no more than four hours per day. Ideally they should do no work at VDU terminals in the three to four months preceding conception, and none during the first twelve weeks of pregnancy. It is also important to remember that the highest levels of radiation occur at the back and sides of the unit, so you must take care in setting up your screen that it is well positioned in relation to units of neighbouring workers.

We are well aware that recommendations to avoid or limit the use of your computer terminal may be unworkable for many of you, so we have included below a few tips which may help to reduce the ill effects of radiation to which you are unavoidably exposed. In Chapter 4, we have listed the herbs and nutrients which you can use to protect yourself as far as possible from the effects of unavoidable exposure. In the Contacts and Resources section we list where to find some of the commercially available antiradiation devices.

To reduce your exposure to radiation, use a laptop *or*:

- Turn off the VDU whenever possible.
- Move away from the screen when you are involved in other tasks.
- Fit an antiradiation (as distinct from antiglare) screen to the front of the VDU.
- Be aware that radiation is emitted in all directions (not just from the front) and the backs and sides of co-workers' screens also present a hazard.
- Put a packet of Epsom salts (in a cotton or cardboard container) in front of your screen. This will absorb a significant amount of emitted radiation. When the crystals have become dry and powdery, the packet needs replacing.
- There are several commercial gadgets that claim to deflect radiation. These are worn by the exposed individual or attached to the computer (see Contacts and Resources).
- Grow green plants in the immediate vicinity of the computer to help alleviate electromagnetic pollution; peace lilies are especially recommended.

Electromagnetic radiation is generated along with electricity and therefore occurs in the vicinity of electric powerlines. There is still considerable debate about the effects of strong electromagnetic radiation on health and reproduction. However, it is interesting to note that in Russia the time farmworkers can spend in close proximity to high voltage powerlines is limited, and in the United States, no homes are allowed to be built near such powerlines.

The use of a number of other common devices has been linked to various health problems. These devices include electric blankets, sunbeds, transformer generators and motors. We recommend that you particularly avoid the electrical fields which are generated in your bedroom while you sleep. This means turning off, or preferably unplugging, electric blankets, water beds and clock radios when you switch off the light. Avoid sleeping near a fuse box.

The debate on the effect of microwaves is conflicting but some research suggests the possibility that the radiation has adverse effects on chromosomes. Since we have already given reasons for avoiding microwaved food we trust you won't be using these devices in your kitchen anyway! To sum up, a sensible general rule would be for you to keep your exposure to all radiation sources as low as possible during the period preceding conception, and also during your pregnancy, particularly during the first three months.

We should also mention, for those of you who are interested in the cosmic picture, that the times when the sun and any of the major planets are in opposition, are also times of increased sunspot activity, magnetic storms, shifts in magnetic fields and an increase in cosmic radiation. All of these may have subtle (or perhaps not so subtle) deleterious effects on germ cells and on the newly fertilised egg. These findings were part of the work carried out by Dr Eugen Jonas, a Czech psychiatrist who was also responsible for the discovery of the lunar cycle affecting fertility (see Chapter 7).

Many of you will no doubt feel that you have plenty to occupy and concern you right here on this planet, without worrying about the 'bigger picture'. But if you feel comfortable with the fact that not only the moon, but the sun and all the planets, both large and small, influence, in some way, what happens here on earth, then you may like to have a chart drawn by a professional astrologer (see Contacts and Resources). This can show auspicious times for your preconception preparation and conception, and can also indicate those times which may not be quite so favourably regarded.

4

HOW TO DETOXIFY

DO YOU DRIVE EVERY day in heavy traffic,
or live or work near a busy road?
Do you ever eat foods that contain additives,
or were grown (or fed) using chemicals?
Do you sometimes take medical drugs
(prescribed or otherwise)?
Do you (or did you) smoke, or drink alcohol,
or caffeine in some form?
Do you use a personal computer or VDU
for several hours each day?
Have you had any X-rays lately?
Do you live near a source of
environmental pollution?
Do you work with chemicals?
Do you clean or fumigate your house
with chemicals?

Do I really need to detoxify?

Unless you managed to answer *No* to all of the above questions (and
we can easily dream up some more!) then the answer is emphatically
Yes!

Even if you are dedicated to organic eating and to leading a healthy, chemical-free life, you've probably often cut corners with the purity of your food, you may have sometimes resorted to drugs (medicinal and recreational), and you have certainly been unavoidably exposed to pollution and radiation. However careful you are, and however pure the life you lead and the food you eat, it is virtually impossible to avoid toxins of some sort. Environmental pollution is ubiquitous, and impossible to avoid entirely. However, you *can* make a difference! *You can protect yourself against toxicity and eliminate accumulated toxins from your body.*

In previous chapters we have talked about avoiding toxicity. In this chapter we will look at some of the ways in which you can *detoxify* (or how you can rid your body of accumulated toxins). Some of these methods require the help of a practitioner, and others you can use on your own. For instructions on preparing herbal remedies, see Chapter 6.

Some of the diagnostic procedures set out in Chapter 9, including hair trace mineral analysis, will give precise information about levels of various toxins (such as heavy metals), in your body. Armed with this information you can be more specific in your use of remedies and can track down the likely sources of these pollutants. If you and your partner show, for example, similar hair trace mineral analysis patterns for heavy metals, this will give you a clue as to their source.

The following symptoms may also indicate a level of internal toxicity (although, of course, there may be additional reasons for these ailments):

- Constipation, diarrhoea, irregular or sluggish bowel movements, flatulence or bad breath.
- Frequent inexplicable headaches.
- Skin rashes, boils, pimples.
- Frequent viral infections/lowered immunity.
- General aches and pains.
- Low energy levels.
- Allergies.

Natural vs unnatural

Now that you have read this far, you will probably not be surprised that we recommend only natural methods of detoxification. There are drugs that can be used to eliminate toxins, but these are employed in acute poisoning cases. They deplete the body of essential nutrients, along with the toxins, and have the potential for side-effects as well as nutrient losses. The difference between drugs and natural remedies, such as anti-oxidants, is that drugs overrule the body's functions, whereas nutrients normalise them.

There are a great many ways that you, with the help of a natural health practitioner, can set about detoxifying your body, as well as a number of preventive measures you can employ in your daily life. Certainly don't attempt to follow *all* of these recommendations. Choose those that you can put into effect easily and that seem appropriate to your particular situation.

All detoxification programs involve the release of toxins from organs and cells. These toxins are then eliminated through various organs and systems. If this release is too sudden or extreme, your symptoms may worsen. If this happens, you may be moving too fast. You need to take it slowly or work with your practitioner. Since you need to be completely detoxified at least four months before conception, and since some detoxification programs (such as those for heavy metals) can cause temporary problems, detoxification is one of the first steps in preconception care.

How to detoxify

Detoxification takes place through, or by, the following body systems. These need to be operating at full efficiency, so many of the remedies for detoxification also restore healthy function to these organs:

- Digestive system—including the bowel and the liver.
- Urinary system—including the kidneys.
- Lymphatic system.
- Circulatory system.
- Respiratory system.
- Skin.
- Immune system.

There also needs to be, in the body, a plentiful supply of all those substances that protect against, or neutralise, the action of toxic products.

NUTRITION

Many nutrients (there's that word again!) are essential to protect the body against the activity of toxins as well as to remove them. We have already mentioned many of these, but here we will look specifically at nutrients which will help you detoxify.

Anti-oxidants

Anti-oxidants are perhaps the most important detoxifiers. They protect against the damaging effects of oxidation in the body, which occurs when oxygen loses an electron, and becomes toxic, grabbing the nearest available electron to replace the one which has been lost. Oxygen without an electron is called unstable (which is not a reference to its antisocial behaviour, but to its chemical status) and unstable oxygen molecules are called free radicals (which is not a description of their politics!). We also call free radicals oxidants.

These free radicals can hit and damage, among other things, your DNA (and do so approximately 10,000 times daily per cell), your proteins (including essential enzymes) and polyunsaturated fats, which make up the membranes that surround your cells and that normally regulate the nutrients and toxins that flow in and out.

Oxidants, and conditions which encourage oxidative stress or free radical damage, include:

- Drugs—including tobacco and alcohol.
- Food additives.
- Excessive iron or copper levels in the body.
- Sunburn.
- Radiation—particularly ionising radiation such as X-rays.
- Stress.
- Pollution.
- Excessive exercise—moderate exercise is helpful, we're talking marathons here.
- Metabolic by-products.

However, some metabolic and immune processes are actually dependent on oxidative reactions. Oxidants therefore don't only have negative effects, but are essential to the body. In fact, there is a fine balance required, and this balance is disrupted by the entry into the body of toxins, such as drugs, additives, pollution and radiation.

The agents that control this fine balance are bacteria in the gut, which control and decompose some of the precursors to oxidants (see Chapter 11), anti-oxidant nutrients that enter as part of the food supply, or as supplements, and enzymes created in the body.

Healthy bacteria in the gut can be increased through the use of *Acidophilus* and *Bifidus* which can be taken as powder, capsules or tablets.

Anti-oxidant nutrients include *Vitamin C* and the *bioflavonoids, Vitamin E, Vitamin A* or *beta-carotene, zinc* and *selenium.* Other nutrients, such as *Vitamins B6* and *B12, manganese* and certain *amino acids,* assist anti-oxidant activity. Practically all dietary nutrients are closely related to, or involved in, various stages of the anti-oxidant defence system. Some of these anti-oxidants are water soluble, such as *Vitamin C,* and others, like *Vitamin A* or *beta-carotene,* and *selenium* are fat soluble. They work in different areas of the body, and even anti-oxidants which work within the same area, do so in different ways, so they complement each other. Using, for example, *Vitamins C* and *E* together, produces an effect which is greater than using each separately.

Enzymes. Another important nutrient is *cysteine,* an amino acid, which is a direct precursor of glutathione peroxidase, an enzyme which has been manufactured by every living thing, plant or animal, since the beginnings of life on earth, billions of years ago. It's one of the most powerful anti-oxidants present in your body, and detox-ifies pollutants and drugs, and the sulphur compounds which it contains bind to heavy metals to prevent oxidation. It also boosts your immune system and the health of your red blood cells. *Zinc* promotes the conversion of methionine (an essential amino acid) to cysteine, and *selenium* is also essential for adequate levels of gluta-thione peroxidase. The herb *St Mary's Thistle* increases glutathione production.

Food and nutrient sources of anti-oxidants include:

- *All fresh fruit and vegetables*—especially citrus, berries and grape seeds (for Vitamin C and bioflavonoids), and all vegetable juices such as carrot, beetroot, broccoli and red and green capsicum).
- *Garlic*—an age-old detoxifier of particular potency, which con-tains sulphur.
- *Coenzyme Q10*—can be taken as a supplement.

- *Green tea*—contains bioflavonoids.
- *Onions*—contain bioflavonoids and sulphur.
- *Apples and pears*—especially if stewed with their pips which release pectin.
- *Spirulina*—can be taken as a supplement.
- *Cold-pressed olive oil*—eaten cold.
- *Nuts and seeds*—especially brazil nuts and pumpkin seeds, but only if uncooked and unsalted.
- *Soya beans*—and all other varieties of beans as well as other legumes such as lentils and peas.
- *Wheat and barley grass and wheat germ*—high in many anti-oxidant nutrients.
- *Fish*—especially deep-sea/ocean, cold-water fish.
- *Red wine*—although this is not appropriate in the preconception period, and the alternative non-alcoholic grape juice is rather high in sugar.
- *Seaweed*—contains algin.
- *Yoghurt*—if it contains Acidophilus and/or Bifidus.
- *Lecithin*—can be taken as a supplement.
- *Papaya*—contains bioflavonoids.
- *Bass, mackerel, cod, trout, perch, flounder*—contain methionine, a precursor of cysteine.
- *Turkey*—also contains methionine.

Herbs that contain anti-oxidant vitamins, minerals and bioflavonoids:

St Mary's Thistle	*Alfalfa*	*Ladies' Slipper*
Rose Hips	*Chaparral*	*Blue Cohosh*
Red Raspberry leaves	*Capsicum*	*Black Cohosh*
Red Clover	*Nettle*	*Valerian*
Hops	*Dandelion*	*Barberry*
Gotu Kola	*Eyebright*	*Bayberry*
Peppermint	*Ginseng*	*Marshmallow Root*
Lemon Balm	*Baical Skullcap*	*Bilberry*
Uva Ursi	*Hibiscus*	*Hawthorn*
Parsley	*Catnip*	*Nasturtium*
Turmeric	*Lemon Grass*	*Salvia (Dan Shen)*

Herbs that can act as an anti-oxidant, by scavenging free radicals through active principles other than vitamins and minerals, include: *Ginkgo Biloba, Schisandra Chinensis, Scutellaria Baicalensis (Baical Skullcap or Scute)*, and many other members of the mint family, including *Self Heal Rosemary* and *Marjoram*. These contain rosmarinic acid, which has similar anti-oxidant properties to Vitamin C.

An extract from the *Maritime Pine* tree, known as *Pycnogenol* is also an extremely potent anti-oxidant, and has been shown to be even more effective, in some cases, than Vitamins C and E.

It should be stressed, however, that many herbs have quite considerable physiological effects, and are better taken only on the advice of a medical herbalist. Exceptions would be those herbs used traditionally in culinary activities, and sold as herb teas, which have an obvious history of safe use.

All anti-oxidants will help to remove toxins and pollution from the body, but there are other nutrients, apart from anti-oxidants, which are protective against toxicity, and some anti-oxidant nutrients also have other actions.

Other detoxifying nutrients and foods

Calcium—helps prevent absorption of lead, cadmium, aluminium and excessive copper, and also helps to remove lead from the tissues. Calcium citrate is the preferred supplement.

Zinc—is particularly important in lowering lead and cadmium levels, as well as elevated copper and aluminium.

Chromium—aids detoxification, specifically of cadmium, lead and excess iron.

Magnesium—cleanses aluminium and excess iron from the body.

Silica—helps to eliminate aluminium (it's present in *Horsetail* and *Nettle* herbs).

Iron is antagonistic to mercury.

Manganese—reduces lead, excess copper, iron and aluminium.

Selenium—specific for heavy metal and pollution detoxification (binds with mercury).

Vitamin C—reduces lead, aluminium, mercury and cadmium levels, and excess copper and iron.

Vitamin D—helps calcium to do its work, and displaces lead from the bones.

Vitamin E—reduces the effects of lead poisoning.

Vitamin B1 (taken with B-complex)—provides protection against lead damage.

Vitamin B5—protects against radiation and excess copper.

Vitamin A—activates enzymes needed for detoxification.

Adequate *copper and iron*—(not in excess) protect against cadmium and lead.

Molybdenum—helps reduce high copper levels.

Reiishi—a Japanese mushroom which protects against the effects of radiation.

Garlic and onions—are specific for cleansing mercury, cadmium and lead from the tissues.

Legumes—are specific for mercury detoxification.

Algin—binds lead in the gut and helps eliminate it (found in seaweed).

Citrus fruits—cleanse carcinogens and lead from the liver (citric acid aids excretion of heavy metals).

Bananas—have antitoxin qualities.

Apples and pears (especially the pips)—help to reduce absorption of toxins, as well as aid detoxification.

Black tea—helps the detoxification of lead (drink in moderation because of caffeine).

Wheat germ—also helps to detoxify lead.

Eggs—protect against lead and mercury.

Asparagus—detoxifies lead and mercury.

Brussel sprouts and cabbage—also protect against lead and mercury.

All cruciferous (cabbage family) vegetables—inhibit carcinogenic effects of chemicals.

Suggested extra nutrient doses for detoxification

In addition to the supplement dosages in Chapter 1, if you have been exposed to a significant level of toxins, you can add the following additional nutrients:

Cysteine—500 mg daily.

Garlic—equivalent of 2,000 mg fresh garlic daily in tablet form (take separately from Acidophilus and Bifidus).

Vitamin C—2–5 g daily, or to bowel tolerance. That is, you increase the dose daily (in *divided* doses) until you suffer diarrhoea, and then you back off to the highest dose that you can tolerate with normal bowel motions. The amount that you can tolerate will increase with the level of toxicity or disease. Studies have shown that this is a good indicator of the body's need for this nutrient. Doses over 3 g daily may interfere with conception.

Silica—best taken as a tissue or cell salt (1 tablet 3 times a day), or through *Horsetail* or *Nettle* herb teas.

Please note: Although the dosages given above are a reasonable general anti-oxidant and detoxification nutrient formula, it should be stressed that your individual need is unique, and will vary according to the oxidative stress or toxicity that you are exposed to on a daily basis.

Two other nutrients also require attention. Those vital for life, oxygen and water, also have a role in detoxification.

Stabilised oxygen

Oxygenation, as opposed to oxidation, refers to the beneficial, detoxifying effects of stabilised oxygen. Oxygen is, of course, an absolutely vital nutrient, without which we cannot survive. Unfortunately, because of our polluted atmosphere, our oxygen intake is compromised. Stabilised oxygen, in liquid form, is now available to be taken as a nutritional supplement, and has been shown to be extremely effective as a detoxifying agent and as a protective measure against all pollutants.

It also seems to have therapeutic effects against intestinal Candida and can help to resolve allergic reactions. It will also, of course, protect against the action of anaerobic bacteria (those that survive in the absence of oxygen).

Water

Water provides a simple method of detoxification that everyone should be able to manage. We recommend that you drink 10 to 12 glasses, daily, of purified or bottled spring water. Unfiltered water may be full of herbicides, pesticides, fertilisers, fluoride and heavy metals, which are precisely the toxins you are trying to avoid. Copper levels in water are frequently excessively high where copper pipes are in use, and similarly in lead, if lead piping is present.

Filtered or spring water, on the other hand, has traditionally been used to flush toxins from the body, via the kidneys. Next time you're thirsty, instead of reaching for coffee, tea or a soft drink, have a glass of water! It's even preferable to fruit juices. It's remarkable how quickly most people become aquaholics, and get used to, and dependent on, frequent water intake.

YOUR DIGESTIVE SYSTEM

You need a healthy gut to absorb all the nutrients you will need for detoxification purposes. The bowel and liver also play an essential role in eliminating poisons from your body. It is normal, and healthy, to have a minimum of one, and preferably two or more, bowel motions daily. This cuts down on transit time, so that toxic matter is not sitting in the bowel, putrefying, fermenting, and polluting your body. Your motions should be easy, should float in the toilet bowl, should not smell foul, and should not be accompanied by mucus.

If *constipation* is a problem, it is preferable to use fibre supplements rather than irritating laxatives. Fibre supplements provide bulk and moisture for smooth elimination. *Wheat bran* is often used, but can become irritating to the intestines, and the phytate in wheat bran reduces the absorption of iron and other minerals. *Oat bran* is preferable. *Pectin*, from apples or citrus fruits, also detoxifies the gut, and lowers cholesterol levels, as does *guar gum*. These three are all good sources of soluble dietary fibre, that complement insoluble fibre such as *psyllium husks*. These act gently, form soft, bulky stools which are easy to pass and are effective detoxifiers. Freshly squeezed *lemon juice*, taken in filtered water, first thing in the morning, is also an excellent remedy for constipation.

In contrast, *laxatives* do not address the underlying problems. They work through an irritant action on the bowel, which will eventually compromise healthy bowel function. Their overuse can also result in depletion of potassium and other nutrients. If a laxative must be used, we recommend *aloe vera juice, butternut bark,* or in more severe cases, *senna.*

Acidophilus, available as a powder, or through live yoghurt, is also extremely useful in keeping the gut healthy, since it provides beneficial intestinal flora. *Slippery Elm* powder assists the smooth flow of the faeces, as does any mucillagenous herb, such as *marshmallow root, barley, liquorice* or *plantain leaves. Zinc* is an important mineral for bowel detoxification.

Roughage (or fibre) can also be obtained from most vegetables and fruits, which should preferably be eaten raw. *Figs*, both fresh and dried, are particularly helpful. However, remember that the sugar content of fruits, especially dried ones, is high, so restrict yourself to 2 to 3 pieces (or their equivalent, juiced) daily. Other high fibre foods include whole corn and brown rice, lentils, beans, peas, sprouts, seeds and nuts.

Adequate *water* intake is important to keep the faeces liquid, which will help to prevent constipation. *Olive oil* has long been used for cleansing the gut and improving digestion. It promotes bile secretion in the liver, stimulates bowel contraction, and soothes the mucous membranes. It is best taken in cold-pressed form, and not heated. *Linseed oil* (also cold-pressed, and not the highly toxic variety used for furniture or cricket bats!) is an excellent alternative, as are *flax seeds*.

Other ways of cleansing the bowel include colonic irrigation, enemas and fasting.

Colonic irrigation is a particular form of *enema*, which uses water that is under pressure, and which therefore penetrates further into the colon. Colonics cleanse from rectum to caecum. They eliminate toxins and putrefactive matter, and can be combined with herbal remedies which will loosen the more stubborn waste that sticks to the wall of the intestine. Both colonics and enemas need to be followed by administration of Acidophilus, to reline the gut with healthy flora. Slippery Elm can also be helpful. Both enemas and colonic irrigation must be carried out by trained personnel only.

Parasites can be eliminated using herbs such as *Wormwood, Black Walnut, Citrus Seed, Cats Claw* and *Pan D'Arco* and infections in the bowel can be treated with an extract of the whey fraction of milk (see the section on 'GUIs' in Chapter 8).

Fasting should also be supervised by a professional, although one day of fasting per week may be undertaken quite safely on your own but only if you are absolutely sure that you are not pregnant. During fasting it's important to clear the gut of old food, as with no new matter entering the system, it will become sluggish. Enemas and colonics can be helpful adjuncts to fasting, and if you are fasting, always drink a liberal supply of fresh (purified) water or vegetable juices.

Exercise will also improve your digestion, and stimulate peristalsis (the motion of the large intestine which passes the food along through the gut), and massage of the abdominal region can have the same effect.

Bowel detoxification should be followed by detoxification of the liver. The *liver* is perhaps the most important detoxification organ of all, and there are many foods, nutrients and herbs which help it to function well. *Zinc, selenium, the B-complex vitamins* (including *choline, folic acid* and *biotin),* and *Vitamin E* are all important for liver function, but most benefit is derived from herbal medicine. The herbs are best administered by a qualified herbalist.

Herbs which stimulate liver function:

St Mary's Thistle	*Golden Seal*	*Barberry*
Dandelion Root	*Wild Yam*	*Turmeric*
Yellow Dock	*Greater Celandine*	*Bupleurum*
Centaury	*Fringe Tree*	*Salvia (Dan Shen)*
Burdock	*Globe Artichoke*	*Schisandra*

Dandelion tea or coffee, made from the ground root, is an effective and safe remedy. Otherwise, herbs should be administered by a herbalist, unless they are eaten as foods (for example, *Globe Artichoke*).

An easy self-help remedy for liver function is the juice of a freshly squeezed lemon, diluted in (purified) water, and drunk first thing each morning, before breakfast.

YOUR URINARY SYSTEM

The main detoxifying organs in this system are the *kidneys*. Our advice about drinking plenty of fresh water is necessary for the proper functioning of these organs. Otherwise, unless you have a kidney disease, they shouldn't need special treatment. However, there are some herbs which will assist elimination, including:

Corn Silk	*Parsley*	*Juniper*
Couch Grass	*Buchu*	*Dandelion leaves*
Uva Ursi	*Horsetail*	*Celery seed*

These herbs (some of which can be found as teas in your health food shop), are soothing diuretics and urinary antiseptics, and much better than chemical diuretics if you suffer from a problem with fluid retention. Chemical diuretics may cause severe potassium loss, as well as depleting magnesium, zinc and possibly chromium. *Vitamin B6* may also be used to prevent fluid retention.

YOUR CIRCULATORY SYSTEM

The blood carries the waste away from all the cells in the body, via the various detoxification organs. *Blood cleansers* are these days called *alteratives* or *depuratives* by herbalists. These are all herbs that, over a period of time, gently expel toxins from the body. Most of these can be taken as tea. *Burdock, Red Clover* and *Nettles* should all be available through your health food store.

Red Clover	Nettles	Cleavers	Yellow Dock
Blue Flag	Queen's Delight	Poke Root[1]	Echinacea
Yellow Dock	Thuja[1]	Violet Leaves	Calendula
Burdock	Figwort[1]	Astragalus	Sarsaparilla
Dandelion	Guiacum	Oregon Mountain Grape	

[1]   These herbs should only be taken on the advice of a medical herbalist.

Circulatory stimulants may be required if the circulation is sluggish. These include *Cayenne, Ginger, Cloves, Prickly Ash* and *Ginkgo*. At least the first three of these can be used in your kitchen.

Chelation can be used in situations where there is a high concentration of heavy metals, such as lead, in the blood. However, even when hair trace mineral analysis shows high levels of these toxins in the tissues, blood levels may not be high. Chelation cannot rid the organs, bones or tissues of toxicity, only the blood. In chelation therapy, agents that bind to toxins and remove them, are passed through the bloodstream. *Vitamin C*, administered intravenously in this way, is an excellent remedy if serum lead levels are high. Chelation and any intravenous therapy must be administered by a medical doctor. For a homoeopathic version, see Contacts and Resources.

YOUR SKIN

Elimination of toxins also occurs through the *sweat glands*. The skin is, in fact, the largest organ of elimination in the body. It has been estimated that the skin eliminates over half a kilo of waste per day! There are various ways in which its function can be assisted.

Brushing your skin with a stiff brush, when it's dry, helps to open pores and stimulate circulation. It removes the top layer of dead skin, with its build up of dirt and acid, and deeply cleanses the pores without removing protective acid and oils. It also improves lymphatic circulation. Use a softer brush on your face, and don't brush harder than is required to produce a slight pink flush.

Saunas, especially after dry skin brushing, will encourage elimination through the skin, but should not be used if you suffer from a cardiovascular condition or hypertension. Sweat lodges and steam baths have a similar function.

WARNING: *Saunas and the like are not to be used during pregnancy*, as excessive heat can damage the foetus, nor should they be used during the four months' preconception preparation. This is especially important for men to remember since sperm are also very vulnerable to heat damage. Sperm are in the scrotum, outside the body, for the simple reason that they must stay cool!

Epsom salts baths can be easily used at home, if you do not have access to a sauna, or steam bath, or if you need to control the temperature. Add half a kilo of Epsom salts to a warm bath, and soak for ten to fifteen minutes. This will draw waste fluid out through your sweat glands.

Daily showers and baths. Although it might seem unnecessary to remind you, the daily use of showers or baths and essential hygiene is necessary to clear the skin of stale sweat, dirt and bacteria.

Sunlight. A daily dose of full spectrum sunlight (best taken in the morning and evening when UV levels are low and always avoid the middle of the day when the sun is hottest) has been shown in animal experiments, to help the removal of toxins.

YOUR LYMPHATIC SYSTEM

Lymph circulates around your body, carrying away toxins and debris. *Exercise*, especially the type in which the arms and legs are pumped up and down, stimulates the flow of the lymph, which is not pumped, like the blood. *Lymphatic massage* is a delightful way to encourage lymphatic drainage and relaxation, simultaneously. Most therapeutic masseurs can do this for you. There are also some wonderful *herbs* that stimulate the flow of lymph:

Calendula (Marigold)
Cleavers (or Clivers, Goose-grass)
Figwort (contra-indicated if suffering from tachycardia)
Sweet Violet
Queen's Delight
Nettle
Bittersweet

Poke Root is also an excellent remedy, but can be extremely toxic and should only be used under supervision.

YOUR RESPIRATORY SYSTEM

Waste is eliminated as you *exhale* (and toxins are *inhaled*). For pollution-free air in your home or work areas, you can use an ioniser or air purifier. With these devices, negative ions attach to airborne pollutant particles and remove them. Ionisers can also improve your mood and help to reduce stress, since negative ions (which are also prevalent after a storm or near the sea), cause a feeling of physical and psychological well-being. On the other hand, positive ions, which build up before a storm, are notorious for their deleterious effects on mental and physical health, causing headaches and a stuffy, faint feeling of listlessness and unease.

Breathing techniques are helpful for improving respiratory function. Breathing deeply will not only help to reduce stress levels, and increase oxygen intake, but can also help to clean out the deeper recesses of the lungs, which are often untouched by the shallow breaths which most people take. Exercise also helps to stimulate deeper breathing, and yoga uses it specifically.

Practising deep breathing

Hold your hand on your tummy, and feel it expand as you pull the diaphragm down and the air into your lungs. As you exhale you can feel the air being pushed out of your lungs as the diaphragm pushes up and your tummy pulls in. It may help to imagine your lungs as two balloons, inflating and deflating. Breathe in through your nose and out through your mouth.

YOUR IMMUNE SYSTEM

The *immune system* is your deepest line of defence against toxins and pathogens. It is dependent on good nutrition (but you've got the hang of that by now!) and there are also several herbs which assist its healthy functioning, though these are best professionally pre-scribed, as some are appropriate for acute conditions, and others for chronically depressed immune states:

Echinacea   Lomatium (Biscuit Root)
Astragalus   Schisandra
Ginseng (Siberian or Korean)   Phyllanthus
Picrorrhiza   St John's Wort
Bitter Melon Vine

A WORD OF WARNING: During any detoxification program, there will be a release of toxins into the body, which may increase symptoms temporarily. To keep this at a minimum, detoxification should be undertaken gradually and gently, and *well before concep-tion*, so that the toxins are safely eliminated, and optimum health *restored and maintained* for at least four months before a conception. *Detox programs are not appropriate during pregnancy.*

Example of herbal formula for detoxification

Red Clover (blood cleanser (alterative), eliminates toxins, expectorant).
Astragalus (immune stimulant, alterative, expels toxins, improves kidney and liver function).
Calendula (lymph cleanser, antiseptic, circulatory tonic, assists digestion).
Dandelion Root (stimulates liver function, assists digestion, blood cleanser, diuretic).
Burdock (blood cleanser, stimulates digestion, expels toxins, diuretic and mild laxative).
Cornsilk (soothing diuretic, aids elimination through kidneys, loosens stagnant material in bowel).
Many other formulae, using different herbs with similar func-tions, could also be effective.

SUMMARY OF SPECIFIC REMEDIES

Radiation—Vitamin B5, Astragalus, Burdock, Ginkgo, Ginseng, Green tea, Grapeseed, Reiishi mushroom, anti-oxidants. There are also flower essence and phenolic remedies specifically formulated for radiation effects. Use protective screens for VDUs. You can also place a packet of Epsom salts in front of your VDU screen to absorb radiation, (replace when powdered). See Contacts and Resources for a list of protective devices' suppliers.

Pollution—all anti-oxidants especially Vitamins C, E, and A (or beta-carotene), zinc and selenium, stabilised oxygen, use of ionisers.

Pesticides—Schisandra, St Mary's Thistle, Rosemary.

Alcohol (liver damage)—Schisandra, St Mary's Thistle, Green tea, Salvia (Dan Shen).

Lead—zinc, calcium, Vitamins B, C, D and E, selenium, manganese, chromium, adequate (not excessive) iron and copper, algin (from seaweed), citrus, black tea (in moderation), wheat germ, high fibre diets, eggs, onions and garlic.

Aluminium—Vitamin C, zinc, magnesium, manganese, selenium, silica, calcium, Vitamin D.

Mercury—garlic, selenium, Vitamin C, eggs, legumes, onions, asparagus, brussel sprouts, cabbage.

Cadmium—chromium, adequate (not excessive) copper and iron, zinc, calcium, Vitamin C, eggs, onions, garlic.

Copper (excess)—Vitamin C, zinc, manganese, selenium, calcium, molybdenum, Vitamin B5.

Iron (excess)—chromium, zinc, manganese, magnesium, Vitamin C, Green tea, Rosemary, Grapeseed, St Mary's Thistle, Schisandra.

LIST OF POSSIBLE MUTAGENS/ TERATOGENS TO AVOID

- Nutrient deficiencies.
- Green potatoes.
- Nitrosamine (formed in the stomach after ingestion of delicatessen meats).
- Food additives.
- Fluoride.

- Excessively high doses of Vitamin A (beyond 25,000 iu daily).
- Alcohol.
- Nicotine.
- Caffeine.
- Drugs and medicines.
- Heavy metals—mercury, aluminium, lead, cadmium and excess iron and copper.
- Spermicides (especially those containing mercury).
- Pollutant gases.
- Environmental and ingested chemicals.
- Herbicides, pesticides, insecticides and fungicides.
- Dioxin.
- Organochlorines.
- DDT.
- X-rays.
- Recent use of oral contraceptive pill.
- Age greater than 40 years of parents (chromosomal defects only, often offset by good nutrition).
- Ageing sperm/ova (prevent with good conception timing, see Chapter 13).
- Birth spacing interval less than 2 years (to avoid nutrient depletion).
- Pre-ovulatory phase greater than 20 days (see Chapter 13).
- Genito-urinary infections/sexually transmitted diseases.
- Parental allergic reactions (can lead to nutrient loss through malabsorption syndrome).
- Rubella.
- High temperatures e.g. saunas/fevers.

ADDITIONAL SELF-HELP MEASURES CHECKLIST

- Eat nutritious food.
- Drink fresh vegetable juices daily, especially carrot, beetroot, broccoli and red and green capsicum.
- Supplement wisely (see Chapter 1, and this chapter for recommended doses).

- Wash foods carefully in a solution of 1 tablespoon of vinegar to 500 mL of water (this will help to remove surface lead). Do not soak as this will leach nutrients.
- Avoid green potatoes.
- Avoid tinned foods, especially unlined or old tins, and *never* leave tins open in the fridge (transfer contents to glass or plastic containers).
- Avoid fish caught in contaminated rivers, harbours and lakes, bottom-dwelling fish, crustaceans and tuna, shark and swordfish (high in mercury).
- Buy organically grown, and fed, foods. Especially avoid organ meats (if animal was not organically fed) and mince/sausage/delicatessen meats.
- Avoid additives in your food. Read labels carefully.
- Use a water filter for all water that will be ingested.
- Don't microwave your food.
- Avoid aluminium and copper cookware and kettles, and avoid cooking or storing food in aluminium foil or cling wrap (use baking paper instead).
- Avoid tetra packs (often containing fruit juices) which are lined with aluminium.
- Don't cook high acid foods (e.g. tomatoes, rhubarb) in metal or ceramic dishes. Use heat-proof glass instead.
- Avoid foods and drinks containing caffeine.
- Avoid all drugs, medicinal (whenever possible) and recreational, including alcohol and nicotine.
- Avoid passive smoking.
- Avoid anaesthetic gases (whenever possible).
- Avoid amalgam dental fillings, flouride treatments and tooth pastes.
- Avoid carbon tetrachloride (as it damages the liver).
- Avoid antiperspirants containing aluminium (check labels of all toiletries).
- Avoid antacids, baking powder, and powder (such as salt) containing aluminium.
- Avoid vaccines, preservatives, colouring agents, pickles (all may contain aluminium).
- Use alternative 'green' cleaning products whenever possible.

- Don't treat your house for pests or dry rot, and be wary of all chemical treatments.
- Check all chemicals you are exposed to at work. Use whatever safety/protective precautions you can.
- Don't handle lead storage batteries.
- Avoid pollution where possible. Close car windows in heavy traffic/tunnels. Put net curtains over windows facing busy roads and wash them frequently.
- Use unleaded petrol and make sure your exhaust system is intact.
- Avoid renovations to houses especially where lead-based paints have been used.
- Avoid all pesticides, herbicide, insecticides, solvents, glues, etc.
- Avoid oral contraceptives and IUDs.
- Avoid electrical gadgets in your bedroom.
- Turn off your water-bed heater or electric blanket before getting into bed.
- Don't sit too close to the television.
- Fit an antiradiation screen to your computer, and avoid extended exposure, by moving away, or turning off screen when possible. Place a packet of Epsom salts in front of the screen (it will absorb radiation). Replace when the crystals have powdered. See Contacts and Resources for list of devices which may reduce exposure to radiation. Laptops do not radiate, but should not be placed on your lap.
- Avoid X-rays.
- Don't stand by the photocopier for extended periods.
- Don't shun sunlight. Simply take care with extended midday exposure, use hats in place of sunglasses except in cases of high ultraviolet exposure, and avoid tinted windows.
- Limit use of mobile phones, use protective covers and carry away from pelvic area.
- Avoid flights if possible and wear protective devices (see Contacts and Resources).
- Avoid an over-acidic diet (see p. 25) as this increases your susceptibility to radiation and heavy metal toxicity.

5

GETTING FIT

IT'S VERY IMPORTANT TO commence an exercise program at
least four months before you plan to conceive. There are three
types of exercise which are beneficial—*aerobic exercise,
strengthening exercise* and *exercises to increase flexibility*, and an
appropriate program needs to combine elements of all three.

AEROBIC EXERCISE

This form of exercise should be undertaken at least three or four
times each week. This exercise can be walking, jogging, cycling,
swimming, rowing or aerobics.

Benefits of aerobic exercise

Aerobic exercise improves your cardiovascular fitness, or, put more
simply, it improves the efficiency of the pumping action of your heart
and also increases the number and size of the blood vessels which
transport oxygen and other substances throughout your body. This
means that your conditioned (or fit) heart does not need to work as
hard as it would were it unfit, and also means that delivery of oxygen
and other nutrients through the bloodstream to all your body organs
and tissues will be more efficient. Among other things, this will
improve the delivery of those nutrients which are needed by sperm

and ova. Regular aerobic exercise can also lower cholesterol levels, enhance your immune function, reduce stress and lead to increased production of endorphins which are well recognised as mood enhancers.

If you have established a pattern of regular exercise before your pregnancy you can expect to have improved stamina and endurance, a great bonus when you are carrying around an extra 15 kilos or so by the end of nine months. You will also experience less fatigue, feel less stressed and sleep better. Both you and the baby (as well as your uterus and placenta) will benefit from your improved cardiovascular and pulmonary fitness. Aerobic exercise is great for improving peristalsis, or the motility of the gut, which helps to prevent constipation, and because of the improvement in your circulation, haemorrhoids and varicose veins are less likely to occur. Aerobic exercise also causes your body to use up any excess calories and if the exercise is weight bearing (unfortunately swimming is not) more calcium will be retained in your bones. Moderately strenuous physical exercise has also been shown to have a significantly lowering effect on elevated blood pressure which may be important in preventing toxaemia (or the high blood pressure of pregnancy).

The benefits of regular aerobic exercise will obviously extend to the birth as well. It has been calculated that the energy that you use during labour is similar to that expended during a 6-kilometre hike. Increased stamina and endurance mean that you tire less readily, but also that you will be much more able to participate actively in the birth of your baby. A good level of fitness means that you will also make a rapid recovery after the birth as well.

Heart rate during aerobic exercise

Aerobic exercise occurs when your resting heart rate is elevated to approximately 70 per cent of its (age adjusted) maximum capacity and is maintained at that level for at least 20 minutes. Aerobic exercise is most beneficial if you do it on at least three or four occasions per week.

Following is a chart which shows you the target heart rate zone (per ten seconds) for your age group. To take your heart rate, find your pulse at a point such as your inner wrist, your throat, or at your temple. Count the number of beats in ten seconds. Until you are reasonably familiar with how hard you need to walk, or how fast you need to cycle or run, it is a good idea to check that your heart rate is in the target zone (and that it stays there for the appropriate length of time) whenever you exercise.

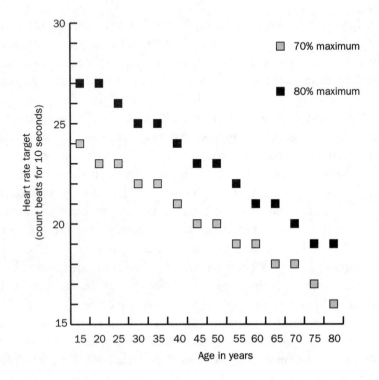

Graph showing heart rate target zone vs age

Getting started on exercise

Get advice

If you have never undertaken any type of physical activity whatsoever, then you should ask your doctor to complete a basic medical examination before you embark on your exercise program. This examination may be done as part of your full pre-pregnancy checkup. If you suffer from any medical conditions or injuries (old or new) which you feel may limit your ability to exercise—get some advice from an expert before you begin. This means seeking help from someone who is trained in exercise physiology or has a special interest in sports medicine and sports injuries. Heed their advice.

Enjoy it

Choose an exercise which you enjoy. If you think that enjoyable exercise is an oxymoron, then at least choose an activity you feel reasonably comfortable with. If you seem to lack the coordination needed for a choreographed step routine, or if you are not yet ready to confront yourself in leggings and leotard, swimming might be a good choice. Conversely, if counting the tiles on the bottom of the swimming pool seems like an absolutely mind-numbing activity, you might be happier exercising your brain as well as your body on the aerobics floor. This may be stating the obvious, but an exercise program which you dislike, one with which you feel uncomfortable, or one which you find totally tedious or boring is unlikely to be successful.

Set aside a regular time

If you don't make time for your exercise, it is unlikely to happen. Whether you choose early morning, lunch hour or evening, set aside a regular time and don't be tempted to abandon it because you're too busy. Once you have got into a regular routine, you'll have more time to spare, simply because you will find that exercise has made you feel better and more productive.

Exercise with a friend

Your partner might seem a logical choice as a companion—after all ideally you will be embarking on this program of exercise together. However, a partner is often not the ideal motivator, and if neither of you has exercised in the past it can be very easy to find reasons to stay at home. A reliable, and perhaps already exercising friend or neighbour, might be a better choice.

You might consider the option of hiring a personal trainer—it's difficult to excuse yourself from an exercise session if someone, for whose services you have paid, is waiting outside your door. This might be a good option for getting you both started—once you're up and well into the routine, you may be able to go it alone. Just make sure that your trainer has the necessary qualifications before you sign up.

Take it easy at first

If you have never exercised before, then you must begin slowly. If you attempt too much too soon, all those muscles which are completely unaccustomed to activity are going to complain, and you will probably give the whole thing away as a bad job.

Warm up . . . cool down . . . stretch out

Remember to warm up before you begin your period of aerobic exercise, then cool down and stretch out afterwards. In other words, don't leap from your bed first thing in the morning and set off around the block at a gallop. Walk for five or ten minutes before you start to increase your pace, then follow a similar period of walking, followed by stretching before you hit the shower. These are very important steps if you want to avoid sore muscles and injuries. Remember too that good aerobics instructors will always include these segments in their classes—be very wary if they are not a regular part of their routine.

Don't ignore pain

If you come from the 'no pain, no gain' club, you are headed for trouble. When your body says to you, 'that hurts' the message should be clear. It means 'stop!' If you grit your teeth and keep on going, you may aggravate an injury. Remember, however, that sustaining an injury does not necessarily mean that you have to stop exercising completely—you may simply need to modify your activity and give yourself a chance to recover and heal. But whatever you do—seek professional advice and treatment.

Try walking or cycling to work

You can actually achieve a reasonable level of aerobic fitness by simply leaving the car at home and walking or cycling to work or to the shops, on a regular basis. However, if this journey involves several kilometres along a major traffic artery, forget it. It might improve your cardiovascular fitness, but it won't reduce your exposure to chemical pollution and to heavy metals such as lead. If you are walking, and can use the back streets, make sure that your footwear is appropriate—you will be unlikely to get your heart rate into the target zone if you are teetering along in the shoes that you normally wear to the office. If you decide on the walking to work option, you will need to spend some time each day improving your strength (carrying all the shopping home can help) and flexibility.

A structured exercise program

You may like the idea of joining a gym because there you can have a personal program designed to combine the three elements of exercise in one workout. Remember that aerobic activity might include an aerobic floor class, an aerobic circuit, or time spent on an electronically monitored exercise machine. Your weight training might include work with free weights or could involve a circuit class. Stretching should follow both types of activity.

The electronic exercise machines which you find in well-equipped gyms can be a great incentive since they can monitor your heart rate, calories used, distance travelled, and so forth. They can also monitor improvements in your fitness level. Working out in company is also a motivator for lots of people.

However, before you join a gym, make sure that it has well-qualified staff who can guide you through a program appropriate for your age and level of fitness. It is also important that you advise your program supervisors of an intended pregnancy, and even more important that you tell them when you do become pregnant, so that they can make any necessary modifications.

Good aerobics instructors will usually ask if there are any pregnant participants in their class. Don't be afraid to raise your hand and tell them. When the rest of the class does an exercise which may be unsuitable during pregnancy, the instructor can show you an appropriate alternative. You may even be fortunate enough to have a gym in your area which offers special classes for pregnant women.

Don't overdo it!

Too much exercise, involving significant loss of body fat, can affect female fertility. You need about 25 per cent of your total body weight as fat if you are to have a normal menstrual cycle. Excessive exercise, combined with stress and concern about body weight, can shut down the control centre in the hypothalamus, leading to amenorrhoea (lack of periods).

Prospective fathers: stay cool

Research has shown that high temperatures can have adverse effects on sperm health so if you are a prospective father, avoid those tight-fitting cycling or jogging shorts and wetsuits while exercising.

Always wear loose-fitting clothing and be cautious about the use of saunas, spas and very hot baths.

Other options

Yoga is a very different form of exercise and may be more suited to your temperament. Yoga exercises are best taught by an experienced teacher, as there are some postures which may be unsuitable during pregnancy. Yoga can induce a very profound sense of calm and well-being as well as bestowing a number of more readily measured benefits on both the mother and the developing foetus. These benefits include improved fertility, improved circulation and consequently improved delivery of oxygen and other nutrients to all organs systems including the placenta, greater flexibility and increased energy. The relaxation techniques which are a regular part of yoga practice will reinforce your goal of achieving an environment for the developing foetus which is free, not only of chemical stressors, but of psychological stress as well. You will find some helpful yoga poses in the Flexibility section later in this chapter.

Rebounding on a mini-trampoline promotes excellent lymphatic and circulatory stimulation and tones the pelvic organs without jarring. A rebounder can be used in the privacy of your living room while you stay tuned to your favourite television program. There is no need to go anywhere or even to change your clothes. If this option appeals to you, make sure that the model of rebounder you buy is strung in such a way that it gives you full support.

Remember that if you want to combine the stimulatory and toning effects of rebounding with the many additional benefits of aerobic exercise, you need to use both your arms and legs as you would when jogging, and you must ensure that your heart rate reaches the target zone and stays there for the appropriate length of time. Remember to stretch out afterwards.

STRENGTHENING EXERCISE

This type of exercise involves a weights program, or total body, bodysculpt, circuit class 3 to 4 times per week, also strengthening exercises for the abdominals, lower back, buttocks, pelvic floor—do these daily.

Benefits of strengthening

If all your muscles are strong then you will be better equipped to tolerate physical stress and better able to carry loads without tiring. These are important factors to consider. You may be surprised at how much extra physical work, particularly of the lifting and carrying variety, that you will be required to do when you become parents. If you jog or cycle you might consider that sufficient, but primarily these exercises are strengthening your leg muscles. Conversely, swimmers frequently have very well-developed muscles in their arms and upper body but less well-developed muscles in their legs. Make sure that your exercise program works to strengthen all major muscle groups.

Strong back, buttock, and abdominal muscles are particularly important for prospective mothers. These muscles form a supporting and protective girdle around your lower body. If all these muscles are strong, the increasing size and weight of your baby will be far less likely to cause backache which is frequently due solely to weak musculature. Sometimes the abdominal (rectus) muscle separates during late pregnancy or in the postnatal period. This allows the abdominal contents to bulge through, so if you want to avoid this happening, you will need to do some prior strengthening of this muscle too.

Prospective fathers should not exempt themselves from muscle-strengthening exercise. If your abdominal muscles are weak your belly will sag, if your back muscles are weak, you are a great candidate for back pain. If you want to take your turn at caring for your baby, then you need to work at strengthening all these muscles along with your partner.

Pelvic floor (Kegel) exercises

The pelvic floor muscles are a sling-like band which surround and form the base of the vagina, anus and urethra. They also support all the abdominal contents and your baby will pass through the pelvic floor muscles as it is born. It is important that you strengthen these muscles along with the abdominals, buttock and back muscles, for a weak pelvic floor is a common cause of incontinence after a pregnancy. Incontinence means that you will wet your pants every time you laugh, sneeze, cough, jump or run.

To identify these muscles, you can try this exercise. Next time you urinate—try to stop the flow in mid-stream. Then relax the muscles—you have just exercised your pelvic floor. Now that you are familiar with the sensation, you can repeat this exercise any time you like. Try to increase the number of times you contract and release these muscles, and also increase the time for which you hold the contraction. Try to repeat the exercise at least five times every hour or so and hold each contraction for at least five seconds.

You can try another version of the pelvic floor exercise. Think of the muscles as a lift—try taking the lift up several floors, stopping at each floor, then go down again, stopping each time. When you reach the ground floor, continue to the basement, releasing the pelvic floor muscles completely. This is what you do when you urinate or empty your bowels. This is exactly how you will use those muscles in the second stage of labour.

You can also exercise your pelvic floor muscles when you're making love. Work hard at contracting and relaxing them—your partner is sure to enjoy this exercise.

FLEXIBILITY

Exercises for flexibility can be done on a daily basis and include stretching and yoga.

The benefits of being flexible

If you are flexible, your muscles will be supple and ready for activity and movement. If you increase your flexibility you will be able to experience the full range of motion for which your body was designed without experiencing tension or stiffness. Improved flexibility will make it far less likely that you will sustain an injury when you exercise. You should do appropriate stretching exercises at the end of every exercise session, but feel free to do them more frequently. Stretching and yoga are also great ways to relax and reduce tension.

Yoga poses

The following yoga poses are relatively simple, and can be relaxed into day by day. They are easy to do at home, though you may benefit more from attending a class where an instructor can attend to your individual needs, particularly if you think you might be pregnant.

Even these few postures, practised regularly, can make a profound difference to your hormonal and reproductive health. If you find a position too hard or too uncomfortable to hold for long, release and try again tomorrow.

For many of you, your work posture, general postural habits and emotional stresses may cause constriction in your pelvic cavity and lower back. These yoga postures open up this whole area, greatly enhancing circulation. A little practice done every day will be more effective than a longer session once a week. The postures will benefit male, as well as female, fertility and reproductive health.

Cat pose This pose is also ideal as an antenatal exercise. It is good for your spinal flexibility and for relieving lower backache and tension (so it can relieve period pain). This soothing exercise stimulates internal organs, and is performed rhythmically on the in and out breaths.

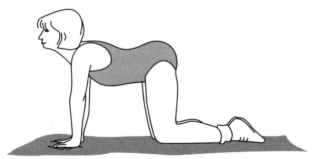

Cat pose 1

(1) Kneel and lean forward slightly. Your hands should be about 35 cm apart, your palms flat on the ground. Breathe in, lift your head and bottom and hollow your back.

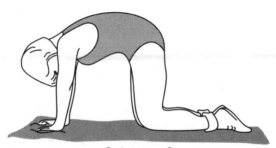

Cat pose 2

(2) Breathe out and arch your back, into a hump. Keep your arms straight and drop your head.

Pelvic stretch This position enhances the circulation of the blood in the whole pelvic area, stretches the muscles and ligaments of the inside thigh, hips and back. It tones all the pelvic organs and is a good prenatal exercise.

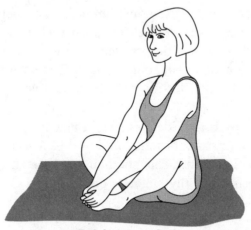

Pelvic stretch 1

(1) While sitting on the ground, with your back against a wall if you need support, bend your knees and draw the soles of the feet together close to your groin. Clasp your feet with your hands. Let gravity pull your knees down to the ground, stretch gently up, and breathe rhythmically and deeply. You can remain in this pose for as long as it is comfortable. Before rising, place your hand under each knee and gently lift, as your hips may have become locked. This is a great posture for meditation and relaxation. Hold the position for 5 minutes, before releasing gently.

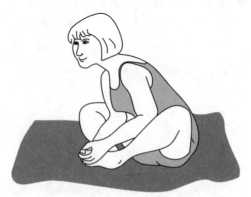

Pelvic stretch 2

(2) Let your knees drop further down towards the ground. Pull your body forward, keeping your back straight. Repeat several times.

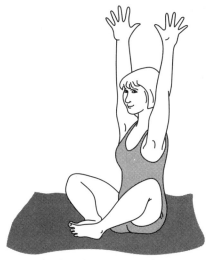

Pelvic stretch 3

(3) While in the same sitting position, stretch your arms up above your head, breathing deeply and rhythmically. Hold for 3 minutes. Release as you exhale.

Three other variations of this posture are:

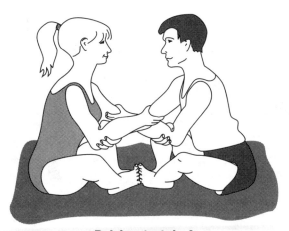

Pelvic stretch 4

(4) You can also practise this posture with a partner. Face each other in the posture with the underside of your toes pressing against those of your partner. Keep the soles of your feet together, cross your arms and hold each other's elbows. Pull against each other, stretch out your hips and bring your chest forward. You can also perform this pose with your toes against a pole or table leg. With your hands around the pole, just above head height, gently pull yourself up. Hold for 5 minutes, before releasing carefully.

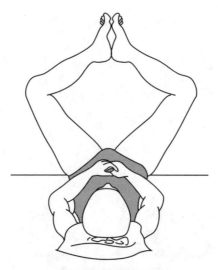

Pelvic stretch 5

(5) Lie on your side with your knees bent, and place your buttocks right up against a wall. Then turn onto your back so your legs rest against the wall, bend your knees with your feet together and let gravity pull your legs further apart and down. Your hands can clasp your feet, ankles or knees, or be placed gently on your tummy. Stay there as long as you need to relax.

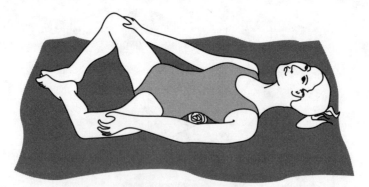

Pelvic stretch 6

(6) A variation of this pose is to assume the same sitting pose as variation (1), and lie down gently. Keep your knees bent and soles together. Relax, gravity will do the work for you. Your hands may rest on your knees, helping to pull them down, or on your stomach. If your back feels uncomfortable in any way, experiment with a folded blanket under your back, placed down, or across, your body. When ready to rise, lift one knee over the other, with your hand as for the sitting pose. Turn on to your side and rest for a few moments before rising up on to your hands and knees. This pose is great for calming the mind. Hold this pose for 5 to 20 minutes.

Inverted pose This position will bring blood to your head and brain, feed your pituitary gland, and, in the splayed variation, also loosen your hips. Do it on a soft surface or a blanket.

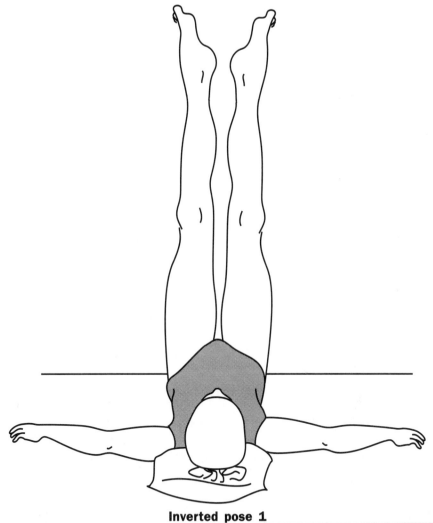

Inverted pose 1

(1) Lie on your side with your knees bent, and your buttocks firmly against the wall, then roll on to your back and straighten your legs up the wall. If you can, stay in this position for 5 to 10 minutes. To make yourself more comfortable, and aid relaxation, put a blanket over your legs, or a cushion under your head and neck. Breathe gently.

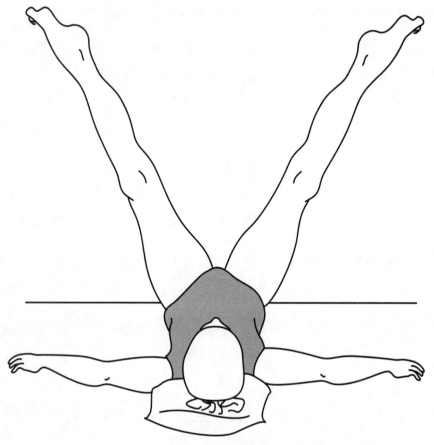

Inverted pose 2

(2) Remain in the previous position, and gently allow your legs to find their natural splayed position. Keep your legs straight, and allow gravity to pull them down the wall gradually, keeping both feet at an even height. Soften and relax your tummy. Build up to 5 minutes for this pose.

Hero pose This one is for heroines too.

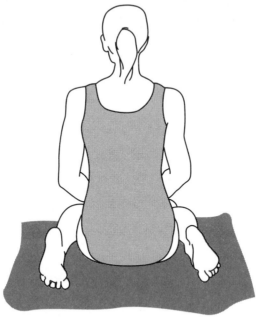

Hero pose 1

(1) Sit with your feet beside your buttocks, which should be on the ground. If you can't get your buttocks to the ground, support them with a cushion or folded blanket, so that you have a firm surface to sit on. Aim for your shins to touch the ground, and stretch your feet back. This may feel like a very slight movement, but it is valuable, nevertheless. Place your hands, palms down, on your legs and keep your knees together. Look forward, with your chin down, and breathe rhythmically. Hold this pose for 5 minutes if you can.

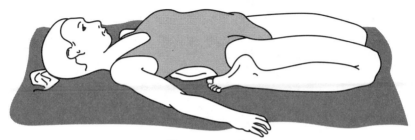

Hero pose 2

(2) Take a break if you need to. Then, from this seated position, lie back gently on a pillow, rolled blanket or bolster, placed lengthwise. Place folded blankets over the bolster if you need greater height in order to lie down comfortably.

Posterior stretch and Wheat grinder This pose increases blood flow to the lower regions of the abdomen, especially to the reproductive organs, as well as stretching the backs of the thighs and calves.

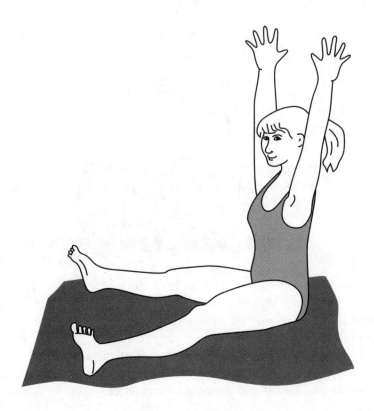

Posterior stretch 1

(1) Inhale, and stretch your arms above your head, sitting as straight as possible. You may find it easier to sit against a wall. Stretch your legs as far apart as you can, without bending your knees.

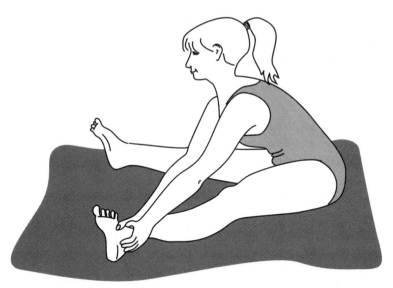

Posterior stretch 2

(2) As you exhale, stretch forward and clasp your hands around one of your feet (or ankles or whatever you can reach). Keep your back low and straight, your chest close to your thighs, your head up.

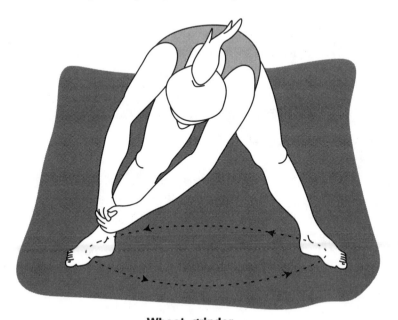

Wheat grinder

(3) Clasping your hands together, move them to the other foot, then back towards your body, completing a circular motion (as if grinding wheat). Keep this movement going rhythmically, clockwise and anticlockwise.

Cobra pose This pose tones the spine and back and expands the chest, improving breathing. It stimulates kidney and adrenal function and tones all abdominal organs, including the reproductive system. It helps to regulate digestion, bowel activity and menstrual/hormonal health.

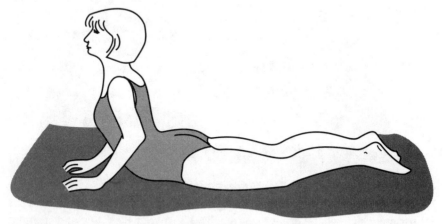

Cobra pose 1

(1) Lie on the floor on your tummy. Extend your legs, feet together, and put your palms flat on the floor next to the middle of your chest. As you inhale raise your body, resting your weight on your hands and legs. Keep your shoulders down and your elbows bent, tense your buttocks and thighs and continue to arch your back and bend your head back as far as possible.

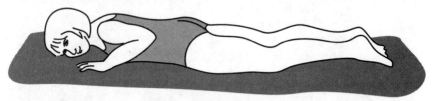

Cobra pose 2

(2) As you exhale, slowly lower your body back down to the ground. Repeat several times, breathing easily and rhythmically.

Bow pose This posture tones the adrenals and kidneys. It also stretches the abdominal muscles, tones the internal organs, and stretches the spine. *Note*: this pose should not be done by those with an ulcer or hiatus hernia.

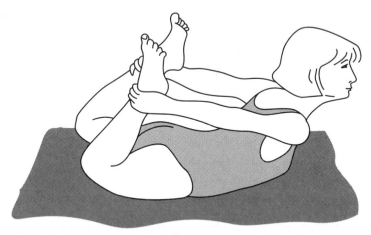

Bow pose

(1) Lie on your tummy with your forehead on the floor. Reach back and grip your ankles. As you raise your head and legs from the floor, pull your legs towards your head. Slowly let yourself back down as you relax. Inhale, and repeat.

(2) When you are in the stretched position, gently rock backwards and forwards, breathing easily.

6

STAYING POSITIVE AND
STRESS-FREE

So you're planning to conceive a baby? Do you
want your baby to be beautiful, healthy, emotionally
stable and intelligent? Do you believe that you can
contribute to the mental, emotional and physical health
of your child? Are you willing to do whatever is
necessary to achieve this?

If the answer to all of these questions is a resounding *yes* then
you have already started thinking positively! This is important, since
a positive attitude, or a strong belief in your own ability to have a
'better baby', may actually be just as important as all the other
preparation that you do.

Don't be tempted to disregard this part of your preconception
care, because current research in the field of psychoneuroimmunology shows that your mind is extraordinarily powerful. Although the
way in which it works is still unclear, it is apparent that whether you
maintain a predominantly positive or a negative attitude has a profound bearing on every aspect of your being. Most particularly, the
effects of a positive state of mind will be reflected in your health
(and consequently in the health of your child).

As we have said, if you answered yes to all of the above
questions, then you are well on the way to achieving your heart's

desire. However, for others, a positive frame of mind may not come quite so easily. There may be special reasons why you need a little help to achieve an optimistic outlook.

You may be impatient to conceive. Now that you have decided to go ahead and have a baby, you will probably want to start trying to conceive immediately. There may also be further imperatives. For example, if you have left parenting until later in life, you may fear that your fertility is declining.

To help you overcome your impatience, it may be useful to start thinking of this preparatory period as the *first step* of your involvement in an exciting, positive program that will result in the birth of the healthiest baby possible. Think of conception as the *second step*, pregnancy the *third*, birth the *fourth*, breastfeeding the *fifth*—all of these steps culminating in an exceptionally healthy life for your child.

Bear in mind too, if this is your second or third child, that the physical body needs a minimum of two years between conceptions to recover full nutritional status, especially if there has been a considerable period of breastfeeding, with the previous baby/babies. All too often second children are not as healthy as the first, and in large families there can be a deteriorating trend.

You may have already started trying to conceive. This could present you with two problems. Firstly, you may feel that you are involved in a continuing process, and don't want to lose momentum. Secondly, you may, if the attempts have been going on for some time, have doubts about your fertility.

To overcome the first problem, hopefully the material in this book will generate enthusiasm for the benefits of a few months' preparation. Enthusiasm brings its own momentum.

If you have been trying to conceive for some time, then your involvement in measures such as those described in the previous chapters, which have been proven to improve fertility, should make you feel much more secure. It is also empowering to know that you are able to exert some control over, and can enhance, fertility through simple, self-help methods.

We realise that it's disheartening when you don't immediately achieve your aims. However, setting yourself a new goal—to conceive only when both of you are enjoying absolutely optimal health, and thus to give your children the best possible start in life, will allow you to refocus your attention and energy.

Given that the recommended *minimum* preparation period is four months, an added benefit of this will be the break you have from repeated efforts to conceive. This will liberate your sex life from the monthly expectation roller-coaster, and give you some respite from any urgency that has developed.

You may have already experienced a difficult pregnancy, miscarriage, prolonged labour, premature birth, stillbirth, or have had a child with health problems. In the light of past experience, you may be fearful of what another conception could mean. If you can let go of these fears, and embrace the possibility of using simple self-help measures as we have described, to directly, and positively, affect the outcome of your next adventure into parenthood, confidence and motivation will replace the uncertain hope that 'we will have better luck next time'. This step alone will have a direct bearing on the success, or otherwise, of your next pregnancy.

You may be apprehensive about conception. You may have developed a 'contraceptive attitude' to sex, during the years when you chose not to have children. This can be difficult to reverse. In some situations, where pregnancy would be traumatic, fear of conception can be deeply ingrained. Even though circumstances change, and you now feel that the time is right to have a child, your emotional response may take a while to catch up with your mental attitude. This could make it hard to enthusiastically or wholeheartedly prepare for your child's conception.

Try to clarify why you may have had these feelings, and on what they were based, then think about how your life has since changed. The following techniques of visualisation and affirmation should help your feelings to become more appropriate, as long as you are sure that your decision is the right one.

You may be unsure if you really want to have a child. Perhaps you are less certain of wanting a child than your partner, or your family, or your partner's family, or even your friends. Maybe you have simply assumed that your priorities are the same as those of other people around you. You may need to distinguish *your* needs from those of others who are close to you.

If you do want a child, it's important to be doing this for your own reasons, not because of pressures (perceived or not). If you are only trying to conceive because you feel that you ought to, it is unlikely that you will be motivated to follow the recommendations in this book.

You may be unsure of your ability to cope with pregnancy, childbirth, breastfeeding or parenting. Many of your beliefs may have been formed as a result of information you received in your childhood, when the role models and experiences you were exposed to were beyond your comprehension or control. You may have been deeply affected by stories of horror labours, or have experienced only extremely dysfunctional family situations. You may have little or no experience of babies or children.

It could be helpful to demystify the process of pregnancy and birth by reading, talking to physicians, friends or midwives, or even attending a birth. Childbirth, under the right conditions, is a fundamentally positive experience. It's also quite natural to be anxious about it. You could try developing your maternal/paternal or nurturing self by offering your services to friends or family as a babysitter (they're sure to say yes!), or by volunteering to help in the local kindergarten.

You may be fearful of repeating the same mistakes your parents made, and in some cases this can become quite disabling. All parents make mistakes (you will too!) and if you can forgive those made by your mother and father, you will free yourself to do your best.

This, of course, can be a difficult and long process for some people, and we are not pretending to have all the answers right here. However, what can often occur is that, as you consciously focus your attention on your preparations for pregnancy, and perhaps use some of the visualisation and affirmation techniques that follow, you will find yourself becoming aware of subconscious problems. Then you can decide what to do about them.

You may be unconvinced that anything you (or your partner) can do will affect the outcome of your pregnancy. Hopefully, by the time you have finished reading this book, you will have changed your mind.

We believe that it is important for each of us to take responsibility for our own lives and health and, as prospective parents, for the lives and health of our children. We hope that the information in this book will not only enable you to do so, but will fill you with enthusiasm for the wonderful possibilities that it opens up for you.

THINKING POSITIVELY

As tools to harness the great power of your mind, to improve confidence, motivation and outcomes, visualisations and affirmations are extremely effective and simple to use.

Visualisations

Here is an example of a visualisation that both prospective parents can use, to assist in overcoming any of the doubts we have already mentioned. It can make it easier for you to carry out the ideas in this book, and greatly increase your chances of a healthy pregnancy, easy labour and birth, and a better baby!

Visualisations are best done when lying down or sitting in a comfortable place, where your whole body, including your head, is well supported, where there is no light shining directly into your eyes, and where you are unlikely to be disturbed. Make sure that you are wearing loose clothing and that your arms and legs are uncrossed, take off your shoes—then just close your eyes—and relax.

You may choose silence, or relaxing music (ambient or classical). If you can't fulfil all of these conditions, don't feel that you have to miss out. Relaxation can be done anywhere, anytime, sitting, standing, and even with your eyes open. In fact, it's a great way to pass the time while you're on the bus or the train. However, we would like to warn against using any of these routines while you're driving or when doing anything that could be dangerous if you get drowsy (such as using sharp knives or machinery). Use any moments that are available to you. The more regularly you use these techniques, the more effective they will be.

Your own special place

(Where you clear away any negative thoughts/habits/beliefs.)

First of all, clear your mind and relax. If you find your thoughts straying to the business of your life, just acknowledge this, and return to the pictures that you are creating, or to something steady and simple, such as the rhythm of your breathing, or an affirmation, until you are ready to continue.

Focus on your breath. Feel your lungs expand and contract as you draw the air in, and release it again. With each breath in, draw in new possibilities, new energies and new realities. With each breath out, let go of old problems, difficulties, limitations, stresses and tensions. You're moving forward, in time, with each inhalation and exhalation, releasing the past, relaxing in the present, and renewing for the future. Imagine that you're filling your mind and body with relaxed, healthy energies.

Focus on the rhythm of your breathing. Let your mind travel down into your body with each breath, gathering together your mental, physical and emotional energies. Get right down to the base of your lungs, around your stomach and diaphragm, where so much tension can gather. Let these tensions go, allow this area to relax. Relaxation is easy, you don't need to do anything, it happens all by itself.

Become aware of your heartbeat. As well as the rhythm of your breathing, pay attention to that other physical rhythm, your heartbeat. Imagine your blood as it is pumped by your heart through your lungs. See it gather oxygen, and distribute that and other essential nutrients to every part of your body, including your reproductive system.

Become aware of the movement and changes happening in your body. See the lymph flowing, detoxifying the tissues and organs. See your body renewing itself, moment by moment, changing and moving, right down to the cellular level, in the endless rhythm of life.

Clearly see your skeleton. Imagine the bones in your toes. Move up from the bones in your feet, to your heels and ankles, then up to the bones in your lower legs. See your kneecaps, then let your mind's eye travel up your thighbone to the place where it rests neatly in the hip socket. Here is your pelvis, sitting like a giant butterfly at the base of your body. Arising from this you can see your spinal column.

Move up your spine. In your mind, ascend your vertebra, one at a time, to where your rib cage is floating. Move up your ribs and backbone to your shoulders, visualise your collarbone and shoulder-blades, and the sockets from where the two bones of your arms hang down.

In your mind, move down your arm bones. Visualise your elbows, the bones in your lower arms, those in your wrists and all the bones in your hands and fingers.

Let your imagination move up your neck to your skull. Imagine each bone, and then see your skull floating like a balloon at the very top of your spine.

Feel your breathing to be easy, relaxed and rhythmic. Flow with the easy rhythm of your breathing. In, out, in and out—stay focused on every aspect of your physical being. *Inhabit your body.*

Imagine now that you are standing at the top of a small staircase of ten steps.

At the bottom of this staircase is a door. Start to walk down this staircase slowly, one step at a time.

Become more relaxed with each step.

With the *first* step—feel your body getting heavier.

With the *second* step—feel your mind floating free, deep down inside yourself.

With the *third* step—your body is getting heavier and heavier.

With each step, your mind is floating deeper and deeper down inside your consciousness.

With the *fourth* step—every breath is relaxing you more and more deeply, as you let go of all other thoughts and go deeper down inside, to the place where you are calm and confident.

With the *fifth* step—any noise from the outside world is just washing over you, as you become more and more internally centred.

With the *sixth* step—become aware of your own deepest needs and desires.

With the *seventh* step—become confident of your own ability to fulfil these needs and desires.

With the *eighth* step—feel extremely quiet, peaceful, calm, confident, relaxed and centred.

With the *ninth* step—make contact with the place deep inside where you are all of yourself, and only yourself,

and . . . with the *tenth* step—you reach the bottom, and open the door facing you. (If you are a smoker, you might like to see a no-smoking sign on this door.)

Step into your own special room.
It's the most beautiful room you've ever seen. It's full of light, colours, flowers and tantalising fragrances. The furniture is attractive and pleasing to the eye.
You feel instantly at home.
Feelings of comfort, rest and security fill you.
Look around the room.
There is nothing you would change. However, you notice a few piles of dirt or rubbish, so you fetch a dustpan and brush, and approach the first pile, to sweep it up.
Recognise the rubbish for what it truly is.
This will depend on your own needs. It could be any of the things in the following list. As you look at it, you acknowledge, experience, and remember the feelings associated with it. Then you sweep it up, and carry it to a chest in the corner of your room, which is a magic disposal unit.

As you tip the pile of rubbish into the chest you feel the negative emotions leave you, being replaced by their positive counterparts. Close the lid of the chest, knowing that next time you open it, the rubbish will be gone. Allow strong, positive feelings to sweep through you.

Dispose of negative emotion	*Replace with positive emotion*
Fear (e.g. of conception, childbirth, parenting, repetition of bad experience).	Peace, security.
Anxiety (e.g. for age, fertility).	Calm, confidence.
Impatience.	Patience (to wait until best possible time for conception).
Lack of control, victimisation.	Empowerment, responsibility.
Resentment (e.g. of previous bad experience, lack of conception, other's success or perceived 'fault' of partner).	Commitment (to the future).
Frustration.	Acceptance, hope, faith, joy.

Grief (at previous bad experience).	Happiness.
Ill health.	Health.
Doubt (e.g. of ability, or of need to prepare for conception).	Certainty, commitment, motivation.
Difficulty.	Ease.
Old habits (e.g. smoking, drinking, coffee etc).	Chance to start again.
Old beliefs (restricting of possibilities).	New beliefs (liberating of possibilities).

Sit in the most beautiful chair in the room.
This is your chair of empowerment. Sit in it. The instant that you do, strong, positive feelings fill you, and you experience an enormous sense of well-being. You feel capable of being or doing absolutely anything that you choose. You know that you can conceive a healthy child, give birth with ease (if you are a woman) and experience the joys of parenting. You are filled with determination to do whatever is necessary to achieve this.

Experience any of these feelings as they fill you.
You can feel them enter your body from your contact with the chair. You know that you are capable of anything!

- Energy
- Health
- Commitment
- Enthusiasm
- Peace
- Strength
- Confidence
- Hope
- Faith
- Motivation
- Security
- Joy

Visualise the successful outcome.
You may also, while full of positivity, like to visualise the conception and growth of your child in the womb, and the successful delivery and birth of a beautiful, healthy, robust and very intelligent baby.

Get up from the chair.
Still filled with all your positive energy and new resolve, move towards the staircase. You are going to bring all these new feelings back up into your daily life with you.

Start to come back up the stairs.
Feel your physical and mental energies start to rise, with each step that you take. Pull strong, wakeful energy into your body and mind with each breath you take. As you climb to the top of the staircase, feel your normal body muscle tone and circulation return, and be aware of your mind coming back to normal consciousness and wakefulness.
Reach the top of the staircase.
Open your eyes! Feel fully awake, alert and full of energy, but remain relaxed and confident. Know that all the transformations that have taken place will stay true for you.
Take a big stretch and a yawn.

You can repeat this visualisation, with whatever variations seem appropriate, whenever you like. Sometimes you may only have time to imagine certain segments, or you may prefer to replace it with something shorter, which can be used easily and quickly, whenever you feel the need.

You may, of course, create whatever other images are appropriate to your current needs. As you approach delivery, you may find it helpful to visualise an easy and successful labour, birth and breastfeeding experience. If you are having difficulties conceiving, try 'seeing' the sperm swim up through the cervix and uterus to fertilise the egg in the Fallopian tubes, which then implants in the womb and grows into a perfect child.

You may even like to record some ideas on tape so that you can just lie back and listen. But only do this in a situation where becoming drowsy won't be dangerous, and stay aware of anyone within earshot. Relaxation tapes can act through the subconscious on those who aren't even aware of listening. Take care to avoid using them in situations where anyone is driving, or using machinery or sharp knives.

There are, of course, many relaxation and positivity tapes available that may be appropriate or useful. If you order one of our 'Natural Fertility Management' kits, for conception, a relaxation/suggestion tape will be included. Books on, and courses in, meditation techniques can take this a step further, and will be helpful for you long after your children are grown. See Contacts and Resources for details of Natural Fertility Management kits and other sources of relaxation tapes.

Affirmations

Sometimes, to finish a visualisation, or to take its place, you may like to use affirmations of your beliefs and intents. Here are some possibilities:

'I am bringing my body and mind back to health, harmony and balance.'

'My fertility is increasing every day, and my reproductive system is getting healthier and healthier.'

'I am in control of my own life, health and fertility.'

'The eggs/sperm that I am producing are healthy and full of nutrients to create a very healthy child.'

'I am finding it easy to do all that is necessary to achieve a healthy conception, pregnancy and birth.'

'As I relax more each day, my confidence grows.'

'I can, and will, conceive a healthy baby.'

'I am joyfully anticipating the birth of my child.'

'I am confident in my ability to give birth easily and successfully.'

'I am confident in my ability to adequately nurture my baby.'

'I am happy to wait until my body is ready to conceive.'

We're sure you will find other affirmations that deal with any issues that are relevant to you. Sometimes a poetic image can be very evocative. Here is one that comes from Africa, and was told to us by one of our clients:

> *'On your way,*
> *On your way,*
> *Child be on your way to me here.*
> *You whom I have made new.'*

COPING WITH STRESS

Do you consider yourself stressed? Do you have a stressful lifestyle? Do you feel an urgency about your life? Are you experiencing any of the following in your life at present, or have you experienced them in the recent past?

- Heavy workload.
- Career path/job change.

- Conflict at work.
- Conflict with partner/relationship.
- Change in partner/relationship.
- Change in residence.
- Holiday.
- Engagement.
- Wedding.
- Birth of a child.
- Financial problems.
- Long-term illness in family.
- Death of family member/friend.
- Difficulty conceiving.
- Infertility.
- Participation in an assisted reproduction program.
- Miscarriage.
- Stillbirth
- Birth of child with health problems.

If you answered *yes* to any of the foregoing questions (and once again we can dream up some more), then you will definitely be experiencing stress. It is also important to remember that pleasant, or much anticipated, life events can be just as stressful as negative ones. Although there is often dispute about the extent of the role of stress in causing health problems, enough is known about its physiological effects to justify paying considerable attention to the reduction of stress levels in the preconception period. There is no doubt that *stress is a significant causative factor in reproductive and sexual problems.*

It's not so much the stress itself that is the issue, but how well you deal with it. Different individuals can tolerate different levels of stress, and problems only arise when you are under too much stress, and your coping mechanisms break down. That's why it's so important to have access to self-help techniques or professional help, and to have the support of groups and organisations as well. In the following pages we will show you ways in which you can help yourself to reduce the ill-effects of stress.

Some level of stress in your life is inevitable. It can actually be enjoyable, and of course it is necessary, to provide motivation and challenge. This aspect of stress is called 'eustress' ('eu' being a Greek prefix meaning 'good', as in euphoria).

You rely on eustress for excitement, and if you never got excited, conception might never occur at all! Symptoms that can indicate distress, such as a fast heartbeat, a quick pulse and heavy breathing are also clear indications of sexual arousal.

However, if your stress levels are too high, or if you're not dealing with them successfully, then none of these things may occur at all, and indeed there may be no erection, no response, or you may both have a headache! One of the reasons often cited for declining sexual activity is that couples are simply too tired and irritable. Ask any man who has had to produce a semen sample in a doctor's surgery what stress does for sexual performance!

Stress not only affects sexual performance, but fertility, conception and all other aspects of reproduction. As well as physical hindrances to conception there are very real psychological blocks, some of which we explored in the last section. As we pointed out, expert help can sometimes be needed to unravel and alleviate these.

Now we want to detail some of the ways in which excessive or unresolved stress can compromise your fertility and the health of your child.

Stress and nutrition

One of the principle factors that increases your body's need for nutrients is stress, both psychological and physical. *Physical stress* includes levels of pollution in your environment, ill health and toxic overload from ingested drugs, chemicals and additives. *Psychological stress* also takes its toll. Among its nutritional victims are:

All the B-complex vitamins	*Zinc*
Vitamin C	*Potassium*
Vitamin E	*Sodium*
Calcium	*Stress also increases*
Magnesium	*copper levels*

Many nutrients require the presence of adequate hydrochloric acid in the stomach for their proper absorption, and production of this acid is reduced by stress. Stress also affects eating patterns, causing you to undereat or overeat, and to generally pay less attention to the quality of your food (at exactly the time when you are most in need of its help).

Levels of other nutrients are also affected by excessive adrenal activity (which occurs in stressful situations). Nervous tension leads to an overproduction of adrenal hormones, such as aldosterone, which hinders the absorption, and increases the excretion, of certain nutrients such as magnesium. These nutritional losses mean you will be less able to deal effectively with stress, and so a vicious cycle is established. Therefore, when you are stressed, increase your intake of threatened nutrients. This will help you deal with the stress more effectively, as will the other techniques we look at in this chapter.

Stress and conception

If either of you experiences high levels of stress at the time of conception, your sexual performance will be affected, as will the physiological processes necessary for fertilisation to occur. If a stress response is too severe, its effect on the pituitary can inhibit the process whereby sperm are added to the seminal flow, and the prospective father may have little or no sperm in his semen.

The stressed female partner may experience chemical alterations in the uterine and vaginal secretions which normally facilitate the movement of the incoming sperm, and cause the release of enzymes necessary for a process called 'capacitation'. Female hormonal secretions cause the release of two enzymes from the sperm, which enable it to break through the egg's two outer coatings. Without this process the sperm literally bangs its head against a brick wall (just like its stressed owner!).

If there are sufficient motile sperm, and capacitation takes place successfully, another stress hazard lies in wait. The fertilised egg needs to be transported down the Fallopian tube to its implantation site in the uterus. This transport is achieved by the action of the cilia (hair-like projections) that line the tubes, and by the rhythmic contractions of the tubes. This process, which normally takes about a week to complete, can be severely disrupted by stress.

Sexual activity is an excellent stress reducer, so your conception attempt may have its own built-in remedy. But you may need other treatments during the preceding few days, if you are using abstinence as a way of building sperm count, or if you are timing your attempt to ensure fresh eggs and sperm (see Chapter 13). You may also be feeling especially tense if conception has been difficult to achieve, and for subfertile or infertile couples, stress can become an intractable problem.

Stress and infertility

Sometimes it's difficult to tell whether the stress precedes the fertility problem or vice versa. It's usually a bit of both. The longer it takes you to conceive, the higher your stress levels, and the more detrimental their effects on both your peace of mind and your potential fertility.

Studies show that infertile women are twice as likely to suffer from depression as fertile women, with the depression peaking 2 to 3 years after the initial diagnosis, and a higher level of depression in those cases where both partners have problems and where the cause of infertility is known. Infertile women have been assessed as being as depressed as those with cancer or heart disease.

Sometimes, a previously physiologically based fertility problem, which may have been resolved, can become a psychological fertility problem, which can be just as intractable. All holistic treatments for infertility will acknowledge and address this difficult problem and will give you a much greater chance of conceiving. Although some studies show that stress does not, in itself, cause infertility, it can contribute greatly to other causative factors, and other studies show a clear link between stress and fertility problems such as difficulty in conceiving and miscarriage, and poor sperm count and sperm health.

Many reproductive functions are affected by stress. We have mentioned the effects on conception itself, and the effect that lowered nutrient status has on the production of hormones, and on the health of ova, sperm and the reproductive organs, but there are also other pathways of cause and effect.

The adrenals are intimately connected to stress response, and also play an integral part in hormonal activity. Stress, therefore, can frequently delay ovulation, and affect your cycles' regularity, even leading to amenorrhoea (absence of menstrual periods) or anovular cycles (those in which no ovulation has taken place). Even a slight disruption in your cycles' regularity can create a problem with fertility, as a delayed ovulation may not produce a viable egg (see Chapter 13). An ongoing, elevated stress response has also been known to contribute to premature menopause, which will bring an end to any hopes of a conception at all.

In clinical practice, the stress of the attempt at conception may be enough to delay ovulation. This is due to the effect which stress has on the hypothalamus gland (which regulates appetite, temperature and emotions). The hypothalamus in turn affects the pituitary gland, which can then delay or prevent ovulation, sometimes through raising prolactin levels, and stimulating lactation. (This is the reverse effect of stress during breastfeeding, when prolactin levels are lowered.)

We have often noticed that, after years of regular cycles, and a happy and effective preparation for pregnancy, as soon as the designated cycle for an attempted conception arrives, there can be a significant delay in the release of the egg. This may indicate some deep disquiet or anxiety about pregnancy, childbirth or parenting. In these situations it becomes even more important to employ stress reduction techniques in the lead up to the conception attempt.

With couples who have been trying for some considerable time to have a child, many other issues may impact on the situation. These all compound the stress issue, and make it more difficult to resolve. They need to be addressed directly, once they are discovered or recognised.

Has your sex life become a duty? If you have experienced fertility problems, sex has probably become inextricably bound up with conception, and you may have lost your ability to enjoy the sexual act as it was intended to be enjoyed. Negativity and pessimism sometimes take the place of personal pleasure and loving communication. This attitude simply adds to your stress levels, since the stress-reducing effect of a normal loving sex life is missing.

It's important to learn to take pleasure in sexual activity, for its own sake, and to use the infertile times in your cycle, when no conception can occur, for healthy sexual expression of your love and care for each other. Otherwise you lose not only the prospect of a family, but also your continuing good relationship. When there is sexual activity that is distinct from attempts at conception, the emotional support of your loving relationship, combined with the destressing effects of the sex act itself, can help you through this difficult time.

Are you on an emotional roller-coaster? Do you set yourself up each month for a fall? Convincing yourself that you've conceived each cycle isn't quite the same as thinking positively. It's better, when you're fully prepared and ready to conceive, to celebrate the fact that you've a chance (and a good one) to succeed, and give your attempt all the energy you can, rather than create a make-or-break scenario. The average time taken by all couples (with or without fertility problems) to conceive, is six months, so give yourselves some leeway, and set about improving your chances by paying attention to your preconception care.

Are you scared of being childless? Maybe you've always wanted children, and have never given any thought to other possible futures. Maybe you've never experienced the frustration of a major aim before. Maybe you consider childlessness a failure and won't even entertain the thought.

Well maybe you should! Suppressed fears are dangerous and need to be expressed and shared. There is always the possibility that your infertility will be overcome, but also always the possibility that it won't. The rest of your life needs to be as fulfilling as it can be, either way.

Although the initial reaction to infertility problems is naturally one of shock and denial, if the problem has been a long-standing one, now may be the time to take the dread out of the situation by facing it, dealing with it, and looking for its positive aspects. This will effectively defuse the stressful effect of the fear, and will, in fact, actually increase your chances of conception.

There are many things you have to give up for children, and though you may be more than willing to do so, there are many and real advantages to a life without the responsibilities and demands of a family. Just try listing them, sharing them with your partner, asking some parents (they'll know) and seeing them as real, enjoyable and viable alternatives. Perhaps you can create a whole new exciting identity for yourself. If you find this too hard, but acknowledge that your fear of being childless is a problem, find a good therapist to help you.

Do you feel a loss of self-esteem and sexuality? This is an issue people have been battling with for centuries. In days past, when an heir was a social requirement and children cheap labour as well as insurance against old age, the stigma of infertility was much more relevant than it is today. Then, there were reasons (however uncompassionate) to replace barren wives, and men, mindful of their virility, seldom accepted, or even entertained, responsibility for the sterile state.

These days childless couples are no longer outcasts in the literal sense, but if you are infertile you may feel excluded from the family culture, which is often portrayed, somewhat unrealistically, as essential or the norm by over-romanticised advertising campaigns.

Your sexuality may also feel threatened. Although sex and reproduction are inevitably linked, sexual attractiveness and involvement are certainly not dependent on fertility. This fear of loss of sexuality also needs expression, and there may be a lot more reassurance available than you realise. Your partner may be feeling just the same. You may need to reassure each other.

Do you talk with each other? Since you're both in this together, you may as well give each other some support, and you can't do this if the subject has become taboo. Rather than assuming that you know how your partner feels, and that conversation on the topic will only rub salt in the wound, why don't you try to talk things over regularly? You may be surprised at how constructive this is for both of you, and how much less stressed you feel afterwards. Loving communicative relationships are not only less stressful and more likely to support conception, they're good training for healthy family life!

If you find it difficult to break long-standing habits of avoiding the topic, you may find it easier to discuss the issue in a group situation. There are many good support groups for infertile couples, where you can find out about possible treatments, and where you can also learn to share your concerns (see Contacts and Resources).

Have you devoted your recent life entirely or largely to conception? You may have responded to this life crisis by putting the rest of your life on hold. This will only feed feelings of envy, resentment, jealousy and anger. These feelings really have no reasonable target and can be difficult to express.

Maybe it's time you had a break. You might need a holiday! If nothing seems to lift your spirits, let your attempts at conception go for a while. Give yourself a specific timeframe for a complete rest, and you can focus on other aspects of your life, knowing that you will renew your attempts when you are refreshed.

Many couples experience the benefit of this sort of break accidentally, for example, when they concentrate on adoption procedures, and divert their attention from their own attempts to conceive. These situations are famous for producing a pregnancy. Recent studies show increased conception rates in couples applying for adoption.

Even greater benefit was obtained by those who applied early. The couple's sense of being in control of the situation was interpreted as the reason for the increased pregnancy rate. This is exactly what our intention is with this book—to give you a healthy sense of empowerment and control.

Do you feel guilt about some action in your past? You may, for no good reason, blame yourselves, or some past action, for your infertility. You may feel that you are being punished for acts such as terminations, (which may have been undertaken for the soundest reasons and may have had no adverse effects on fertility), unusual sexual practices, masturbation, or even for resentments and jealousies you may have experienced towards friends who have children.

These understandable feelings usually have no rational foundation, and cause a great deal of harm. Certainly they are easier to resolve if general stress levels are reduced by some of the methods outlined, but in some cases their resolution may need in-depth psychotherapy. Problems such as these do not need to be borne alone. There are people and groups who can help.

Stress and reproductive technology

We would like to emphasise that orthodox methods of fertility treatment tend to exacerbate stress levels, both physical and emotional. They are notorious for producing anxiety, rather than allaying it. Holistic, low-tech, naturally based approaches, on the other hand, use remedies that are relaxing to both your mind and your body.

Although the prospective father may have ample evidence, as he attempts to produce his semen sample over a *Playboy* magazine, that stress and fertility do not mix, there are much graver threats to emotional well-being ahead. One of the main problems is the tendency for conventional medical treatments to de-personalise the patient. We feel that you should be treated as an equal partner with the health professional in all aspects of the fertility quest. Conversely, of course, you need to take responsibility for your own health. You must ask questions, do the research, seek advice, make appropriate changes to your diet and lifestyle, and employ self-help measures whenever possible.

Although it is tempting to hand over responsibility to specialists, then sit back and wait for a miracle, this is not only disempowering and eventually frustrating, but unfortunately it is also unrealistic. Medical answers to infertility, regardless of the high levels of funding and attention given to them, are not very successful.

Many of the diagnostic techniques employed to ascertain the reproductive health of the hopeful mother-to-be are quite traumatic, and involve full anaesthesia and surgery. Then treatment often proceeds immediately to assisted conception technologies. In its least invasive form, assisted reproduction may involve artificial insemination (by partner's or donor sperm). One study found that the stress, fear and embarrassment associated with this procedure during each woman's first try was enough, in many cases, to stop ovulation in women who were normally quite regular.

Often there is no recourse to artificial insemination, but the woman is straight away given a course of fertility drugs or referred to an IVF/GIFT/ZIFT program. Use of these drugs is stressful since there are frequently both psychological and physical side-effects and many couples' experience of the IVF/GIFT programs is extremely traumatic.

One of the main problems is due to the fact that so much attention is placed on each single attempt, whereas the chance of success from a single attempt is, not surprisingly in most cases, lower than that of a single, well-timed natural act, given good preconception care. We rarely improve on Nature, though we can certainly learn to make the best of her.

There are also the unavoidable stresses of having to attend the clinic on a daily basis, take time off work, travel (sometimes long distances), and take large quantities of drugs. Add to this the great expense normally involved, and no wonder both stress levels and expectations run high. These days there is some attempt to give counselling to assisted reproduction patients, but the programs offer essentially negative, rather than supportive, experiences.

We hope that the ideas in this book may render it unnecessary for you to resort to these programs, but in some cases there may be a particular problem which justifies assisted reproduction. In these cases you would do well to employ some of the stress reduction techniques mentioned in this chapter, as they may very well improve your chances of conception. They will certainly make the whole experience a great deal less traumatic!

Stress and miscarriage/stillbirth

In the previous section on thinking positively, we gave some simple self-help ideas that can help you move on from these experiences. The evidence also shows that the probability of a recurrence will be much reduced if you both attend to your preconception care.

While unhappy experiences may contribute to your stress levels, you also need to understand that stress, from any cause, may increase the likelihood of your experiencing, for example, a miscarriage. By its action on nutritional status, stress can also contribute to a possible congenital deformity or stillbirth. Therefore, it becomes important to address this issue, whether or not you have previously experienced any of these traumatic events.

The emotional response to a miscarriage may be just as intense as that experienced after a stillbirth, and the degree of trauma does not necessarily seem to be in direct proportion to the duration of the pregnancy, but rather to the degree of attachment and involvement of the parents. There may also be the cumulatively stressful effect of grieving for repeated miscarriages.

Certain psychological traits have been noted as being typical of women who have suffered multiple miscarriages. Whether these are causative, or the result of the experiences is not clear. Chronic depression and anxiety, loss of self-esteem, distorted body image, anger, decreased libido and guilt, all too often follow for both parents, especially if no effort is made to resolve these feelings (through counselling, for example). Unfortunately, there may also be a breakdown in communication between partners. Each may, in part, hold the other to blame for the loss(es).

However, studies show that counselling of some kind, even simple reassurance and support from an understanding physician, can have a considerable impact on the probability of miscarriage recurring. Studies indicate that psychotherapy, including relaxation therapy and hypnosis, is the most significant factor in reducing the incidence of recurrent miscarriage.

Grief counselling is another, obvious, recourse for those who have experienced some loss, when typical responses will be shock, denial, anger, anxiety, guilt, depression, apathy and blame (of self, partner and others, including health-care givers). However, reduction of stress may well help to prevent the event in the first place, and some of the simple self-help techniques we outline here are best used as preventative measures rather than treatment.

Making your conception attempt stress-free

Each conception attempt should be as special, joyous, and optimistic as possible. This might be the one! You want your child to enter on a positive note, and you also want to be able to remember the occasion as a very happy one.

Spend the day or evening in ways that you both enjoy. Set aside the time for relaxing, supportive activities. If you have had previous failed attempts, it may help to change the circumstances. Try a different location, vary the time of day, experiment with your sexual technique, use fantasy, do something romantic, decorate your bedroom with candles, flowers, or sweet-smelling oils, and arrange to have time off from other responsibilities. Not only will this create a more supportive environment in which a conception may occur, but, even if you aren't lucky this time, you can look forward to the next attempt!

You may be practising abstinence for a few days, to build sperm count, and time conception accurately, but it's not necessary to shun each other in bed! There is a great deal of sexual contact that doesn't involve ejaculation, and this is a time to express love with kisses, cuddles and caresses.

Touch and massage are excellent ways of expressing affection and relieving stress, and you don't have to be a trained masseur to give pleasure and induce relaxation. Neck, shoulders, face, head, hands, feet, back and tummy are all sites where tension collects, and even an untrained touch can work wonders, and be an especially helpful part of preconception foreplay. During this time you can restate, in these and other ways, your attraction for each other, which will boost your self-esteem and confidence. Above all, be tolerant of each other's flaws and difficulties, and avoid blame and guilt if the occasion doesn't measure up to expectations. You can always kiss, go to sleep and try again another time.

Coping with stress in your daily life
Massage and bodywork

There's no need to restrict massage to your conception attempts. A regular full body treatment, or attention to the pressure points throughout your body (*shiatsu*), or specifically in your feet (*reflexology*), are some of the most enjoyable and effective ways of reducing stress, and of making you feel pampered.

Both expert treatments and friendly exchanges can be helpful. If you find it too expensive to go to a trained masseur, find someone else who is stressed (shouldn't be difficult!) to share at least a neck and shoulder rub with you—it's almost as enjoyable to give a massage as it is to receive one.

Peristaltic massage (which releases abdominal tensions) is particularly appropriate, and there are many other forms of energy balancing, such as pulsing, applied kinesiology and Reiki, all of which can help. Aromatherapy introduces helpful essential oils, whose fragrances have a specific effect on the nervous system, and if you have really stubborn muscular problems, osteopathy or chiropractic where there is soft tissue and skeletal adjustment, may be necessary. These can all have the effect of toning the circulation and nerve supply to the reproductive system, and can be extremely effective adjuncts to fertility treatment.

Acupuncture

An acupuncturist will focus on the same pressure points that are used during massage, shiatsu or reflexology, to bring relief for specific complaints. The theory behind acupuncture, which has been in use for hundreds of years in China, is that energy flows through the body along specific pathways, and any blockage of this energy flow brings disease. As these blockages are released, and the 'Chi', or life force, flows freely again, health returns. There may well be some correlation to nerve pathways, or other physiological processes which are closer to our Western understanding of health and disease, but no really satisfactory parallels have yet been drawn.

Acupressure

In shiatsu, or acupressure, the masseur uses pressure to release these blocks. The acupuncturist traditionally uses needles, but these days laser, ultrasound and electronic pulses often replace them. Any stimulation to the point has a similar effect, and these treatments can be useful, not only as a remedy for disease, but also to alleviate stress, and to treat an exhausted nervous system.

In order to have a treatment with needles, laser or ultrasound it is necessary to visit a practitioner, (laser and ultrasound should be used with caution, especially if pregnant), but the other techniques can be employed at home. There are also available on the market some neat little gadgets which deliver a small electronic pulse to the appropriate spot. Some even indicate when the correct pressure point has been found. These are, of course, also useful for the treatment of other diseases, and in Chapter 8 we look at some helpful pressure points.

You can use acupressure on a point without special gadgets or without professional training (though it will be more effective to visit a trained practitioner). The advantage of self-help is that you can use the techniques frequently throughout the day. If you choose to do it yourself you should follow these guidelines:

How to stimulate an acupressure point
- First, find the point as accurately as you can.
- Apply pressure in the appropriate way (as directed below).

Calming—Cover the point with the palm of your hand, or gently stroke, for about 2 minutes.

Tonifying—Apply stationary (or clockwise) pressure for 2 minutes. This pressure can be slowly increased as your tolerance to any discomfort increases (points relating to an organ or condition in need of treatment may often be tender). Pressing too hard straight away can cause you to tense. Gradually increased pressure can be better tolerated, and therefore more easily built up to effective levels.

Dispersing—Apply moving pressure, such as a circular anticlockwise motion, or a pumping action in and out on the point. This pressure can be begun fairly deep, and then brought up to the surface. Take care to keep the area relaxed, and increase the pressure on successive treatments as you learn to tolerate it.

Acupressure points for relieving stress/tension

Note: All treatments for stress will use the 'calming' technique and, except for points on the mid-line, always treat both sides of the body.

Conception vessel 12—on the mid-line of the body, equidistant from the navel and the solar plexus.

Conception vessel 15—on the midline of the body, at the level of the solar plexus.

Conception vessel 17—on the midline of the body, at the level of the nipples.

Colon 4—see Chapter 8 (Acupressure points for the digestive system) and

Liver 3—see Chapter 8 (Acupressure points for allergic reactions), should be calmed and used together for stress reduction.

Stomach 36—see Chapter 8 (Acupressure points for irregularity and hormone imbalance) should be calmed for stress reduction.

Pericardium 6—see Chapter 8 (Acupressure points for allergic reactions) should be calmed for insomnia

Stomach 45—bottom outer corner of nail bed of second toe on the side nearest to the third toe, should be calmed for insomnia.

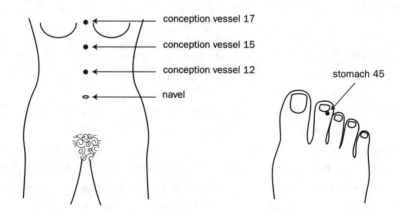

Finding Conception vessel 12, 15 and 17   **Finding Stomach 45**

Herbs, homoeopathy and flower essences

There are many herbal, homoeopathic and flower essence remedies available to treat stress. You may go to a practitioner and get expert advice, (this alternative would be most effective), or you may find some help in your local health food shop.

All the *flower essences* work to shift emotional blocks and negativity in a gentle but powerful way. There are several traditions, some old, some new.

Bach flower remedies are based on the work of Dr Edward Bach, an Englishman working in the 1930s, whose remedies have been used worldwide. Some of the Bach flower remedies we would recommend include:

Gentian—for discouragement.
Gorse—for hopelessness and despair.
Impatiens—for impatience.
Willow—for resentment.
Crab Apple—for a sense of physical unhealthiness.
Wild Oat—for uncertainty re path in life.
Pine—for self-reproach and guilt.
Larch—for lack of confidence.
Oak—for despondency though struggling on.
Mimulus—for fear of known things.
Walnut—for protection against outside influences.
Sweet Chestnut—for extreme anguish.
Honeysuckle—for living in the past.
Heather—for obsession with own health.
Wild Rose—for resignation, apathy.

There are also Australian bush flower essences, created by Ian White, an Australian health practitioner.

Bottle Brush—for major life changes.
Sturt Desert Pea—for deep hurts and sorrows, emotional pain, or anger from grief.
Wisteria—for tension about sex and effects of sexual abuse.
Sturt Desert Rose—for lack of self-esteem, guilt, peer pressure.
Southern Cross—for victim mentality.
Dagger Hakea—for resentment, bitterness towards family, close friends.
Kapok Bush—for resignation, apathy, being easily discouraged.
Banksia Robur—for loss of drive and enthusiasm, frustration.
Old Man Banksia—for weariness, being disheartened.
Illawarra Flame Tree—for a sense of being left out, rejection and fear of responsibility.
Billygoat Plum—for sexual revulsion, disgust at aspect of self.

She-oak—for distress associated with infertility.
Black-eyed Susan—for stress, rushing, constant striving, impatience.
Boronia—for obsessive thoughts.
Sunshine Wattle—for struggle, being stuck in the past and anticipating a grim future.

Flower essences are in homoeopathic dosage (that is, the remedy contains only a trace of the active element) and do not rely on physiological actions.

Homoeopathy is a whole tradition of treatment which offers care of body and mind. Each individual is treated separately, and the remedy used will depend on your total circumstances. For homoeopathic treatment for stress to be effective, you should see a trained practitioner.

Herbal remedies have been with us since time immemorial and are still the most widely used form of health care in the world. Many plants have long been known for their ability to calm and restore, assist sleep, and cure anxiety and depression.

Medical herbalists are fully trained in both the traditional aspects of their lore, as well as in the ever-growing body of scientific research into the active constituents of plants. They also have a thorough grounding in, and understanding of, physiology, biochemistry, diagnostic techniques and disease processes. If you have a chronic problem resulting from stress, a herbalist can usually help.

In your health food shop you will find many herbal remedies in tablet form (when they may be combined with certain nutrients), or as a dried herb, which should be taken as an infusion or herbal tea (tisane). These can be taken safely, although treatment from your health practitioner may be more effective.

How to make an infusion For every 30 g (2 tablespoons) of the herb, pour on 500 to 600 mL of boiling water.

Let it steep (infuse) for at least 15 minutes, to get the full benefit of the active ingredients of the herb.

Then strain, and drink a teacupful, three or four times daily. (The last dose to be at bedtime, if sleep is a problem.)

Make a fresh brew every day, use within 24 hours, or refrigerate.

If you use herbal teabags, leave them to steep in the water for a similar period of time.

Herbs to calm you
Chamomile
Lavender
Vervain
Wood Betony
Schisandra
Lime Flowers (Linden)
Lemon Balm
Motherwort
Kava Kava

Herbs to help you with stress
(adaptogens)
Ginseng
Withania
Liquorice
Gotu Kola
Astragalus
Oats

Herbs to lift depression
St John's Wort
Damiana
Rosemary
Basil

Herbs to help you sleep
Hops
Skullcap
Valerian
Passionflower

Seek professional advice if there is any chance of conception occurring.

Aromatherapy

Essential oils can be used in a number of ways to help you relax. We have mentioned that they can be used to increase the effectiveness of massage. They can also be used in an oil-burner or in the bath. Oils which you can use include:

Oils for relaxation
Lavender
Neroli
Rosewood
Myrtle
Geranium
Marjoram

Oils for stress
Ylang Ylang
Rose
Clary Sage

Psychotherapy

There are numerous practitioners available to help you through stressful times in your life, and who may well offer the most appropriate remedy for any intransigent problems. Some of these will be health-care personnel within orthodox medicine, such as psychologists, counsellors and psychiatrists.

Counselling is employed to some degree by all health professionals concerned with emotional distress, and can be one of the most constructive methods of dealing with stress. However, even by talking, you can get further into distress rather than out of it, and a trained counsellor or therapist is the best person to assist you. He or she will help you come to your own conclusions and decisions, rather than attempt to give you advice.

Other psychotherapeutic modalities could include Gestalt and Somatic therapy. These should be undertaken with the help of a trained professional.

Drugs

We would warn against the use of psychotropic drugs (drugs which alter mental function), before conception or during pregnancy, unless completely unavoidable. Some of these drugs are known to affect the unborn, through either the mother or the father, and all drugs are suspect during pregnancy as we have already mentioned. Natural remedies are generally to be preferred.

Antidepressants. Known problems occur with the use of antidepressants which are monoamine oxidase inhibitors. These decrease sperm count and motility. Tricyclic antidepressants do not have the same effects, but should still be used with caution, and only as a last resort.

Tranquillisers and sleeping pills. Benzodiazepines, often prescribed as tranquillisers, have been linked with visible malformations, functional deficits and behavioural problems. They can disturb the formation of the central nervous system, including the brain, if taken in the early stages of pregnancy. Some studies suggest that cleft palate and hare lip occur three times more frequently in babies whose mothers took these drugs in early pregnancy. Instead of using tranquillisers, try giving up caffeine and other stimulants, make certain that levels of nutrients, such as zinc, magnesium, calcium and B-complex vitamins are adequate, and try natural and herbal alternatives.

Breathing, music and water

Breath therapy (or Rebirthing), where breathing is used to release tension and psychological blocks, often makes use of water immersion, and its calming and supportive properties. Another popular use of this combination for relaxation is with *float tanks*, where highly salted water allows you to float with no effort. Soothing music which is certainly a marvellous aid to serenity, is often played while you float.

Ambient music, on tape or CD, has gained great popularity in recent years, where subtle musical compositions, often combined with natural sounds, take place at slower, more relaxed tempos than the frenetic pace of popular modern music. *Classical music*, acoustic or choral, secular or sacred, may be more to your taste, and can bring great peace and joy.

Relaxation or auto-suggestion, hypnotherapy and meditation

Other tapes or CDs, which can be found in bookstores, health food shops and other outlets, use suggestion to release tension, and increase optimism. These may use overt or subliminal affirmation, which is similar to a gentle form of hypnosis or meditation.

Hypnotherapy merely takes this a little further (or deeper), but should only be practised by qualified therapists. It may be used by psychologists or psychotherapists as part of an overall treatment, or on its own. It is a prerequisite to the state of hypnosis, that you enter into deep relaxation, and so, apart from any specific therapy that may be undertaken to address particular problems, the relaxation alone will always be of benefit in tension and anxiety states.

It is often thought that, in hypnosis, a trance state is entered, where the therapist has some kind of control over you. In fact nothing could be further from the truth, and hypnotherapy will, and can, only work with your complete cooperation. At no time is there loss of consciousness, and you can end the treatment at any stage, and receive only those suggestions to which you are amenable. Hypnotherapy is, however, a powerful tool in the hands of a good therapist, for overcoming emotional blocks and trauma, and for inducing optimism, confidence and motivation. Self-hypnosis can also be taught by your therapist.

Meditation is similar to hypnotherapy in that a state of absolute calm is induced, as you focus on one particular stable event, thought or word. As with self-hypnosis, meditation is usually self-induced. The techniques for doing this are easily learnt and there are many excellent courses and teachers available (see Contacts and Resources). Meditation can be done on a daily basis, alone, or in group situations, and brings undoubted benefit and peace of mind. You do not need to be religiously inclined to practise meditation.

Meditation, contemplation and prayer are traditionally part of religious life, and if you are of a spiritual persuasion, religious groups such as churches, ashrams and other congregations can be very supportive.

Exercise

Exercise is a great de-stressor, and also helps to 'tone' reproductive function. The endorphins released during normal exercise will make you feel much more positive. Studies have confirmed that moderate exercise can increase the effectiveness of other treatments for depression. However, excessive training can cause disruption to body fat levels and hormone production, so you should beware of becoming too zealous.

Swimming and brisk walking are good non-violent forms of aerobic exercise, which can be continued throughout your pregnancy. Non-aerobic exercise can include gentler forms which are specifically focused on relaxation. Yoga and Tai Chi are enormously calming to the mind, and are sometimes thought of as a physical form of meditation.

Good nutrition and sleep

By now, having read this far, you should be able to say nutrition in your sleep! We've certainly stressed the idea of good nutrition, though if you've heeded our words you shouldn't be so stressed yourself, and you certainly won't be if you get a good 6 to 8 hours of sleep each night! Having made a play with these words, we should just say simply that stress, nutrition and sleep are fundamentally and inextricably intertwined, and none of these other techniques or methods will work very effectively for you if you don't sleep and eat well.

If you have difficulty sleeping, try the ideas we gave you on herbal remedies to take internally, or buy a pillow stuffed with soporific herbs such as hops and lavender which smell delightful. Tapes containing suggestions or soothing music, specifically designed to get you off to dreamland, can be helpful. Take a warm bath with soothing essential oils, or use an oil-burner in your bed-room. You can also profitably spend a few minutes relaxing each body part, toes to head, or repeating a favourite affirmation.

Sleep should be undisturbed, in a darkened room, on a supportive mattress, away from technologies, telephones, intrusive noises and electromagnetic fields (see Chapter 3).

Lighting

Full spectrum lighting (as in daylight) is used as an essential nutrient by your endocrine system. It is taken into your body largely via the optic nerve, and partly through the skin, and a lack of it causes stress. Studies have shown that if people are deprived of full spectrum light, for example if they work in a factory which has only fluorescent lighting, stress indicators such as sick leave go up, and productivity goes down.

Use daylight as much as possible in all your activities. Where this is not possible, incandescent light (as in normal light bulbs) is preferable to fluorescent light, which is extremely deficient in the spectrum, and also flickers, which is disturbing to your brain. Unfortunately, environmentally friendly long-life fluorescent bulbs are no better than the tubes. There are, however, full spectrum fluorescent tubes available (see Contacts and Resources).

Full spectrum light reception is also affected if you frequently wear sunglasses, shaded lenses or sit behind tinted windows. Deal with the UV light with hats and shades, and remember that sunlight still has many important properties, but exposure should be limited to small doses in the early morning or late afternoon.

Order

Keep your life and environment in order, and reduce chaos where you can. Complete tasks that you undertake, so they don't hang over you, and try not to make commitments that you can't fulfil. Where possible, surround yourself, at work and at home, with cleanliness, order and beauty, and these properties will spill over into your feelings about yourself and your life.

Leisure

You're less stressed if you're happy and involved in activities which are fulfilling and rewarding. Taking time out from work, family, domestic commitments and your usual routine is essential, and making room in your life for activities and hobbies outside work and domestic duties will bring its own rewards. Especially helpful are activities which bring you into contact with nature. This contact can be relied upon to lift your spirits and soothe your soul.

7

NATURAL BIRTH CONTROL

WERE YOU THINKING OF coming off the pill (or
having your IUD removed) in order to conceive?
Are you aware that these contraceptive methods
could affect your fertility and/or your baby?

YOU MAY THINK IT'S strange to have a chapter on contraception
in a book about conception. However, avoiding and achieving pregnancy are not really always so separate, and both can be furthered
by an understanding of fertility. It is this understanding which forms
the basis of both natural contraception and conscious conception.
Natural methods of contraception are important because they are an
essential part of your preconception care.

The adverse effects of orthodox methods of contraception, especially the oral contraceptive pill (OCP), on any pregnancy started too
soon after their use, can be considerable. There is, therefore, a need
for you to stop using OCPs (or IUDs) and to make sure that any
treatment to reduce these adverse effects is carried out, and that any
nutritional deficiencies are corrected, before any attempt at conception is made.

In order to avoid a pregnancy before all of your preconception
care is complete, you will need to be confident that your contraception method is reliable, and that it poses no threat to your future

pregnancy. Therefore we strongly recommend that you start, as soon as possible, to learn the methods outlined below.

NATURAL CONTRACEPTION

Well, for a start, we are not talking about the notorious rhythm method! Although the rhythm calculations can be quite helpful if you have regular cycles, the method is not reliable if you experience any unexpected changes in your cycle, and, at best, relies on large safety margins, or an extended fertile time, during which you must avoid unprotected intercourse.

However, what we are advocating is an informed assessment of the symptoms which you experience, which will tell you when you are fertile, whether or not these come when expected.

All that is required to use natural contraception methods successfully are:

- A healthy curiosity on the part of the woman (or, better still, both partners) about her own body and its functions.
- Commitment and motivation to observe, record and interpret the symptoms and signs of fertility and their cyclical patterns.
- A good teacher or reliable method of learning.

You do *not* need:

- To have regular cycles (although it would be healthier if you did—see Chapter 8, section on 'Female Reproductive Health').
- To abstain from sexual activity for long periods of time.
- To have a degree in anatomy/physiology/probability theory!
- A cooperative partner—though it would obviously be preferable.

These methods *can* be used by a woman on her own.

Natural methods work!

Despite the jokes that prevail about natural contraception (holding an aspirin between your knees!), natural methods these days are updated, scientifically researched and validated, and extremely effective and easy to use.

There have been many surveys showing effective rates, and, as with all methods of contraception, there is a difference between the *theoretical* rate (that which pertains if the methods are used correctly) and the *user* rate (which includes user errors). One of the latest surveys, based on couples with high motivation and good teaching, gave a result of 99.8 per cent—a rate equal to the combined contraceptive pill's best effective rate (surveys of success rates for the pill vary too).

The table in the Appendix shows the effective rates for contraception methods. These are based on a number of surveys, and therefore show a range of results for each method.

Choosing the right time to conceive

Although you may be planning to conceive soon, it's important that natural contraception methods work effectively for you so you can complete your preconception care. You will also then be able to use these methods during breastfeeding, and when you need to avoid using chemicals or devices before you conceive your next child (or until your fertile life is over). It has been shown conclusively that second and subsequent babies can be less healthy than the first, as the mother's nutritional status has not recovered from the demands of the previous pregnancy (ies) and lactation—so preconception care is even more important if this is not your first child.

However, you need to be aware that *spacers*—those people who use natural methods of contraception between children, or as a waiting device for the *right* time to conceive an already desired child—are not usually as successful in their avoidance of pregnancy as those who have a strong desire not to conceive.

If you are reading this book, then you have probably already decided to conceive—so take care! In order for your preconception care to be effective, your method of contraception must be effective too. Therefore, we suggest that every time you menstruate, you seriously consider whether the subsequent cycle is the one during which you wish to conceive, or whether you still have some preparation to complete. Maybe even do some meditation to help you decide. A *conscious* decision can then be made to practise contraception until the time is right, when you can switch to *conscious conception*.

For those of you who are impatient, we suggest that you see these months of preconception care as the first step in your program, with intercourse for conception as the second step. In this way you can see these preparation months, during which you practise contraception, as a positive step towards the healthiest possible conception, and not just as a waiting time.

Continuing use of natural contraception

These methods offer so many advantages, that we're sure you will continue to use them as your method of choice, after the birth of your baby and until you are ready to conceive the next (or until you are no longer fertile, if you are planning no more children). Because they are based on understanding the way your body works, they are an excellent way of interpreting fertility during confusing times such as breastfeeding and during the approach to menopause, and can be used effectively right throughout your fertile life.

We know of no woman who cannot use these methods effectively, given commitment, motivation and good teaching.

More advantages

Using natural contraception methods as part of your preconception care allows you to:

- Become confident in their use, so that, after this baby is born, you can effectively avoid conception until you are ready to have your next child.
- Time your conception attempt to coincide with peak fertility and avoid any ill-effects from ageing eggs or sperm (see Chapter 13, for more on this).
- Avoid any adverse effects on your pregnancy or child that may result from the use of the pill, IUD or spermicides (see section 'Effects of unnatural contraception' later this chapter).
- Confidently avoid conception until your detoxification, dietary modification, nutritional supplementation and all other preparatory measures are complete.
- Become much more informed about, and in control of, your reproductive processes. You will be amazed at how much information is right there in your own body, and how exciting it is to discover the significance and implications of changes and patterns that you may have been subliminally aware of since puberty. For women, this is a profound affirmation of their *cyclical* nature, and a chance to become aware of the implications of this for their whole being.

- Make contraception a mutual responsibility, involving both partners.
- Only use contraception for the few days each month when conception is actually possible, thereby freeing up most of the month for sexual activity during which you won't need to worry about conception.
- Be self-sufficient, and not dependent on devices, drugs, prescriptions and medical resources. This means, of course, that it is much cheaper to use natural methods.
- Diagnose, with the help of a health practitioner trained in the use of these methods, hormonal and nutritional imbalances or deficiencies which could affect your pregnancy. The charting of temperature, mucus and other cyclical changes that you do when using these methods for contraception will show how you can be treated more effectively during the months preceding conception, and will also indicate if extra care or treatment during pregnancy is likely to be necessary. During charting it will become apparent if you suffer from an overly long pre-ovulatory phase, or a post-ovulatory phase which is too short. Both conditions can cause problems which should be acted on now. If the pre-ovulatory phase of the cycle is greater than seventeen days, use natural remedies to attempt to shorten your cycle (see Chapter 8, section on 'Female Reproductive Health').

Temperature and mucus readings can also pinpoint exactly when ovulation occurs. *The optimum time for ovulation is on day 14, or earlier*, when the chances of fertilisation producing healthy offspring are greater than 90 per cent. If you ovulate on day 15, or later, your chances of a viable conception drop to 43 per cent. Remember, these statistics are taken from women and couples who were unaware of the importance of preconception care, so were not necessarily taking care of their health. Your chances of a healthy conception, if you have prepared well, are considerably higher. However, these figures do show the relative rates.

Long pre-ovulatory phases (greater than seventeen days) have been associated with changes in the corpus luteum, and the efficiency of progesterone secretion, which is necessary to maintain the pregnancy.

If ovulation occurs very late (day 20 to 25), there is a higher risk of miscarriage and abnormal eggs. This has to do with the size of the follicle at different times in the menstrual cycle. On the first day of the menstrual period it is about 2 mm. Over the next 14 days, it grows to 25 mm, before it begins to shrink back to its original size. This increase in size is the fastest growth observed in any human tissue during the normal life cycle, apart from the initial development of the embryo. When the follicle is at its maximum size it will release the healthiest egg, and the ensuing corpus luteum will be large enough to produce adequate progesterone.

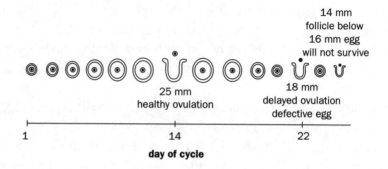

Size of the follicle at different stages of the cycle

Delayed ovulation, which could be the result of smoking, alcohol excess, drug use, environmental toxins, ill health, hormonal imbalance, fasting or nutritional deficiencies, may occur when the follicle is, for example, at about day 22, only 18 mm. If the follicle measures below 16 mm, the egg will not survive.

A post-ovulatory phase that is too short (below ten days) is also infertile, because progesterone levels are too low for the endometrium to be properly prepared for the fertilised egg. Progesterone levels need to be peaking adequately about a week after ovulation, as the egg takes this long to travel down into the uterus. Good nutrition, calcium, magnesium, zinc and Vitamin B6 supplements and herbal medicines can usually remedy this condition. See section on 'Female Reproductive Health' in Chapter 8 for more on hormone balance.

HOW TO USE NATURAL CONTRACEPTION

Natural contraception methods rely on being able to determine when you are fertile. As you go through the hormonal changes associated with your menstrual and ovulatory cycle, there are several symptoms, caused by these changes, which can help you to determine exactly when you are fertile mid-cycle. You can then make decisions as to how to avoid conception at this time.

There are three ways to determine mid-cycle fertility. One of these is by calculation (*rhythm method*). This is not sufficiently accurate, and it is far preferable to be guided by the indications of the other two, which are:

- *Cervical mucus observations.*
- *Body-at-rest (basal) temperature observations.*

We will give a brief outline of what is involved in these methods, though their effective use requires more specialised and extensive information than we have room for here. However, don't be concerned that this means using them is difficult. It's not! In Third World countries, where teaching methods have to be adapted for a largely illiterate population, these methods can be learnt extremely successfully. A World Health Organisation survey of five countries, including undeveloped Third World societies, showed that 95 per cent of women were able to return an interpretable chart of the changes in their cycle in the first month. Of course, the methods become easier to use over time, and the first three months are usually considered a learning period. After this, most women are confident that they can clearly tell when they are fertile. Luckily for us, this coincides neatly with the minimum interval required for your preconception care, so by the time you are ready to conceive you will have sufficient experience to time your conception attempt accurately and to use natural contraception after the birth of your child. See the section in Chapter 8 on ovarian hormones for more on the symptoms caused by hormonal changes experienced through the monthly cycle.

Changes in the cervical mucus

You may already be aware of these changes, though not, perhaps, of their significance. Although the observations will require some focused attention on your part for the first few cycles, your awareness of these changes will soon become automatic, and you'll probably wonder how you could ever have ignored them.

The important thing to realise is that the changes are learnt experientially, through observing, charting and interpreting, preferably with the help of a good teacher or teaching aid. You will soon become aware of the significance of these changes, and of when you are fertile and when infertile.

The mucus is produced by the cervix (the neck of the womb), in the 'crypts', which are little pockets opening into the cervical canal. There are special cells inside the 100 or so gland-like crypts, which produce mucus constantly. This changes in quantity and quality throughout your menstrual cycle. The crypts also provide a haven for the sperm that are migrating from the vagina to the uterus in search of an egg to fertilise. When the sperm are in these crypts, they are safely sheltered, nourished, and then, over a period of hours, or even days, released into the uterus.

The mucus produced by the cervical crypts is controlled by the level of hormones present:

- Low oestrogen levels, as at the beginning and end of the cycle, result in scant amounts of sticky, or tacky, mucus which is usually opaque.
- As the levels of oestrogen rise, and ovulation approaches, the mucus becomes more profuse, thinner, wetter and clearer.
- When oestrogen levels peak, just before ovulation, the mucus becomes jelly-like (still wet), resembles raw egg-white and can be stretched between the fingers (see diagram opposite).

It is these changes which enable the sperm to survive and travel and which are your body's way of preparing for conception, that you can learn to recognise. They clearly define the approach of fertility, or lack of it. Every woman will experience some changes in her cervical mucus as she progresses through her hormonal cycle. You can learn to recognise them. They do *not* mean that you have an infection.

If your mucus discharge changes in quantity and quality, it is probably your natural cervical mucus, produced in response to hormonal messages. If your mucus is constant, and does not go through changes, has an offensive smell, or causes irritation, itching or burning, then you may have an infection. See Chapters 8, section on

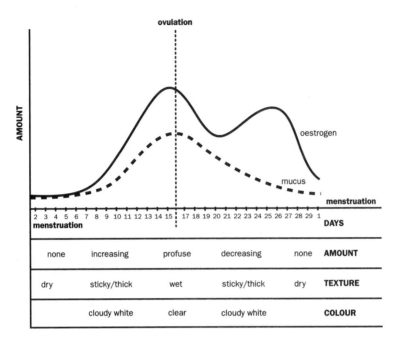

none	increasing	profuse	decreasing	none	**AMOUNT**
dry	sticky/thick	wet	sticky/thick	dry	**TEXTURE**
	cloudy white	clear	cloudy white		**COLOUR**

Hormone levels and mucus changes

'Female Reproductive Health', and 10 for more information on these and how to treat them.

A great many drugs can also affect mucus production. We have seen how the pill causes the mucus to become infertile, but this is not the only medication which causes problems. Some antibiotics, antihistamines and, ironically, some drugs used to treat infertility, can have effects on the production of fertile mucus.

Other conditions which can affect mucus production include:

- D and C (dilation and curettage).
- Thyroid dysfunction.
- Stress.
- Cervical problems (erosion, dysplasia, harsh treatments, see section on this in Chapter 8).
- Vaginal lubricants, deodorants, douches, sprays or spermicides of a chemical nature, which can cause inflammation of the vaginal lining, or an allergic reaction, resulting in discharge.
- Retained tampons.
- Ovarian disease.

Mucus and fertility

Change in the cervical mucus is the only observable symptom that precedes ovulation and, therefore, gives reliable warning of approaching fertility.

Without this change, there is, indeed, no fertility. Even if ovulation occurs, if there is no fertile mucus the situation is infertile, because the sperm cannot stay alive.

In favourable circumstances, *sperm can live for up to three days.* They have even been found alive after five, though this is extremely rare, and they are generally considered to be non-viable at this advanced age. Three days is usually considered to be their maximum viability. Sperm life reduces by one-third each day, and 16 to 18 hours is an average life span. The number of sperm (sperm count) also drops each day and, even in a favourable environment, falls below a viable level after three days.

However, acidity immobilises sperm, and vaginas are naturally acidic. Fertile mucus provides protection for the sperm from this acidity, it nourishes them and guides them up into the uterus. Mucus present at other times in the cycle (if any) is unable to provide the sperm with this protection and is, therefore, infertile.

Four different types of mucus have been identified—the G-type, L-type, S-type and P-type—and they all have different functions, repelling the sperm in the infertile phases, filtering out the defective sperm, guiding and channelling them into the cervix and uterus just before ovulation, and alkalising the normally hostile acidic vagina.

These different types of mucus can all be identified under a microscope, but luckily, the significant changes can also be differentiated by appearance and sensation. Gravity does the work for you and brings the mucus down to the mouth of the vagina, where changes in quality and quantity can be seen and felt.

One very important aspect of mucus observation is its capacity to warn of the approach of ovulation. This is essential for both contraception and conception purposes.

If you are trying to avoid conception, and are aware that you are ovulating, it may be too late, if you had unprotected sexual intercourse up to three days before. Luckily, mucus can give you ample warning, and can help you identify approaching ovulation, if you observe changes in quantity and quality.

A typical cycle progresses as follows:

- After bleeding, there may be some dry days, when there is no apparent mucus at all. The mucus at this time is completely infertile and forms a plug across the cervix—this may come out as a blob of sticky mucus. Other women will experience small unchanging amounts of this thick, pasty, infertile mucus.
- Then you may start to feel the presence of some possibly infertile or slightly fertile mucus. This is usually a damp or sticky feeling.
- The water content then rises and the mucus becomes wetter and more lubricative. This is the change to fertile mucus. It is also more profuse.
- Most, but not all, women then experience the 'spinnbarkeit' or 'spinn' mucus that resembles raw egg-white, while remaining wet to the touch.
- After ovulation there is, sometimes quite suddenly, a return to the thick, infertile mucus or to none at all.

All women do not experience all of these stages. They vary with the length of the cycle and the amount of mucus produced.

If you are using these methods to avoid conception, then *three days* must be allowed after the mucus has ceased to be fertile in order to be sure that ovulation is over.

How to check your mucus

Mucus is usually observed while seated on the toilet, before urinating, by collecting some from the vulval area (the mouth of the vagina), and assessing the texture and amount. These changes can then be charted, and patterns will quickly become apparent.

These patterns will not only enable you to determine when you are fertile, but will also give clues to you or your practitioner about your levels of oestrogen, and the effects of this on your fertility. If necessary, treatment can then be initiated (see section on 'Hostile' mucus in Chapter 8).

Simplicity itself

As you can see, with proper tuition, the mucus method is really very simple. Fertility is defined as starting as soon as the mucus changes, and lasting until three days after the last day of any type of fertile mucus. For contraceptive purposes, you must avoid unprotected intercourse on these days. As we shall see in Chapter 13 some refinement of this definition is helpful to optimise the chances of a healthy conception.

It has been confirmed in laboratory tests that 'the woman's own awareness of her cervical mucus could indicate ovulation even more accurately than [serum] oestrogen measurements'.

The effectiveness of the mucus method, correctly applied, for contraception is usually assessed as around 98.5 per cent, but, with good teaching and motivation, at 99.8 per cent.

The mucus method is also sometimes called the Billings method, in honour of the two Australian doctors, Evelyn and John Billings, who pioneered the research and use of the method.

Changes in the basal or body-at-rest temperature

Temperature readings, although they do not warn of the approach to ovulation like the mucus observations, can still be extremely useful. This is particularly true while you are learning how to tell when you are fertile, and the method is an ideal back-up if there are times of confusion in mucus checking. You can confirm through *checking your temperature graph* whether or not ovulation has occurred, and if you have entered into the post-ovulatory infertile phase.

Mucus observations, and their usefulness in identifying fertile times, can be compromised in a number of situations, as we saw earlier. Furthermore, even though mucus changes will still be evident, you may be less confident if any of the following occurs:

- Your mucus pattern changes due to hormonal changes.
- Your cycle becomes irregular, or its timing alters.
- You are suffering from an infected discharge, such as thrush.
- Your level of sexual activity increases.

In the first few months of learning, especially if you are recovering from taking the pill, the temperature method can be extremely helpful to confirm that ovulation has taken place, when this occurred, and that the fertile phase is over.

As well as giving you information that helps you to avoid conception, and later to achieve it, these observations can also help you, or your practitioner, to identify hormonal imbalances, and whether there are problems with the length of the pre-ovulatory or post-ovulatory phases. Treatment can then be initiated, to help you optimise your chances of a healthy conception.

Why does your temperature rise?

As ovulation occurs, the increased production of progesterone generates greater heat in the body, and the basal or body-at-rest temperature rises. This is what is measured to ascertain whether or not ovulation is over, and when it occurred.

In a classic graph, the temperature jogs along with small changes in the first half, or pre-ovulatory phase, of the cycle. It drops slightly just before ovulation (this is not always recorded on the graph, as it is a 12 hour drop, and a 24 hour reading), and then rises by up to 0.5° Celsius (Centigrade) or 1° Fahrenheit, and stays up until just before, or during, the menstrual period, when it falls again. If ovulation doesn't occur, your temperature won't go up, and if menstruation doesn't occur, your temperature won't come down again.

If your body-at-rest temperature has been elevated for more than 20 days, you can consider yourself pregnant. Let's hope that you have completed your preconception care, and that this is good news.

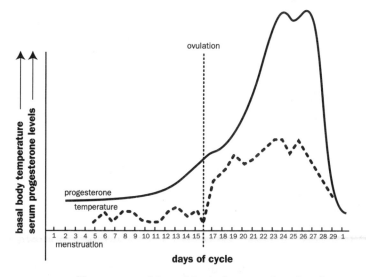

Hormone and basal body temperature levels

When does ovulation occur?

Ovulation is generally considered to have occurred at the beginning of the temperature rise. This is usually also the lowest reading, as your temperature does in fact drop (by 0.12 to 0.3° Celsius (Centigrade) or 0.25 to 0.6° (Fahrenheit) just before ovulation takes place. However, as we have just noted, this drop may not show on your graph. Therefore we define the most likely day of ovulation as being at the beginning of the rise, which is not always the lowest temperature recorded in the cycle.

Although this is the most likely time for ovulation, up to three days prior to the rise is reasonably common, and it is possible for the egg to have been released up to five days before the rise, during the rise, or up to two days after. A late rise may indicate a sluggish progesterone response, which should be treated (see Chapter 8, section on Female Reproductive Health). Here is a diagram showing the possibilities.

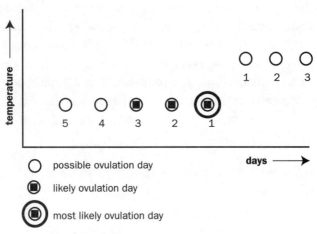

Likely day of ovulation

Given good tuition, temperature graphs are easy to interpret after a little experience, and most people can tell from their very first chart when they have finished ovulating, and are therefore infertile.

How to take your temperature

- Use a mercury thermometer (they are more reliable for small changes than digital), and take your temperature in the mouth (we usually find taking your vaginal temperature to be unnecessary).
- Your temperature should be taken before undertaking any activity.
- At least four hours sleep is required to reach the body-at-rest state required.

- Your temperature should always be taken at the same time of day as the basal temperature rises through the day.

The temperature method is really very simple to use and can give you some idea of what is going on while you learn to distinguish mucus changes, or if these are unclear. It will also give you information about the timing of ovulation and whether or not this is, in fact, occurring. This information will be invaluable in helping you to achieve good reproductive health as part of your preconception care, as well as helping you to avoid conception until you are ready. You cannot, however, use the temperature method to warn of the approach of ovulation and, therefore, used alone, it has limited application, for either contraception or conception purposes.

The effective rate of the temperature method for contraception correctly applied with abstinence in the pre-ovulatory phase has been assessed as 99 per cent.

If you are using a combination of mucus and temperature observations, which may be further combined with the recording of other cyclical symptoms, the method is called the Sympto-Thermal method. There is one other method that you may also be interested to learn about, and use for avoiding or achieving conception. This is the observance of a biorhythm, called the lunar cycle, which affects fertility.

The lunar cycle

In the 1950s a Czech doctor, Eugen Jonas, identified and assessed a biorhythmic cycle as having an effect upon fertility. Through extensive research and thorough testing, he concluded that a woman is fertile during the same phase of the lunar month that was present when she was born, regardless of whether she is at her mid-cycle ovulation.

This seemingly impossible finding has been extensively tested both by Dr Jonas and many other practitioners and researchers, and some possible answers as to why this may be the case have to do with the moon's relationship with, and effect on, gravity, ionisation, electro-magnetic fields and light, and the effects these have on a woman's reproductive system.

Several researchers have established that this bio-rhythm is like a blueprint for the hormonal cycle, and that the more relaxed, and generally and reproductively healthy, a woman is, the more likely she is to experience her mid-cycle ovulation at the same phase of the moon that was present at her birth. Furthermore, it appears that if this is the case, then her fertility is enhanced, and she is more likely to conceive.

This synchronisation of the hormonal and lunar cycles appears to occur even more readily in women who are aware of their bodies, such as those who are checking their mucus symptoms, or those who are trying to conceive.

It is not surprising that the hormonal cycle has a lunar beat—the words for menstruation are derived from classical roots meaning month and moon—and many cultures worldwide have a history of acknowledging the connection between the moon, women and fertility in their religious, mythical and social traditions. An average menstrual cycle is 29.5 days long—the length of a lunar month from one new, or full, moon to the next.

However, if your menstrual cycle is not regularly this long, it may not synchronise with this lunar blueprint, and the lunar peak may not coincide with ovulation. In these cases, Jonas found that women were often still able to conceive at the lunar peak.

How can this be so? Although there is, as yet, no definitive research, the indications are that it may have to do with what is called a spontaneous ovulation. Many studies have confirmed that women can ovulate out of cycle as a response to sexual stimulation. Ovulation can be assessed, in a laboratory, by measuring the electrical potential in the body, which increases significantly at ovulation.

Clinical observations also show symptoms normally associated with ovulation occurring at the lunar peak, even though this does not coincide with the regular, mid-cycle ovulation. Many conceptions have also been recorded as occurring as a result of intercourse happening at this time. It may be that this biorhythm, starting at birth, is creating peaks of fertility when, if the mid-cycle ovulation is not already occurring, there is the potential, perhaps created through the effects of gravity, electromagnetism, light and ionisation or other associated phenomena, for a spontaneous ovulation to occur.

Although there are many unanswered questions surrounding this biorhythm and its effect on fertility, it is difficult to ignore the extensive findings linking it to fertility, and therefore the need to take it into account both for contraception and conception. The angle between the sun and the moon present at the time of the woman's birth needs to be calculated, and then the dates of the return of this angle each (lunar) month must be predicted. These times can then be used as a guide for avoiding or achieving conception given certain guidelines, and for contraception, safety margins for egg and sperm life. If you wish to use this cycle to increase your success, it is obviously preferable, whether you are trying to conceive or not, if the two cycles, biorhythmic and hormonal, synchronise, creating one fertile time per month.

This can be achieved, in many cases, by fulfilling the conditions known to predispose women to ovulating at this lunar peak. These include becoming reproductively and generally healthy, less stressed, avoiding activities (such as international air travel) known to disrupt cycles, and becoming aware of body changes associated with the hormonal cycle. It is also helpful to be aware of the individual lunar cycle, as this will influence the timing of your hormonal cycle, in much the same way as women living together, ovulate and menstruate together. Visualisation and affirmation techniques similar to those suggested in Chapter 6 can be used to great effect.

As we will see in Chapter 8, male fertility can also be affected by the lunar cycle, though the evidence of its effect for men is not nearly as strong. If necessary, the woman's ovulation might be 'influenced' to synchronise with her partner's peak fertile time, rather than her own. In our experience, however, this can disrupt a woman's regularity and should only be attempted with professional guidance.

Back-up contraception

When you have learnt to identify your fertile times, you will then have to decide what action to take (or not!) until you are ready to conceive.

Abstinence is the obvious, (and very effective!) answer, but not necessarily the only one. Indeed it may not be realistic to suppose that at fertile times, when a woman is more highly sexually moti-vated, and even has a sexually alluring smell to attract her partner, that abstinence will be easy to maintain. In order to be sure that you can wait until your preconception care is complete (and, later, to be confident that you will not conceive until, or if, you decide to do so) it is preferable to have some alternative back-up contraception available.

Back-up contraception need only be used on those few days a month you have identified as fertile, and then only if you feel unable, or prefer not, to abstain from intercourse. The most appropriate methods to use are the *condom* or the *diaphragm*.

The diaphragm avoids many of the problems associated with loss of tactile experience, interruptions to foreplay and embarrassment associated with condoms, but condoms have a big practical advantage in that they contain the semen, and therefore interfere less with your mucus observations.

Both the condom and diaphragm are extremely reliable (see table of effective rates in the Appendix) but need to be used correctly. By determining fertile days, the occasions on which barrier methods are required are reduced to only a few days each month, motivation for correct use is therefore high, and user fatigue low. However, it may be useful, especially if these methods have not been used before, or recently, to receive some advice on their use.

How to learn natural contraception

These methods are widely taught. They may be known as Natural Family Planning, Natural Birth Control or Natural Fertility Awareness. We prefer the term Natural Fertility Management, implying the use of the same methods for both avoiding and achieving conception, and for identifying reproductive and menstrual problems, which can then be remedied using natural medicine.

Natural Fertility Management is a system that includes the use of mucus and temperature methods, rhythm calculations (where appropriate) and lunar cycle observance, and is taught by health professionals. It has been developed by Francesca, who trains other health professionals in its use. You can learn to use these methods by contacting us for the name of one of our counsellors, or for a mail-order kit. This kit includes tapes, notes, charts, computer-calculated lunar biorhythms, and Francesca's previous book *Natural Fertility*, which comprehensively explains the use of the methods (see Suggested Reading and Contacts and Resources).

Other ways of ascertaining fertility

There are several aids that can be bought that help you detect your fertile period. Some of these test basal temperature, and some the surge in luteinising hormone that precedes ovulation.

Clear Plan, The Right Day, and First Response are all testing kits, available through chemists, which measure the LH surge, by testing the urine. Most kits come with enough assessment indications to last one or two cycles. They are rather expensive to use on a regular basis, but can be useful if you are confused about your mucus or temperature observations. Baby-comp and Lady-comp are computer-assisted thermometers which build up a record of your temperature observations and claim to be able to predict the fertile time in advance. They will only work for regular cycles.

Another quite useful device is a microscope that lets you see if your mucus is 'ferning', which is the pattern most fertile mucus crystallises to, as it dries on a slide. Since saliva is also affected by hormones, this will show the same effect. You can buy microscopes that are especially designed for the purpose, and, although not cheap, they are re-useable, so the cost may be defrayed over several cycles, and they can provide a helpful adjunct to manual testing and your awareness of the sensation of the mucus. However, in our opinion, they do not replace the look and feel approach.

EFFECTS OF 'UNNATURAL' CONTRACEPTION

Unnatural methods of contraception rely on drugs and devices, which manipulate and suppress reproductive function and which can have devastating effects on reproductive and foetal health. They endanger, rather than enhance, subsequent fertility, and contribute to the ill health and confusion of most women of child-bearing age and their partners. These methods reflect the view of the reproductive cycle as a curse, a nuisance and an embarrassment, something that women are better off ignoring, except for those few occasions on which they wish to conceive a child.

On the other hand, natural methods of contraception aim to understand and tune into natural cycles, and make use of the body's own signs of fertility. They celebrate cyclical activity in the woman, and fertility in both partners, and also give a choice each month as to whether you choose to conceive or not.

Drug-based methods

Rather than list all the possible ways of delivering hormonal drugs to the woman to prevent conception, we will deal only with the most commonly used form, the OCP (oral contraceptive pill). The effects are comparable, whatever the method, though some use greater amounts of drugs, and carry with them the increased likelihood of side-effects. We will also refrain from listing all the possible life-threatening or quality-of-life-threatening side-effects, focusing, for the purposes of this book, on the direct implications for the child conceived within a short period of the use of these drugs.

One of the principal ways in which you are adversely affected by the OCP is through alterations to your nutritional status. Since a large part of your preconception care involves establishing a good nutritional profile, it is imperative that these effects are no longer active, and have been compensated for, by the time conception occurs. Of particular concern are the effects of the OCP on your levels of folic acid and zinc. Both these nutrients are absolutely essential for healthy reproduction and both are severely depleted by taking the pill. However, it is important to realise that nutrients do not occur in isolation, and the complete nutritional spectrum needs to be considered.

Following are some of the ways in which the pill disrupts your nutritional status. See also Chapter 1 for more on deficiency states.

Vitamin and mineral deficiency

Vitamin A (Retinol)—levels in the blood are increased during OCP use, and take approximately three months to return to normal after stopping. Whether this means that the body's turnover of this vitamin is higher, with increased likelihood of a deficiency, or whether, there is greater availability to the tissues, is not yet clear.

Vitamin B1 (Thiamine)—there is a probability that OCP users are deficient in this vitamin, as there is some evidence that the pill interferes with its metabolism, increasing the body's requirements.

Vitamin B2 (Riboflavin)—the body's requirements are increased by the use of the OCP, making a deficiency more likely to occur, especially in those women who have taken the pill for three years or more.

Vitamin B6 (Pyridoxine)—depletion during OCP use varies from marginal to severe.

Folic Acid—the OCP causes levels of folic acid to fall. This is a serious problem if conception occurs during, or too soon after, pill use. Since folic acid is required by the body to facilitate cell division, a process that starts immediately after conception, there is a much higher risk of congenital abnormalities, including spina bifida, hydro-cephalus, mongolism and limb defects if this vitamin is deficient (see Chapter 1 for a more complete list). Deficiencies of folate can also lead to anaemia and cellular abnormalities of the cervix. Women who conceive within six months of OCP use have been shown to have lower than normal red blood cell and plasma folate levels in the first trimester of pregnancy. Zinc deficiencies will also compromise folic acid absorption.

Biotin—levels of biotin are lower in pill-users. This nutrient helps to prevent the overgrowth of *Candida albicans* in the gut.

Vitamin B12 (Cobalamin)—blood levels are lowered in pill-users, especially vegetarians.

Vitamin C (Ascorbic acid)—the pill causes levels to be reduced by up to 30 per cent, since the body's requirements for this nutrient are increased.

Vitamin C is also necessary for the production of the sex hormones in your body. Since this is something that your body has to start doing for itself when you stop taking the pill, a deficiency of this nutrient can make it even harder for your body to resume normal hormone production. However, taking Vitamin C while on the pill can increase the concentration of oestrogen in the body, effectively turning a low dose pill into a high dose one and increasing potential side-effects—so wait until you stop OCP use before supplementing with Vitamin C.

Bioflavonoids (Rutin, Hespiridin, etc.)—body levels are decreased during OCP use.

Vitamin E (Alpha Tocopherol)—the need for Vitamin E is increased while taking the pill (this vitamin helps to normalise oestrogen levels) and plasma levels are lowered by approximately 20 per cent.

Vitamin K (Menadione)—higher levels during OCP use may lead to blood clot formation.

Iron—less iron may be lost, due to lighter periods, although some-times pill-users have lowered levels in their blood.

Calcium—absorption is improved. This may be an advantage (at last!), as long as critical ratios of other minerals are not disturbed.

Magnesium and *potassium*—although there is no conclusive study that we know of linking lowered magnesium and potassium levels with pill use, in our, and others', clinical experience, deficiencies of both nutrients are very common in women who have been on the pill. Deficiencies may affect fertile mucus formation.

Selenium—levels of this essential anti-oxidant are reduced by pill use. Selenium has been shown to reduce the chances of deformity, including Down syndrome. This protective effect is lost in pregnancies commenced immediately or soon after pill use.

Copper—absorption is increased, raising the body's need for Vitamin C, disrupting the zinc/copper balance. Disruption of the zinc/copper balance has serious implications for many aspects of pregnancy and foetal health (see Chapter 1).

Zinc—levels are significantly lowered by the pill. Long-term pill-users may often find it difficult to restore their zinc status to adequate levels. See Chapter 1 for more on this extremely important mineral.

Prostaglandins—levels of certain prostaglandins are lower during OCP use. Prostaglandins are normally made from essential fatty acids (such as those contained in Evening primrose oil and fish), using zinc as a catalyst, and are intricately involved in hormone production, level of pain experienced and clot formation.

Blood Lipids—low density lipids, cholesterol and triglycerides (the baddies) are increased during OCP use, increasing the risks of heart disease.

Birth defects, problem pregnancies and the pill

These various nutrient deficiencies may be a major reason why women experience health problems while on, or after taking, the pill. They are definitely a reason why children conceived too soon after stopping oral contraceptive use may have an increased chance of birth defects. Maternal deficiencies in folic acid, for example, have been linked with an up to five times greater chance of giving birth to a child with limb defects as well as with an increased incidence of neural tube defects, such as spina bifida, and of Down Syndrome.

As we have mentioned in Chapter 1, many reproductive problems, and physical and mental ill health in children may partly be caused by maternal zinc deprivation due to OCP use.

The hormones contained in the pill (oestrogen and progesterone in the combined pill, and progesterone only in the mini-pill) may also have direct adverse effects. These are particularly problematic if oral contraceptive use continues after conception, and ill-effects can include foetal limb deformities and heart defects. Even if oral contraceptive use has ceased before conception, hormonal balance is affected for some time after cessation, as evidenced by the very slow return, for many women, of regular cycles.

There is also a much higher incidence of stillbirths and miscarriages as well as birth defects in pregnancies started within a month of stopping OCP use. Women who have, at any stage, taken the pill, have a 4.3 per cent increased chance of giving birth to a child with an obvious defect.

The mini-pill, which does not suppress ovulation, but causes changes in the endometrium and the cervical mucus, also interferes with the passage of the eggs or sperm in the Fallopian tubes. This may result in a greater likelihood of a pregnancy being ectopic if conception occurs while taking the mini-pill. This form of oral contraceptive also has a much lower success rate than the combined pill, and has the added disadvantage of needing to be taken at the same time every day.

Of course if the mini-pill is taken during lactation, as is common, the breastfeeding infant is likely to suffer from all the aforementioned nutrient deficiencies. Synthetic progesterone is also known to act on the hypothalamus, and may masculinise a female infant, who is forming her hormone receptor sites soon after birth. It may also contribute to neonatal jaundice.

Because there is a link between oral contraceptive use and diabetes, previous use of the pill may well be a contributing factor to gestational diabetes, though we know of no proven connection. There may also be a link between the pill's tendency to increase blood pressure and the toxaemia of pregnancy.

A further contributing factor to nutrient depletion and reproductive failure is the increased tendency of women on the pill to suffer from Candidiasis, allergic reactions and compromised immune response. See Chapters 11 and 12 for more on how these conditions can affect your fertility and reproductive outcomes.

Ironically, there is a distinct chance that the drug that you may have taken to prevent pregnancy when you didn't want to conceive, may also prevent it when you do. A recent study found that nearly 25 per cent of women could not conceive for at least thirteen months after stopping the pill. Only 10.6 per cent of women using other methods of contraception had a similar experience.

We have already mentioned that one post-pill effect is irregularity and hormone imbalance. The pill suppresses ovarian and pituitary function, and this disruption may continue after the pill is withdrawn. This can lead to irregularity, PMS and dysmenorrhoea. Monitoring the cycle, as for natural contraception, will indicate if these conditions are sufficiently problematic to need treatment. In some cases ovulation does not recommence even though menstruation may appear regular.

Inflammatory conditions of all body systems, including the reproductive system, are much more common in pill-users. These conditions can affect fertility. Natural methods are usually successful in restoring the correct hormonal balance and in treating all other symptoms. See Chapter 8, section on 'Female Reproductive Health'.

Several studies have shown there is a link between pill use and cervical erosion or cancer. Less life-threatening but more relevant to our fertility concerns, are the effects of oral contraceptive use on cervical mucus. In this chapter we have seen that this mucus is essential for fertility, providing the means by which sperm survive and swim up the female reproductive tract, and mucus also enables us to tell when a woman is fertile.

This mucus requires certain nutrients, such as calcium, magnesium, zinc and potassium, to enable it to change into its fertile state. As we have seen, these nutrients are depleted by pill use. The pill can also cause atrophy of the cervical crypts which produce the fertile type mucus.

Both nutrient deficiencies and hormone imbalances increase your chances of giving birth to a child with birth defects. They also affect the condition of the cervical mucus, and the effective fertility of all the reproductive organs, including the ovaries, pituitary, uterus and endometrium. You can clearly see that hormonal drugs, such as the pill, can affect your fertility and the viability of your pregnancy and your unborn child in a variety of ways. There is, of course, reason to suppose that the recently developed male pill will have similar problems, since it is also a hormonal drug.

Coming off the pill

Natural remedies are very effective in reducing post-pill symptoms. Treatment should include attention to the following:

- Elimination of chemicals (via the liver).
- Restoration of normal activity to the pituitary and ovarian glands.
- Restoration of normal mucus production.
- Restoration of normal endometrial function.
- Restoration of normal and regular ovulation and menstruation.

Treatment should therefore be continued until:

- There is regular menstruation, preferably not more than 30 days apart, or less than 28.
- There is regular ovulation, as indicated by the temperature rise—see the section on Temperature—which is not more than seventeen days after the last menstrual period and not less than twelve days before the next.
- There is a regular change mid-cycle in the cervical mucus to the fertile state.
- There is an absence of irregularities such as PMS, dysmenorrhoea, clotting or abnormal bleeding.

Much of this will be achieved through good nutrition, and the use of remedies suggested in the preceding chapter. A specific herbal formula for those coming off the pill could be:

St Mary's Thistle—for liver detoxification.

Chaste Tree—for ovarian/pituitary axis, hormone balance, progesterone production and a successful post-ovulatory phase.

False Unicorn Root—to normalise ovarian function, oestrogen production and uterine health.

Wild Yam—to reduce inflammation in the uterus, and assist normal hormonal activity.

Golden Seal—assists liver detoxification, and is a tonic for the ovaries and the mucous membranes.

Ginger—to promote normal reproductive circulation.

Other methods

Here we will concern ourselves with the possible adverse effects of the IUD, and barrier methods of contraception.

Popularity of the IUD has declined significantly because its use is associated with a greatly increased risk of Pelvic Inflammatory Disease (PID). PID has serious implications for fertility, and in the following chapter in the section on 'Female Reproductive Health' we consider this problem in more detail. The scarring to the Fallopian tubes, and their subsequent blockage, are the main concerns. Women who are under 20 years of age, or who have never had children, are at a significantly increased risk of suffering PID if they use an IUD.

One thing that is not commonly known is that the IUD is not a contraceptive at all, but an abortifacient. In most cycles, the eggs will be fertilised if intercourse occurs at the fertile time, and if there are no other reproductive problems. However, due to the inflammation and irritation in the endometrium and uterus induced by the IUD, implantation of the egg is prevented and an early abortion occurs. This inflammation and irritation will need to be treated well before a conception attempt is made, since these conditions are linked with a higher incidence of ectopic pregnancies and miscarriage.

Disruption to zinc levels is another problem which ensues with the use of IUDs made of copper. High copper levels cause zinc levels to fall. This is due to the antagonistic relationship between copper and zinc. Further ill-effects can include damage to the cervix, anaemia through increased blood loss and uterine perforation.

With barrier methods of contraception, the problem lies not with the actual condom or diaphragm, but with the spermicides which are often used with, or are impregnated in, these devices. There is a proven link between the use of spermicides and birth defects. The risk is greatest if the spermicide contains mercury and if its use continues after conception. In America the parents of a deformed child conceived in these circumstances have successfully sued the manufacturer of the spermicide.

PART TWO

- - - - - - - - - - - - - - - -

How your health practitioner can help

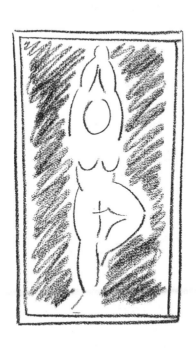

8

IMPROVING YOUR
REPRODUCTIVE HEALTH

ARE YOU AWARE THAT your general health affects
your reproductive health (and vice versa)?

Are you aware that your reproductive health
(before conception) may affect the health of your
pregnancy and your baby?

Are you aware that you suffer from any of the
following conditions?

Women

Irregular Periods—Your cycle is shorter than 27 days or longer
than 31.

Irregular Ovulation—Occasional or frequent cycles that are anovular
(with no ovulation).

Hormonal Imbalance—Including cycles where the pre-ovulatory
phase is longer than 17 days, or the post-ovulatory phase is less
than 12 days.

Amenorrhoea—Total lack of menstruation.

Premenstrual Syndrome—Including sore, swollen or lumpy breasts,
fluid retention and bloating, food cravings, fatigue, digestive
upsets, headaches, aches and pains and premenstrual tension
(PMT).

Dysmenorrhoea—Painful periods, possibly accompanied by nausea or vomiting.

Menorrhagia—Dysfunctional menstrual bleeding which is too profuse or frequent.

Inadequate Mucus—Little or no fertile (wet) mucus present mid-cycle (at or before ovulation).

Recurrent Vaginal Thrush—Accompanied by itching, burning and (possibly) discharge.

OR do you suffer from:

Endometriosis
Pelvic Inflammatory Disease (PID)
Genito-urinary infections (GUIs), including sexually transmitted diseases (STDs)
Blocked Fallopian tubes
Ovarian cysts
Polycystic ovarian syndrome
Fibroids
Cervical dysplasia (abnormal pap smear)
Thyroid dysfunction
Pituitary dysfunction

Men
Low sperm count
Low level of sperm motility
High level of abnormalities
Genito-urinary infections including sexually transmitted diseases
Varicocele (varicose vein in the testicle)
Prostatitis (inflammation in the prostate gland)

Mutual problems
Sperm antibodies
Hostile mucus

MANY OF THE ABOVE conditions can threaten your chances of having a 'better baby!' They may either prevent conception from actually occurring, or they may compromise the quality of your pregnancy and the health of your child.

They must be attended to *well before conception*, and relevant therapy should be part of your preconception care.

Many of these conditions are linked to other aspects of your general health and well-being that are discussed elsewhere in this book. Your endocrine, immune and digestive systems may need attention just as much as your reproductive system.

Many of these conditions can be effectively treated, partially or completely, by natural medicines and/or self-help measures. Some of these treatments have been covered in other chapters, and in this chapter we will look at specific remedies that you or your practitioner can try before resorting to the harsher treatments of drugs and/or surgery.

Many can be diagnosed easily without resorting to invasive tests. For some you will need expert professional treatment. In this chapter we will suggest when this may be necessary, and whether natural or orthodox medicine is more appropriate. If your health practitioner is not conversant with the specific needs of preconception care, you may find it useful to consult this book together.

All of these conditions will heal faster and more effectively if you are generally healthy, nutritionally balanced, non-toxic, non-stressed, have good digestion and regular bowel motions, and get adequate sleep and exercise.

In the following pages we will refer to many remedies, some of which you can administer yourself. Otherwise, you should seek professional help. Many of our suggestions involve the use of herbal medicines or acupressure. For diagnosis you may need the help of your practitioner, who may then prefer to know what self-help measures you are using. Here is some advice on how to prepare or apply these remedies.

NATURAL THERAPIES

Herbal medicine

Herbs have been used safely for centuries to treat all manner of disorders, and are still the most commonly used system of medicine worldwide. However, some herbs are extremely potent and can be toxic in excess, so always use caution and dose only within the given guidelines.

Herbs that are beneficial for the female reproductive system have some wonderfully evocative names such as *False Unicorn Root, Chaste Tree* and *Squaw Vine*, which reflect feminine mythology and fertility. We will also discuss the use of herbs for the male reproductive system, and for digestive and other connected disorders.

Many of these herbs will be on sale at your local health food shop, in the form of loose dried herbs or tea bags, encapsulated dried herbs or herbal tablets. All of these forms can be self-administered with confidence, as long as you don't exceed recommended dosage levels. You may, however get more effective results by consulting with a natural therapist. Follow the instructions in Chapter 6, section on 'Herbs, homoeopathy and flower essences' to make up herbal teas (or infusions). Herbal teas or infusions can be very effective, and in some situations they are the preferred form of medicine. However, if you visit a medical herbalist, you will probably be given fluid extracts or tinctures, liquid forms of herbal medicine which are stronger and easier to combine into individually relevant formulae. Some commercially available teas, tablets or capsules are also made from combinations of herbs for specific conditions, but these are not tailored to the individual.

Acupressure

As discussed in Chapter 6, acupressure can be an effective self-help remedy, although you may prefer to visit an acupuncturist, and benefit from their expertise and diagnostic skills. See Chapter 6 for details on how to stimulate a pressure point.

Other therapies

Other alternative or natural therapies we recommend include:

Osteopathy and chiropractic can relieve congestion, stimulate the body's own healing processes, restore health to the nervous system, as well as correct skeletal problems which can contribute to reproductive disorders.

Massage is soft tissue manipulation which can restore circulation and relax muscle tension.

Homoeopathy involves giving minute traces of substances to stimulate the body's own healing processes. A single remedy is often used to encompass all the symptoms experienced by an individual, although there are remedies which are specific to certain conditions.

Yoga can achieve very powerful healing effects. These may be temporary, for conditions such as menstrual pain, and longer-term, for conditions affecting reproductive and general health. Continual yoga practice can benefit fertility and the childbirth experience profoundly, and can also calm the mind and spirit.

By now you will be well aware that we advocate holistic healing, preferably through the use of natural medicines. Reproductive health cannot be separated from general health, and will be positively affected by those factors which we keep stressing:
• Adequate nutrition.
• Avoidance of toxins and detoxification
• Rest, sleep and attention to stress levels.
• Exercise

NUTRITION

In Chapter 1 we looked at the importance of preconception nutrition, and discussed what you should eat and how to adequately supplement your diet. However, there are specific nutrients required for certain reproductive conditions. Of course, it is essential to seek professional advice if your case is at all unusual or complex!

Swallowing, digesting and absorbing

These are not necessarily the same thing! You need good nutrition for good digestion and good digestion for good nutrition! Even though you may eat well, and take an apparently adequate range of supplements, you may have digestive problems, or suffer from a malabsorption syndrome, and these conditions may affect your nutritional status, which in turn will affect your health.

In Chapter 4, we looked at some ways to relieve constipation, and ensure that you have at least one or two bowel motions daily, but there are some other aspects to good digestion and absorption.

Healthy eating habits

Digestion occurs to best advantage if you chew well, eat slowly, and little and often, rather than all at once. Try to eat in calm surroundings, not on the run.

The mouth

Digestion starts in the mouth, and strong healthy teeth (which depend on calcium and other minerals) are needed to break the food down into small portions which can be digested by the stomach. Bleeding gums can indicate *Vitamin C* and *bioflavonoid* deficiency, and mouth ulcers may be a sign of *iron, Vitamin C* or *B-complex* deficiencies. A white-coated tongue, bad breath, frequent burping and/or a chronically sore throat can be signs of Candida infestation.

Stomach acidity

Contrary to popular belief, lack of acidity in the stomach is a much more common digestive problem than an excess. The digestive processes which occur in the stomach depend on *hydrochloric acid* and *enzymes*. The stomach wall is usually resistant to acid, and is only adversely affected if the stomach lining is damaged. It's more important to repair the stomach lining than it is to reduce the acidity, which is necessary for adequate digestion and absorption.

Excess gas, distension, and the pain and discomfort of indigestion are more often a symptom of too little acidity rather than too much. Hydrochloric acid, usually combined with digestive enzymes, can be taken as a supplement to relieve these symptoms and to improve your ability to digest your food and absorb its nutrients.

Herbs for the stomach

Herbs such as *Meadowsweet, Chamomile, Savory, Tarragon, Sweet Flag* and *Aniseed* are excellent stomach remedies. Many culinary herbs are also excellent aids to digestion, and help to control symptoms such as excess gas and indigestion. *Caraway, Ginger, Coriander, Cumin, Dill, Fennel, Cardamom, Cinnamon, Parsley, Thyme* and *Marjoram* are all helpful, as is *Peppermint* tea taken after a meal.

Bitter tonic herbs (that is, herbs which have an exceptionally bitter taste) trigger the release of gastric digestive juices by their action on the bitter receptors on the tongue, and have been used traditionally for all digestive problems. Excellent bitters include *Barberry, Golden Seal, Gentian, Dandelion Root, St Mary's Thistle, Fringe Tree, Wormwood, Centaury, Agrimony* and *Chicory*. Many of these also have therapeutic effects on other aspects of digestion, such as appetite, gall bladder, liver and pancreatic function, and also aid the restoration of a normal micro-environment in the gut. *Uva Ursi* is a helpful herb for improving pancreatic health.

Digestive enzymes

Some digestive enzymes are present in the stomach, and some are released from the pancreas, which also neutralises any excess acidity from the stomach. They can also be taken in supplement form, usually combined with hydrochloric acid, and are best taken approximately half an hour before main meals.

Candida and anaerobic bacteria

The presence of abnormal amounts of either *Candida albicans* (yeast) or anaerobic bacteria in the gut can contribute significantly to indigestion, and can give rise to symptoms such as excessive flatulence and bloating. The presence of these organisms will also interfere with the absorption of nutrients from the gut.

In Chapter 11 we will give you more information about systemic Candida, including the use of *Acidophilus* and *Bifidus* cultures, both of which help restore a normal micro-environment to the digestive tract. *Citrus Seed* extract can also help to eliminate anaerobic bacteria as well as Candida.

Irritable bowel syndrome

Symptoms which include gas, changes in bowel habits (such as constipation or an increase in frequency with poorly formed motions), abdominal pain, gurgling in the bowel, and an incomplete evacuation, may indicate an 'irritable' bowel, which does not have a smooth peristaltic action. Stress is often a factor in this condition, as is diet, and allergic response. The condition is best treated by a practitioner who has specific experience, as it can be stubborn to treat.

Acupressure points for the digestive system

Stomach 25—three finger widths on either side of your navel (the third finger will find the point). Stimulate with a clockwise or pumping dispersing motion.

Colon 4—in the apex of the 'V' shape formed by the bones of the index finger and the thumb, on the back of your hand. Stimulate with a clockwise or pumping dispersing motion. This point is often very sore, so increase the pressure slowly.

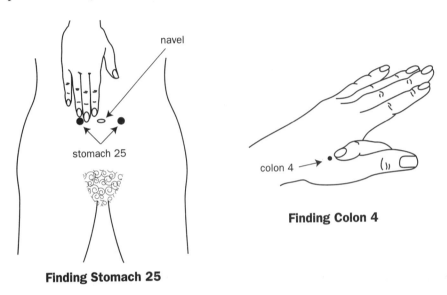

Finding Stomach 25

Finding Colon 4

Do not use these two points if you are pregnant.

Allergic reaction

Many dietary allergies or sensitivities can interfere with normal gastric activity. Common symptoms include constipation alternating with diarrhoea, abdominal pain and flatulence. Food sensitivities or intolerances can also contribute to colic and spastic colon.

Common allergies such as those to cow's milk and cheese, wheat, yeast and eggs can be very irritating to the stomach mucosa and can significantly disrupt nutrient absorption. Once you have identified any allergies, you should seek professional help to boost your digestive and immune systems, while avoiding the offending foods. By doing this, you can, over a period of time, improve or restore your tolerance to the foods, which is preferable to embarking on a long-term restrictive diet.

Acupressure points for allergic reactions

Conception vessel 17—on the mid-line of the chest at the same level as your nipples. Use dispersing pressure. See Chapter 6 (Acupressure points for relieving stress/tension) for diagram.

Liver 3—in the furrow on the top of the foot between the first and second toes, where the bones meet, two thumb widths below the bottom of the toes. Use dispersing pressure.

Pericardium 6—on the inner surface of the forearm between the two tendons, three finger widths (the third finger will find the spot) above the fold at the bend of the wrist. Use dispersing pressure.

Colon 11—at the external extremity of the fold at the bend of the elbow. Use dispersing pressure.

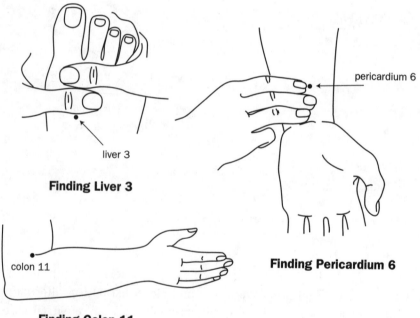

liver 3

Finding Liver 3

pericardium 6

Finding Pericardium 6

colon 11

Finding Colon 11

THE IMMUNE SYSTEM

Lowered immune response not only affects your ability to tolerate foods and environmental pollutants but may also lead to auto-immune disease, which can cause miscarriage and affect reproductive and endocrine health.

Your immune system is under constant bombardment from toxins and pollutants, and often needs support. There are many effective herbs to choose from, including *Echinacea, Picrorrhiza* (both of these are best for acute conditions), *Astragalus, Ginseng (Korean and Siberian)* (use these for chronic, or ongoing conditions) and *Pau D'Arco.* Japanese mushrooms such as *Reiishi* are also excellent. Other herbs such as *Albizzia, Baical Skullcap, Feverfew and Hemidesmus* can reduce the chances of an allergic reaction. Good nutrition is also essential for a healthy immune response, with *zinc, beta-carotene, Vitamin C* and the *bioflavonoids* all having vital roles to play.

STRESS

Whether you are concerned with the health of your reproductive, digestive, endocrine, nervous or immune systems, or with their interaction, you can't afford to ignore the ill-effects of excessive stress.

Today, stress is endemic and can't always be avoided, but you can increase your capacity to cope with it, and reduce its harmful effects. This can make a critical difference to the success of any other therapy you undertake.

TOXICITY

Environmental, dietary and drug toxicity all affect general health as well as reproductive capacity. Detoxification is part of becoming healthy and fertile. None of what follows will be as effective if these issues are not addressed.

Now let's look at some specific reproductive health problems, and what you can do about them. We'll start with the prospective mother, because the female reproductive system is more complex, and has to provide not only a healthy egg, but also the right environment for it to grow into a baby. But remember—it takes two to tango and babies have fathers too! Prospective Dads—your turn will come!

FEMALE REPRODUCTIVE HEALTH
Irregular cycles and hormonal imbalance
Personal assessment of regularity varies enormously. Some women consider themselves irregular if their periods aren't 28 or 29 days

apart. Others think they're fairly regular, but, on questioning we find that their cycles vary from 24 to 36 days or more. However, there's not much dispute that cycles as short as 20 days, or as long as 40, are abnormal.

So, let's define regularity. An average cycle is 29.5 days long, which is the same length as a lunar month (the time between one full, or new, moon and the next) Studies have confirmed that this is the 'norm' rather than the 28 days (a lunar orbit) which is commonly accepted.

There is no real problem if your cycle varies a few days either side of this average—say from 27 days to 31 days, and irregularity due to external circumstances, such as stress, travel, ill health, diet and weight changes, fasting or drug use (medical or recreational), is something you should be able to assess readily enough. These external stimuli will, normally, lengthen, rather than shorten, your cycle, except during breastfeeding, when stress may have the reverse effect.

If your cycles are irregular, you are usually aware of your periods coming too frequently, or not often enough. The problem, however,

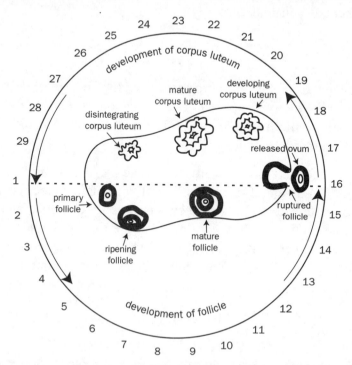

Ovarian activity through average 29-day cycle

is not usually with the process of menstruation, but with that of ovulation. After ovulation, there is, in most cases, a post-ovulatory phase of approximately two weeks, during which time the follicle in the ovary which released the egg becomes a crater on the surface of the ovary. This forms a tiny, temporary, endocrine gland called the corpus luteum, which is Latin for 'yellow body', and which controls the release of progesterone.

This hormone causes, among other things, the endometrium, or lining of the womb, to thicken, so that within 5 to 7 days it is fully supplied with blood and nutrients, and ready for the fertilised egg to implant.

Long cycles are nearly always due to a delay in ovulation, followed by a period two weeks later, and short cycles are usually the result of an early ovulation. By observing body signs such as changes in cervical mucus and basal body temperature (see Chapter 7), you can tell:

- If, and when, you ovulated.
- The length of your pre-ovulatory phase.
- The length of your post-ovulatory phase.
- If menstruation is really late or not.

In Chapters 7 and 13 we look further at how you can determine if and when you ovulate, so you can avoid or achieve conception. We also see why it is best for your baby if you ovulate as close as possible to day 14 of your cycle (day 1 is the first day of your menstrual flow).

Ovulation after day 17 is less likely to lead to a successful conception, and pregnancies started as late as day 20 often result in miscarriage. So it's important that the pre-ovulatory (or follicular) phase is not too long. This phase is usually governed by the hormone oestrogen.

For sufficient levels of progesterone to be generated to prepare the endometrium for the implantation of the egg, it's also important that the post-ovulatory (or luteal) phase of the cycle is not less than 12 days long. (Cycles with post-ovulatory phases of less than 10 days are infertile; this is called a 'luteal defect'.)

To summarise, what we are concerned with for a healthy conception is that:

- You ovulate in every (or most) cycles.
- You have a pre-ovulatory phase of not more than 17 days.
- You have a post-ovulatory phase of not less than 12 days.

These effects are the result of hormone balance. Luckily, natural medicine has many remedies for irregularity and hormone imbalance, including herbs, homoeopathy, acupuncture and soft tissue and skeletal manipulation (osteopathy, chiropractic and massage). Nutrition and stress control are fundamental (you guessed it!) and exercise (not too much or too little, but just enough) can also be a critical factor, as can obesity or too little body fat. Vegetarians, or those on low calorie diets, may find their cycle becomes irregular and their luteal phase defective (see above). Fifty per cent of infertile women with very irregular cycles (oligomenorrhoea) or none (amenorrhoea) have an eating disorder. It's even possible for over-the-counter drugs such as aspirin to delay or prevent ovulation, by inhibiting the prostaglandins which mediate the process. Travel (especially flying) can delay ovulation, so try to limit this to the post-ovulatory phase of your cycle.

Other effects of hormonal imbalance

Most of the common reproductive disorders, if they are not the result of disease (such as endometriosis, pelvic infection or ovarian disease) are caused, or worsened, by hormonal imbalance, either those produced by the pituitary gland or by the ovaries. Therefore, therapy needs to focus on the healthy functioning of these organs.

PMS, dysmenorrhoea, menorrhagia and inadequate fertile mucus are all symptoms of hormone imbalance, and these conditions may correct themselves when the hormonal balance is restored. There are also some other causal factors, and specific remedies (see later).

Pituitary hormones

The pituitary is the controlling and initiating gland (in men too), which sends messages, via hormones, to the gonads (ovaries or testicles) which then manufacture their own hormones (to send messages back to the pituitary). This cycle of hormonal activity prepares your body for conception. The pituitary hormones are unfamiliar to many people, but are an integral part of the menstrual, and indeed of the whole reproductive cycle.

Prolactin—this is the hormone which stimulates lactation after child-birth. If your prolactin level is high at other times it can prevent ovulation taking place (as happens during breastfeeding). This is normally a result of some abnormality of the pituitary gland. Stress can also be a factor, through its affect on the hypothalamus, which usually suppresses prolactin production.

Follicle stimulating hormone—this hormone is commonly referred to as 'FSH'. It is released by the pituitary in response to a signal from the hypothalamus. This special part of the brain is concerned with control of body functions and contains a further specialised section called the 'menstrual clock' which is responsible for the periodic timing of the menstrual cycle. The hypothalamus and pituitary are both responsive to increased levels of light, so it is no accident that menstrual cycles are generally (lunar) monthly.

When FSH reaches the ovary, it stimulates the release of the hormone oestrogen and causes the follicles to ripen several eggs, in preparation for ovulation.

Luteinising hormone—this hormone is commonly referred to as 'LH'. It is released by the pituitary in response to rising levels of oestrogen, and causes the ripest egg to be released from its follicle in the ovary.

Ovarian hormones

The hormones released by the ovaries are more familiar to most women, and are the major female sex hormones.

Oestrogen—is responsible for all sorts of effects, such as the development of female characteristics at puberty, and during the menstrual cycle it causes:

- The cervix to soften and rise, and its opening, the *'os'*, to widen, thus facilitating the entry of sperm.
- The mucus produced in the cervical crypts to change in quantity and quality and become fertile, thus ensuring survival and transport of the sperm (see Chapters 7 and 13).
- The endometrium (lining of the uterus) to thicken and prepare to receive the fertilised egg (if there is one).
- The pituitary gland to release a sudden surge of LH.

Progesterone—is secreted by the corpus luteum, the crater left after the follicle has released the egg. Reduced quantities of oestrogen are also released by this temporary gland. Progesterone causes:

- The body-at-rest (basal) temperature to rise (see Chapter 7).
- The cervical mucus to lessen and thicken and become infertile and hostile to sperm.
- The cervix, to lower, harden and close.
- The lining of the uterus to thicken even more, so that within 5 to 7 days it is ready for the egg.
- The ovary to cease releasing eggs.

Male hormones (in the female)

Testosterone—although this is an androgen or male sex hormone, it is also present in women, and is largely responsible for sex drive (libido). It can be raised in some disease states (notably polycystic ovarian syndrome), and is normally converted by the ovaries to oestrogen.

Diagnosis and symptoms of hormonal imbalance

Medically, a thorough testing procedure can be carried out to determine whether the problem is in the ovaries, pituitary or hypothalamus. This is done through the administration of synthetic hormones. In this way it can also be determined if late periods are the result of a faulty endometrium and not the result of hormonal imbalance. To avoid the ingestion of chemical hormones, much information can be gathered through blood tests. These are a simple way to test hormone levels, but other symptoms may alert you to possible problems. The tests should be carried out at specific stages of the cycle in order to give useful information.

Pituitary hormones, LH and FSH are usually measured at the mid-cycle peak, a few days before ovulation is due. LH is often high if you have polycystic ovarian syndrome, as the pituitary sends out increasing amounts of this hormone to try and stimulate the release of an egg from the unresponsive ovaries (this also happens at menopause). Raised levels of both pituitary hormones can be caused by 'resistant' ovaries, or by the presence of auto-immune disease.

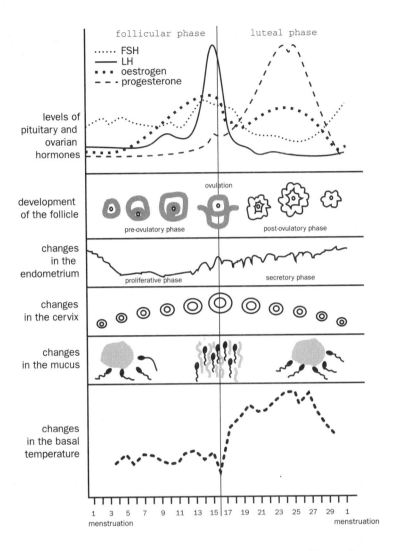

Female hormone levels during a monthly cycle

Prolactin, also released by the pituitary gland, can be measured at any stage during the cycle, though in some women it is only raised nocturnally, and may therefore be missed in tests. If it is raised it may cause some milky discharge from the breasts, irregular or absent ovulation and menstruation, and shortened post-ovulatory phase. This is sometimes the result of disease in the pituitary, possibly a tumour (not necessarily malignant), or decreased function of the hypothalamus or thyroid gland. A CAT scan may be necessary to rule out a pituitary tumour (remember to avoid X-rays whenever possible, and to wait for four months minimum after an X-ray before trying to conceive if you need to undergo this sort of test).

Oestrogen level is usually measured 1 to 2 days before ovulation is due, when it should be peaking. Low levels of oestrogen can be caused by pituitary dysfunction, when low FSH may be a factor, but is more commonly a result of ovarian problems. Symptoms of low oestrogen can include delayed ovulation (which can also be a result of excessive oestrogen levels) and inadequate amounts of fertile cervical mucus, which will be obvious to anyone observing their mucus changes. Excessive oestrogen can contribute to PMS, mid-cycle spotting, endometriosis, uterine fibroids and breast cysts.

Progesterone level is usually measured approximately one week after ovulation, when it should be peaking. Low levels will be reflected in a shortened post-ovulatory phase, inadequate or sluggish temperature rise, and various PMS symptoms, such as sore breasts, fluid retention and PMT.

The important thing to remember is that each hormone is part of an interactive process, and that the key word is balance.

Remedies for irregularity and hormonal imbalance
Remedies for healthy ovarian function

There are two ways in which herbs can help to balance oestrogen. Firstly, through their action on ovarian function, and secondly, through the presence of phyto-oestrogens, which are oestrogen-like substances found in plants.

Phyto-oestrogens are weaker than human oestrogen, and have the overall effect of balancing oestrogen levels, whether they are too high or low. Herbs and food that supply phyto-oestrogens include:

Alfalfa	Sesame seeds	Dong Quai
Soya beans (and sprouts)	Millet	Black Cohosh
Soya milk	Aniseed	Liquorice (not the
Tofu	Parsley	confection)
Tempeh	Red Clover	Sage
Linseed	Saw Palmetto	Fennel
Sunflower seeds	Hops	Cucumber

All sprouted seeds are high in phyto-oestrogens.

Lower levels are present in seaweed; and all kinds of beans, peas and lentils; most wholegrains, notably barley, corn and oats; as well as some fruit and vegetables, notably carrots, apples and the cabbage family.

Though these foods will normally have a balancing effect on oestrogen levels, it is probably inadvisable to eat excessive quantities of them before conception or during the early stages of pregnancy, as very high doses can lower fertility, or cause miscarriage. Also, babies should not be fed excessive amounts of soya milk in the first three months of life, when they are forming their hormone receptor sites.

Other herbs can affect the production of oestrogen through their 'tonic' action on the ovaries. These include:

False Unicorn Root	*Wild Yam*
True Unicorn Root	*Peony*
Ladies' Mantle	*Dong Quai*
Liquorice	*Saw Palmetto*
St John's Wort	*Black Cohosh*

Ginseng has also been shown to increase oestrogen levels, though this may be due to its stimulating effect on the adrenal glands. It increases the output of adrenal hormones, one of which is converted to oestrogen. This may also be one of the mechanisms by which liquorice increases oestrogen levels.

Adequate *Vitamin E* is also essential for correcting oestrogen imbalance, as it helps to regulate its production. The dosage may need to be between 500 and 1000 iu daily. But remember, individual nutrients should never be given in isolation. *Zinc* and *Vitamin C* are also important for all hormone regulation and production. *Dong Quai* is a herb which can guard against *Vitamin E* deficiency.

Medical treatment for hormone imbalances involves taking synthetic oestrogen and/or progesterone. Ovarian stimulants such as clomiphene citrate (Clomid) are used to trigger ovulation.

There are also herbs which contain progesterone precursors. These herbs include:

Wild Yam	*Fenugreek*
Sarsaparilla	*Beth Root*
True Unicorn Root	*Yucca*
Blue Cohosh	*Mistletoe*

The herb which is most useful for raising deficient progesterone levels, however, is *Vitex Agnus Castus* or *Chaste Tree*. This acts on the pituitary, and has an effect on prolactin and luteinizing hormone (LH), and thereby on corpus luteum function and progesterone levels. It can also lower raised testosterone levels in women (though it may be contraindicated in Polycystic Ovarian Syndrome, as it can also raise LH).

Vitamin B6 is the most important nutrient for the treatment of insufficient progesterone. However, this must always be given with the complete range of *B-complex vitamins*. Dosage of B6 is controversial, though levels up to 250 mg daily are very safe. Higher doses are often needed in individual cases, usually up to the level that prevents PMS, but these should only be taken under professional supervision.

Remedies for hormone balance

The ovarian hormones cannot always be treated separately, as it is their balance which is important, though it is sometimes useful to give oestrogen-enhancing herbs pre-ovulation, and progesterone boosters post-ovulation.

Many of the herbs we have mentioned are traditionally used for all types of irregularity. These include:

False Unicorn Root	*Blue Cohosh*
Damiana	*Chaste Tree*
Black Cohosh	*Golden Seal*
Dong Quai	*Sarsaparilla*
Bladderwrack	*Blue Flag*

The ovarian hormones are also, of course, directly affected by the action of the pituitary gland, and the hormones it secretes.

Remedies for healthy pituitary function

Prolactin excess can be treated with *Chaste Tree*, or a Chinese herbal formula called *Rehmannia Eight*. Other useful Chinese herbs include *Peony* and *Liquorice*. This condition also often responds to reasonably high doses of *Vitamin B6* (supervised by a health practitioner) which (like Vitamin C) have the effect of increasing dopamine levels. Any zinc deficiency should also be corrected. *Ergot* decreases prolactin, but has highly toxic side-effects, and should never be self-administered.

Medically the drug used is *bromocriptine*, which is an ergot derivative.

High levels of LH can be treated herbally with *Bugleweed* (which also lowers excessive FSH and reduces thyroid activity), and *Hops*. Low levels of FSH can be raised through the use of *Black Cohosh*, which also lowers raised LH and increases oestrogen. *Chaste Tree* lowers elevated FSH, testosterone, prolactin and raises low levels of LH and progesterone.

Reflexology can help to treat pituitary dysfunction. The area to press is in the centre of the ball of the big toe.

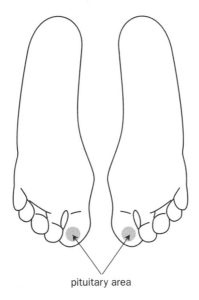

pituitary area

Reflexology area for treatment of the pituitary gland

The pituitary, in its turn, is governed by the hypothalamus, and it may be necessary to distinguish between pituitary and hypothalamic dysfunction using medical tests.

Remedies for healthy thyroid function

The thyroid gland also has an important influence on hormone production. If it is overactive the condition is described as hyperthyroidism, and sufferers are characteristically thin, with bulging eyes and possibly a goitre (which can also be present with other forms of thyroid disease). These individuals are often very nervous, with a rapid pulse. If this describes you, *Bugleweed* is the most helpful herb for you, and you may also respond to *Vervain (Verbena)*. Foods such as soya products, walnuts and the cabbage family may form a useful part of your regular diet.

Persistent problems of an overactive thyroid are treated medically with drugs or by partial removal of the gland.

Hypothyroidism, or underactivity of the thyroid gland, is often a cause of inadequate sex hormone levels. Physical characteristics include obesity, dry skin, hair loss, recurrent infections, susceptibility to cold, depression and lack of energy. If this sounds like you, a blood test for levels of thyroxine can give some indication of whether the thyroid is the problem, though this test is not always a completely reliable indicator of thyroid function.

Another indicator of thyroid function, which may alert you to the problem, is a low body-at-rest (basal) temperature. If you are using natural methods to avoid or achieve conception you will be charting these temperature readings. If these seem to be low (off the chart), it may well be that you have a hypothyroid condition, and the most important herb for you is *Bladderwrack (kelp)*. It is often suggested that this herb is 'tonic' to the thyroid and can also be used for overactive thyroid states, but as it contains iodine, which stimulates thyroxine (thyroid hormone) production, you should take care, and seek professional advice.

Iodine combines with an amino acid, L-tyrosine, to form thyroxine, so this (*L-tyrosine*) can also be taken as a supplement if you are low on thyroid hormone. You should also include all foods from the sea—fish and other seafood, as well as seaweed—in your diet.

Vitamins B6 and *C, zinc, copper, choline, selenium* and *lecithin* are also helpful here, and it's possible to use a thyroid 'glandular' remedy. Other useful herbs are *Coleus, Blue Flag, Poke Root* and *Sarsaparilla. Poke Root* must be used with extreme caution (and not used during pregnancy), and preferably only under supervision, as it is highly toxic in excess, and the therapeutic dose is extremely small.

Celloids, or tissue salts, to try are *calcium phosphate* and *magnesium phosphate*. These are minerals which are already in the biochemical form (which is how they are found in the body), and are more easily assimilated at the cellular level.

Massage of the thyroid area can be helpful (shoulder stands can also help), and there are reflexology areas in the feet, at the base of the big toes, which can be treated with pressure.

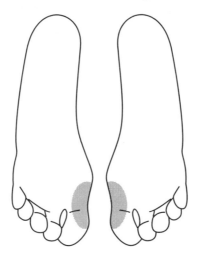

Reflexology area for treatment of the thyroid gland

Drug medication for hypothyroidism is with thyroxine.

Professional help

If all of this confuses you, visit your local medical herbalist or naturopath. If you have been charting your mucus, temperature and other clinical symptoms, your practitioner will be able to diagnose your condition more clearly, and may also order blood tests to verify the diagnosis.

Nutritional supplementation

Nutritional supplementation also has an important role to play in the natural treatment of hormone imbalance. Useful supplements include *zinc, calcium, magnesium, Vitamins E, B-complex and C.* Celloids, or tissue salts, that are particularly helpful are *sodium phosphate* (sometimes called Nat Phos), *potassium chloride* (Kali Mur) and *silica*.

More about nutrition!

Evening primrose oil is another important nutrient, which has beneficial effects on hormone balance, through the action of the essential fatty acids (EFAs) it contains. These affect the balance of prostaglandins in the body, which in turn affect the hormone levels. Essential fatty acid metabolism is adversely affected by saturated fats, so any hormone-balancing program should be low in heated or animal fats such as fried foods, dairy produce and fatty meats.

Sources of these EFAs are *olive oil, linseed, flax seed, borage* and *blackcurrant seeds*. Further important EFAs can be found in *fish*, especially oily fish which comes from cold, deep water. Fish is an excellent food as it's also very low in saturated fats. If you do not eat fish regularly (2 to 3 times weekly is best, but not deep-fried), add *MaxEPA* (fish oils) to your supplement list.

Meat is not only high in saturated fats, but may often be high in chemical hormones, which will further upset your hormone balance. Many animals are fed large amounts of steroids, as well as antibiotics and other chemicals, and their food has often been sprayed with pesticides and grown with chemical fertilisers. The best way to avoid these is to eat only organically fed meat. Ask your local health food shop to direct you to a reliable source, and see Chapter 1 for more on meat.

Acupressure points for irregularity and hormone imbalance

Acupuncture is an excellent therapy for hormone imbalance and irregularity, and combines well with herbal medicine.

Conception vessel 4—five finger widths (the fifth finger will find the spot) below the navel on the mid-line of the belly. Tonify this point to invigorate the blood and regulate menstruation.

Spleen 6—four finger widths (the fourth finger finds the spot) above the interior ankle bone, in the small hollow just behind the tibia. Disperse this point to regulate chi and the blood in the uterus.

Do not use these two points if you are, or may be, pregnant.

If your cycles tend to be short, add:

Spleen 10—bend your leg at a right angle (90 degrees). Get someone to place the fingers of their opposite hand (right on left, and vice versa) along the front of your kneecap, and stretch the thumb backwards towards your groin. The tip of their thumb will be on Spleen 10, 5 cm above your knee. Disperse to circulate chi and blood.

If your cycles tend to be long, add:

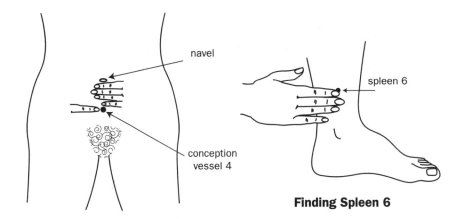

navel

conception
vessel 4

Finding Conception vessel 4

spleen 6

Finding Spleen 6

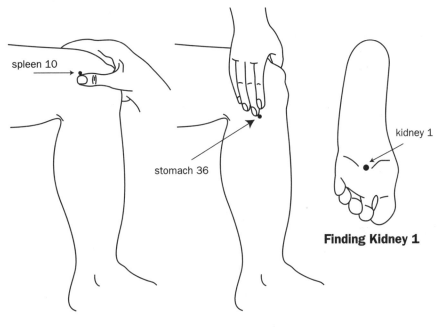

spleen 10

stomach 36

kidney 1

Finding Kidney 1

Finding Spleen 10   **Finding Stomach 36**

Stomach 36—Bend your knee as for Spleen 10. Catch your kneecap between index finger and thumb. The middle finger is on the outside of your shin bone, and Stomach 36 is at the tip of this finger, outside the tibia. Disperse to circulate chi and blood.

Kidney 1—Another important pressure point for fertility is the one at the end of the kidney meridian. In Chinese medicine, the kidney meridian governs sexual energy, and the end of the meridian is a powerful point. This point is at the centre of the ball of the foot. Disperse this point with your thumb for help in conceiving.

Stress control and suggestion

Another important remedy for irregularity, especially delayed ovulation, is stress control, You've been given many techniques to use for controlling stress in Chapter 6, and some of these involve relaxing deeply and using suggestions and visualisations.

As your cycle's timing is controlled by the hypothalamus and the pituitary glands, and as these are very susceptible to external influences, such as stress and other cycles in the environment, you can use this sensitivity to help program yourself to regularity. Women tend to tune into the timing of other cycles in their environment (such as other women's menstrual rhythms, or new and full moons), so that it's common to have whole dormitories in boarding schools bleeding simultaneously. Therefore you can, through suggestion, influence the timing of your cycle.

Instead of cycling with your sister, or work-mate (close physical contact affects the cycle through the pheromones that are given off and which vary throughout the cycle), you can set your own agenda. Strong visualisations and verbal suggestions of regular monthly ovulation and menstruation, undertaken (at best daily) while deeply relaxed, can be a very effective remedy for irregularity, especially if stress of any kind is a causative factor.

In Chapters 7 and 13, we talk of a fertility biorhythm, the lunar cycle. Many women find that they already cycle to this rhythm, and in those chapters we look further at how suggestion can be used to achieve this, and thereby increase your fertility. These suggestions can be used as self-help, through the use of a relaxation and suggestion tape, or with the help of a hypnotherapist.

Yoga for irregularity and hormone balance

Yoga has an important role to play in optimising reproductive health, as well as in preparing the body for the demands of pregnancy and childbirth. Because of the toning effect on all the organs and the circulation, yoga has traditionally been used to regulate cycles and balance hormones. See Chapter 5, 'Flexibility' section, for yoga poses.

Amenorrhoea

If your irregularity involves long cycles, and this extends to several months, you can consider that you are suffering amenorrhoea. This condition accounts for 20 per cent of all female infertility and is manifested by a lack of menstruation (for more than six months). If you haven't had a period for this long, you are also suffering from a lack of ovulation, which is more to the point. You can check if you have ovulated or not by taking your temperature.

Amenorrhoea is called primary, if you have never had a period and are over fifteen, or secondary, if you previously had a (fairly) regular cycle. Occasionally, it is a result of a blockage of the cervix or vagina, or disorders of the uterus. Here, the emmenagogue herbs (which promote the menstrual flow) take priority. Usually, the cause will be a lack of ovulation, which may be the result of disorders in the ovaries, pituitary or hypothalamus. Once the underlying cause is determined, it can be treated accordingly.

First, you must have a pregnancy test. Then, you need to assess whether you could be menopausal (presumably you're not on the pill). All of these could be reasons for lack of ovulation or menstruation. Other reasons could include:

Post-pill (oral contraceptive) sterility
Dramatic weight loss/gain
Fasting
Anorexia
Malnutrition
Eating only raw food (you need to eat some cooked food)
Breast-feeding
Anaemia
Stress
Hypoglycaemia
Excessive exercise
Uterine tumour
Congenital uterine defects
Low body fat
Polycystic ovaries
Endometriosis
Infected ovaries
Ovarian cancer
Hypothyroidism (underactive thyroid)
Illness/severe infection
Drugs (tranquillisers and narcotics)
Disorders of the circulation
Premature menopause
Uterine infection
Auto-immune ovarian failure
Resistant ovary syndrome
Pituitary tumour
Endocrine disorder (including ovarian, pituitary, hypothalamus and adrenal)
Chromosomal abnormalities
Surgery

If the reason for amenorrhoea is high levels of prolactin, it should be treated as for hormone imbalance.

One reason for amenorrhoea can be low levels of body fat, which can be caused by excessive exercise or training, or anorexia. Sudden dieting or fasting may have the same effect. In Chapter 1 we look at why you should try to normalise your weight if you are below the ideal for your height. Remember, to conceive in good health, as well as to maintain oestrogen levels, you need to eat enough! If you need to put on weight, eat more nutritious food only. Adequate protein (a minimum of two servings, or 75 g daily) and unsaturated fats such as those found in avocados, nuts and olive oil are important.

If you are overweight you may also suffer from amenorrhoea, but as small a change as a 5 per cent loss in body weight can be enough to correct this condition. Since anaemia is another cause of amenorrhoea, take care that you have enough iron-rich foods in your diet, and, if necessary, take a supplement (which must be organic and chelated). If you are unsure of your need for iron, have a blood test (serum ferritin or iron stores is the test of choice) to confirm levels, but do not supplement indiscriminately since an excess of iron is toxic. Fatigue may indicate an iron deficiency, but you should always confirm this with a blood test. Iron-rich herbs are *Parsley* and *Nettle*. Vegetarians and those on low calorie diets are also at risk of amenorrhoea.

Since women suffering from amenorrhoea have low levels of oestrogen, their calcium absorption is threatened and the risk of osteoporosis in later life can be increased.

Herbal remedies for amenorrhoea

Useful herbs include all those mentioned in the previous section on hormone balance, as well as:

- General reproductive 'tonic' herbs—*Squaw Vine, Blue Cohosh, Damiana, Golden Seal, Bladderwrack (kelp), Blue Flag* (endocrine tonic).
- Herbs for the effects of stress and tension on the cycle—*Motherwort, Withania, Pulsatilla, Valerian, Green Oats.*
- Emmenagogues—(To promote bleeding if *not* pregnant, and normalise circulation), *Mugwort, Ginger, Pennyroyal, Tansy, Rue, Sandalwood, Wormwood, Yarrow, Prickly Ash.*

Acupressure points for amenorrhoea

Acupressure points are as for Irregularity and hormone imbalance.
If your periods have not actually ceased, but are so light as to be
virtually non-existent, you must first of all check that you are
ovulating. This can be confirmed with basal temperature readings or
through a blood test to measure progesterone. If you are, then treat
the condition similarly, with the accent on the emmenagogue herbs.

If amenorrhoea does not respond to self-help treatment, you
should see a health practitioner.

Menorrhagia

If you are suffering from the opposite condition to amenorrhoea, and
your periods are too profuse, you are suffering from menorrhagia.

Menorrhagia, or dysfunctional menstrual bleeding, is a term
which refers to periods that are too profuse, or occur excessively
often. The causes could be:

Uterine cancer	Intra-uterine Device (IUD)
Uterine fibroids	Ectopic pregnancy
Endometriosis	Spontaneous abortion
Pelvic Inflammatory Disease (PID)	Pelvic circulatory congestion
Underactive thyroid	Capillary fragility
Liver dysfunction	Severe hormonal imbalance

Whatever the cause, excessive bleeding can lead to loss of iron,
fatigue and, eventually, anaemia. If it is caused by any of the more
severe conditions listed above, you must seek the guidance of your
health practitioner. However, before you accept any drastic solution to
this problem (some medical solutions include long-term hormone
therapy, 'painting' the inside of the womb with microwaves (?!) and
hysterectomy), make sure that your bleeding pattern is, indeed, excessive. Subjective assessments vary enormously.

Certainly, it would be best to first attempt the methods outlined
in this book to see if you get some obvious relief. If your dietary
habits have been such as to create a severe hormonal imbalance, it
may be necessary to give yourself a head start by going on a fast
before commencing healthier eating habits.

If you fast, it must be under the guidance of a qualified practitioner.

Herbs for menorrhagia

The hormone-balancing herbs are indicated here, and acupuncture can be helpful. Your health practitioner should be able to help you understand the underlying cause, and choose the appropriate treatment.

If you suffer from anaemia, capillary fragility, and associated vascular deficiencies, then take *Vitamin C* and bioflavanoids in large doses (to bowel tolerance, see Chapter 4, 'Suggested Extra Nutrient Doses for Detoxification') and: *Parsley   Buckwheat   Lime Flowers   Yarrow*

If menorrhagia is due to pelvic congestion, try rebounding, massage, osteopathic adjustments, and: *Cayenne   Ginger   Blue Cohosh   Ginkgo*

For an underactive thyroid, try *Kelp* (a good source of iodine) and: *Blue Flag   Poke Root (see below)*

For liver problems, fast on juices only for one day a week, stay off all alcohol and drugs, and try:

Dandelion Root	*Celandine*
Bupleurum	*Salvia (Dan Shen)*
St Mary's Thistle	*Globe Artichoke*

In order to check the bleeding, use haemostatic and astringent herbs. Try:

Shepherd's Purse	*Raspberry*
Beth Root	*Periwinkle*
Ladies' Mantle	*Black Haw*
Cranesbill	*Squaw Vine*

And to 'tone' the uterus, try the 'organ remedies', such as:

Dong Quai	*False Unicorn Root*
Blue Cohosh	*True Unicorn Root*

Normalise the circulation with: *Ginger   Yarrow*

And, if you suspect that the cause is hormonal, as well as the usual balancing herbs, a very effective herb to use for excessive or frequent bleeding is: *Poke Root*

But be careful. The use of this herb needs to be supervised by a practitioner. It can be toxic if you overdose.

You may also experience relief from massaging the abdomen with essential oils. Use *Cyprus, Geranium* and *Rose* (diluted in a vegetable oil), or add them to a warm bath.

Acupressure points for excessive bleeding

Spleen 1—on the outside corner of the nail bed of your big toe. Use strong tonifying action with your thumb nail. *Do not use this point if you are, or may be, pregnant, except to control a bleeding problem.*

Conception vessel 4—see Acupressure points for irregularity and hormone imbalance for diagram and explanation.

Liver 3—see Acupressure points for allergic reactions for diagram and explanation.

Liver 1—on the inside corner of the nail bed of the big toe, tonify.

Although there is much that you can do for yourself to balance your hormones and regulate your cycle, you may find a consultation with a natural health practitioner helpful.

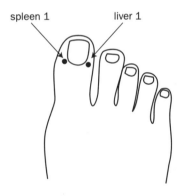

Finding Spleen 1 and Liver 1

Dysmenorrhoea

This disorder, meaning 'painful periods', can be divided into two distinct types. Congestive dysmenorrhoea tends to be associated with premenstrual syndrome, and is often worse before menstruation. The pain is a dull, heavy and dragging ache, and is usually associated with other congestive symptoms such as fluid retention.

Spasmodic dysmenorrhoea refers to the sharp, cramping pains that start with bleeding. This is often also associated with hormonal, prostaglandin and nervous imbalances, or occasionally, can be to do with a tight or obstructed cervix, especially in younger or childless women or adolescents, who are the typical sufferers of this type of period pain.

It is, of course, quite possible to suffer from both types of dysmenorrhoea. If you experience the congestive type, use the suggestions in the next section, Premenstrual Syndrome. In this section, we will be looking at remedies for the spasmodic type.

First, you need to establish that you are not miscarrying. Then you need to rule out any underlying conditions that may be causing or exacerbating the pain and distress. Possible associated diseases could be:

Endometriosis, PID (Pelvic Inflammatory Disease), *Ovarian cysts* and *Uterine fibroids.*

If there is an underlying condition, such as one of the above, then the dysmenorrhoea is called secondary, and will not improve until you have dealt with the associated disease (see this chapter). Naturopathic approaches can be successful, although it's best to consult your practitioner rather than attempt self-help.

Secondary dysmenorrhoea is characterised by pain that often occurs at other times in the cycle, starts before bleeding begins, and often worsens towards the end of the period. It may also worsen from cycle to cycle, there may be pain on intercourse, fever and other symptoms.

If the dysmenorrhoea is *primary* (that is, not a result of some other condition), then the cause is usually a result of nutrient deficiencies leading to the imbalances in essential fatty acids, saturated fats, prostaglandins and hormones that we referred to in the section on hormone balance. These imbalances should be remedied as part of your preconception care to normalise your nutrient status. Symptoms such as dysmenorrhoea are an indication that you still have some work to do in this area!

Nutrients for dysmenorrhoea

Potassium, magnesium and *calcium* are essential for proper muscle contraction. A lack of any of these will cause irritability of the muscles, and will lead to problems when the uterus starts to contract to dispel blood. *Evening primrose oil* or other sources of essential fatty acids, will help to alleviate the imbalance of prostaglandins which is commonly the cause of severe cramping. Saturated fats, on the other hand, should be avoided. Levels of *Vitamins A, B-complex (especially B6), C* and *E* should be maintained (see earlier section on diet). *Vitamin E* is a natural prostaglandin inhibitor, which also increases circulation to, and oxygenation of, uterine cells.

All of the supplements, if they are not taken on a regular daily basis, should be used for at least one, preferably two, weeks before menstruation. It is actually preferable to take them throughout your cycle, and in most cases these nutrients will be part of your general preconception care. You may in some cases need to increase the dose premenstrually.

Herbal remedies should also be taken *before* your period starts, and, in the case of hormonal balancing herbs, may have a progressive effect over several cycles.

Herbal remedies for dysmenorrhoea

- Antispasmodic herbs—*Cramp Bark, Black Haw, Wild Yam, Dong Quai, Motherwort, Skullcap, Pulsatilla, Mugwort, White Dead Nettle, Bilberry, Blue Cohosh*, (especially if the pain is in the cervix), *Black Cohosh* (especially if the pain is in the ovary and radiates down the legs).
- Anti-prostaglandin herbs—*Feverfew, Tansy.*
- Circulatory stimulants (for easy release of blood)—*Ginger, Cayenne, Mugwort, Tansy, Yarrow, Horsechestnut* (also helpful for nocturnal leg cramps).

- 'Organ' remedy herbs (to tone uterus)—*Dong Quai, False Unicorn Root, True Unicorn Root, Blue Cohosh, Squaw Vine, White Dead Nettle.*
- Hormone-balancing herbs—*Chaste Tree, False Unicorn Root, Saw Palmetto, Sarsaparilla, Dong Quai, Liquorice, Squaw Vine.*
- Laxative herbs—*Rhubarb, Cascara, Senna, Psyllium husks.*

Self-help pain relievers

If you do experience cramping in spite of preventive measures, there are several self-help techniques to alleviate pain.

- You can try taking *calcium* and *magnesium* supplements (twice as much calcium as magnesium), every hour or two as soon as cramping starts. The celloids, or tissue salts, are particularly helpful, use *mag phos* (magnesium phosphate) and *cal phos* (calcium phosphate).
- You can try heat—a hot-water bottle on your tummy or back. Try 'Warm ease' briefs with heat-retaining inserts, for use throughout the day.
- You can try having osteopathic treatment of the lower back to ease congestion.
- Any local massage will relieve pain and stimulate circulation and blood flow. Massage over the uterus itself, over the lower back and down the legs is particularly helpful, and essential oils such as *Clary Sage, Geranium, Rose* and *Lemon grass* will increase the effectiveness. Massage to head, neck and shoulders is good for relieving headaches, particularly if you concentrate on the base of the skull and the scalp where there are sore spots. If you can't find a willing partner, do it to yourself.
- Hypnotherapy, either self-induced, from a tape, or with a therapist, can also be very effective in reducing pain. See Chapter 6 for more on this.
- Yoga can also be very effective. Try the cobra or bow poses (see Chapter 5), also this double tuck pose (below) which stretches the lower back and relieves abdominal pain.

All of these measures will also be helpful during childbirth (with the exception of osteopathic treatment). Some of the pressure points listed below may also be helpful.

Double tuck pose—lying on your back, you simply pull your knees into your chest with your arms. It is important to use the arms' strength and allow the lower back to just relax and stretch out.

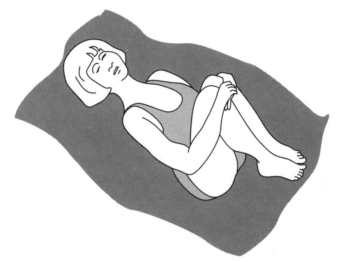

Double tuck position

- Make sure that you are not constipated around the time of your period since this will increase your symptoms. Eat lots of fruit, use herbal laxatives only, avoid smoking and drink plenty of water (see Chapter 4).
- Tampons can increase the pain experienced during menstruation, and with the threat of toxic shock syndrome, it is probably better to switch to pads as often as possible (remember you have at least nine months free of periods coming up—hopefully lots more when you breastfeed!). There is some thought that tampons may contribute to diseases such as endometriosis (by restricting normal blood flow) and they have an abrasive effect on the delicate mucosa in the vagina. Avoid synthetic, bleached or deodorised pads as they can cause reactions, such as thrush (candida) or dermatitis (eczema).
- Natural (recyclable) cotton pads are available. See Contacts and Resources for details of Moonphase and other natural pads. In this section you will also find a reference to 'organic' tampons which contain no chemicals or bleaches. These are preferable if you do need to use a tampon. Loose clothing can also help to minimise reactions to sanitary products.

Acupressure points for period pain relief

Pressure points can be included in a massage, or used independently. For cramping there are several points.

For pain *during* the period try these points:

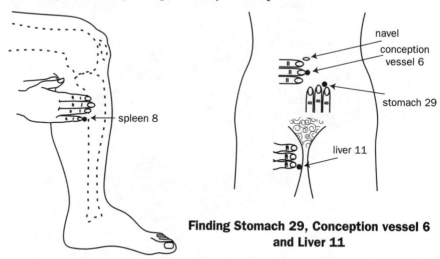

Finding Stomach 29, Conception vessel 6 and Liver 11

Finding Spleen 8

Spleen 6—(see Acupressure points for irregularity and hormone imbalance). Disperse this point.

Spleen 10—(see Acupressure points for irregularity and hormone imbalance). Disperse this point.

Stomach 29—three finger widths down from the navel, and three finger widths to each side (the third finger finds the spot). Disperse this point. *Do not use this point if you are pregnant.*

Stomach 36—(see Acupressure points for irregularity and hormone imbalance). Disperse this point.

Conception vessel 4—(see Acupressure points for irregularity and hormone imbalance). Calm this point.

Conception vessel 6—two finger widths (second finger locates the point) below the navel. Calm this point. *Do not use this point if you are pregnant.*

Colon 4—(see Acupressure points for the digestive system). Disperse this point.

Liver 11—three thumb widths (the third thumb (if you have one!) will find the spot), down from the crease between the thigh and the torso, on the inner thigh. Use dispersing pressure.

For pain *before* the period try these points:

Spleen 8—four finger widths below the inside of the knee joint between the calf muscle and the tibia, up against the bone. Fourth finger finds the spot. Use dispersing pressure.

Liver 3—(see Acupressure points for allergic reactions). Disperse this point.

For pain *after* the period try these points:

Conception vessel 4—(see Acupressure points for irregularity and hormone imbalance). Tonify this point.

Stomach 36—(see Acupressure points for irregularity and hormone imbalance). Tonify this point.

Spleen 6—(see Acupressure points for irregularity and hormone imbalance). Tonify this point.

If all else fails, or if you forget to put your preventive measures into practice in good time, aspirin is the pain reliever of choice, as it will counteract the troublesome prostaglandins. Unfortunately, the natural sources of salicylates (aspirin-like compounds) do not contain enough of the active ingredient to be effective for pain relief, but they are found in *Black* or *White Willow Bark, Meadow Sweet* and *White Poplar.*

If your periods are excessively painful, you should always check with your medical practitioner that none of the more serious underlying conditions are present. A natural health practitioner may be able to guide you to the most appropriate remedies.

Mittelschmerz

This is the German word for ovulation pains, meaning 'pain in the middle'—in your middle, and in the middle of your cycle. These can be sharp, 'twangy' pains felt over short periods such as a few minutes, but they can last longer and be quite severe.

The pain is usually felt on one side or the other, often alternating, since the ovaries generally take turns to release an egg. It can be one way of telling which ovary is active, although if one is defective, the other may compensate, and the defective one may still hurt anyway. A more reliable diagnosis is achieved by noting the swelling of the lymph gland on the side on which ovulation has occurred.

If the pain is severe, or lasts until menstruation, try the following:

Vitamin E—500 to 1000 iu daily

Vitamin C—1500 to 3000 mg daily

Garlic—two capsules, taken three times daily (with food)

If self-help remedies are not effective, seek professional help.

Premenstrual Syndrome (PMS)

PMS is a name that covers a wide spectrum of symptoms. The emotional swings, as well as the physical discomfort, can be extreme. Sometimes a woman's partner, family and friends are more aware of the problem then she is herself. However, for many women, the symptoms are quite debilitating.

The trouble is, when you are cranky, irritable and tense, it's often the external situations that you are irritated with that you blame, and preventive measures are usually far from your mind. However, since PMS is usually due to hormone and nutrient imbalance, it is important to rectify it before conception.

Of course PMT, or premenstrual tension, is only part of the whole syndrome. You may suffer from a few, many, or all (poor you!), of the following symptoms during the week or so prior to your period, usually with fairly instant relief as you start bleeding. However, for some women, the problems continue into the first days of the next cycle.

- Tension
- Anxiety
- Reduced concentration
- Tearfulness
- Aggression and anger
- Depression
- Listlessness
- Confusion
- Fatigue
- Insomnia
- Headache, seeing spots
- Excessive weight gain
- Fluid retention
- Abdominal bloating
- Swelling of hands, feet, legs and face
- Sore, swollen or lumpy breasts
- Backache
- Pelvic pain
- Aching legs
- Ovarian pain
- Sweating
- Bladder problems
- Constipation
- Diarrhoea

- Nausea
- Low blood sugar
- Sugar cravings
- Chocolate cravings
- Food cravings
- Increased appetite
- Thirst
- Itchiness
- Oily skin and hair
- Pimples
- Heart pounding, palpitations
- Dizziness, fainting
- Sore eyes
- Decreased libido
- Highly increased libido (this *can* be a problem!)
- Hives
- Bruising
- Muscular tenderness
- Joint tenderness
- Increased tendency to arthritis, epilepsy, schizophrenia, infections, herpes, Candida, asthma, eczema, hay fever and allergic response.

This (incomplete) list covers over 50 symptoms! Their only common feature is that they all get worse cyclically. Of course, the range of symptoms experienced varies from woman to woman, as the individual hormonal imbalances interact with unique personalities, metabolisms and circumstances.

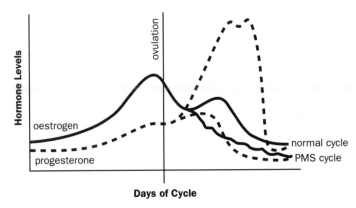

Hormone levels in a PMS sufferer

The imbalance is usually of too little progesterone and/or too much oestrogen, but it varies with each individual, and is critically linked to the availability of certain nutrients. Your efforts to overcome PMS need to reflect this. As well as using self-help techniques to relieve the symptoms, you need to address the underlying causes. This is not, as Hippocrates thought, a wandering uterus, somehow disturbing the brain on its journey around the body. So, you don't need to burn incense at your vaginal opening to entice your uterus back, as he suggested, but here is what you can do:

Self-help for PMS

- Take a good vitamin and mineral supplement which fulfils the guidelines laid down earlier.
- Increase the level of *Vitamin B6*. You can take 250 mg daily very safely. Some women need much higher amounts and there is a precedent for setting the level at that which relieves PMS symptoms such as sore breasts and fluid retention. Higher doses should be supervised by a health professional, though up to 400 mg daily (even in the first trimester of pregnancy) should present no problems The first signs of toxicity will be tingling in the upper lip, fingers and toes. These symptoms are entirely reversible, and will cease as soon as you lower the dosage. Take only with the complete *B-complex* range. These are essential vitamins for anxiety, mood swings and fluid retention.
- *Selenium* is a particularly important mineral for tender and sore breasts. This nutrient is only available on prescription in Australia, though freely available over the counter in most other countries, including America and the United Kingdom.
- *Poke Root* is a specific herb for lumpy breasts, and can be used externally as an ointment. Internal use can also be helpful, but it must *not* be taken if there is any chance that conception has occurred.
- A wet or bruised *cabbage* leaf, applied to the breast, brings fast relief. Maybe you could start a fashion trend!
- Make sure that you have adequate levels of *Vitamin E, Vitamin C, zinc, calcium* and *magnesium*. (See Chapter 1.) *Vitamin E* is particularly helpful for premenstrual headache, sweet cravings, increased appetite, fatigue, dizziness and palpitations. *Calcium* and *magnesium* are important nutrients to stabilise your nervous

system, and reduce irritability, anxiety, depression and headaches. Levels of both these minerals may drop about ten days before menstruation, as do zinc levels which are affected by rising copper levels.

- Take *Evening primrose oil* supplements for the essential fatty acids they contain. Some of these come with *marine fish oil* which is also helpful, especially if you eat little fish. (See previous section on hormone balance for more on EFAs). *Evening primrose oil* can help alleviate anxiety, irritability, depression, headaches, fluid retention and cyclical breast changes.

- *Kelp, spirulina* and *garlic* supplements can be useful (take care with garlic if you are hypoglycaemic, though Candida sufferers will need plenty).

- Some types of PMS may be aggravated by *Vitamin B5, folic acid* and *PABA*.

- Eat well all through your cycle, but pay special attention to your diet as soon as ovulation is over. Research shows that your need for food increases in the post-ovulatory phase, but this may be due to nutrient imbalance. You need to be sure that the quality of your diet does not deteriorate just because the quantity increases.

- Avoid all saturated fats, eat fish rather than meat. Cut out salt, sugar, alcohol and all refined grains such as white bread, pastry, rice, pasta and foods made with white flour. Salt increases water retention, alcohol increases your need for *Vitamins B* and *D, calcium, magnesium* and *zinc*. Although red wine contains valuable *bioflavonoids*, red grape juice will have to do for now! All refined carbohydrates (sugar, alcohol and refined grains) leach *zinc, chromium* and the *B-complex vitamins* from your body, just when you are in particular need of these nutrients. On the other hand, whole grains contain all the nutrients your body needs to metabolise the grain and therefore your own stores are not depleted.

- Don't smoke, and keep tea and coffee intake to a minimum. Tea restricts *iron* and *zinc* absorption, coffee does too, and is linked with breast problems. The caffeine contained in tea and coffee (and soft drinks) is a diuretic, and with increased urination you get increased excretion of minerals (this is not a problem with herbal diuretics, which contain minerals). Water retention is not helped as you will simply want to drink more. Add to this the disturbing effect on anxiety states (caffeine is also a stimulant) and you can see that you will be better off drinking herbal teas and dandelion coffee (see list of helpful herbs in next section).

- Exercise daily for at least 20 minutes to improve circulation to the ovaries and uterus (try rebounding).
- If you suffer low blood sugar levels at this time, with fatigue and a desire for food (particularly sweets), try eating small amounts of nutritious, high energy foods fairly frequently. Complex carbohydrates, almonds and other nuts are best.
- Avoid sugar since it reduces the availability of chromium (and thus lowers your tolerance for sugar). *Chromium* supplementation may help prevent sugar cravings, as can *Vitamin E.* If your cravings are specifically for chocolate, you need more *magnesium.* Chocolate is rich in magnesium, though *not* the best source of this nutrient (since it is also full of saturated fats, caffeine and sugar). Magnesium is actually a very important nutrient for PMS symptom alleviation, and your chocolate cravings may act as a guide as to whether you are getting enough of this mineral.
- Since lowered blood sugar levels increase any tendency to allergies and lower your resistance to infections, you should take extra care at this time not to expose yourself to allergens (substances to which you are intolerant), or to viral or infectious agents.
- If you are a PMS sufferer, check your allergy status. The most common allergens are cow's milk, wheat gluten, yeast, eggs, oranges and house dust mites. Try removing these from your diet or environment and see how much difference it makes.
- Yeast is thought to stimulate oestrogenic activity and may make PMS worse (and you may easily have an allergic reaction to it).
- If one of the reasons for PMS is either excessive oestrogen or an underactive thyroid, you may need to avoid the cabbage family, soya beans, cucumbers, alfalfa, fennel, peanuts and hormonally fed meat.
- Practise massage, yoga, relaxation, meditation or self-hypnosis to encourage helpful habits and a peaceful mind.
- Seek therapy or help for any underlying emotional problems which may only surface at this time.

- Give yourself a break. If it is possible for you, use this time for the less strenuous, less externally demanding activities. Allow your energies to become more inward, and quieter, and don't have expectations of yourself that are unrealistic and unconnected to your cyclical nature.

Acupressure points for PMS

There are some specific pressure points for PMS.

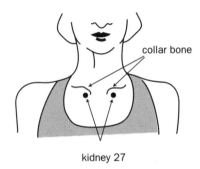

Finding Kidney 27

Kidney 27—two points in the hollows just below your collar bone, in line with the outer edges of your neck. Use tonifying pressure.

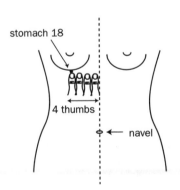

Finding Stomach 18

Stomach 18—under the breast, four thumb widths from the mid-line, between the fifth and sixth ribs, below the nipple. You will need to lift the breast and press right up into the fold between the breast and the chest wall. Calm this point by holding your palm over it, to reduce breast swelling and tenderness, and to reduce bloating.

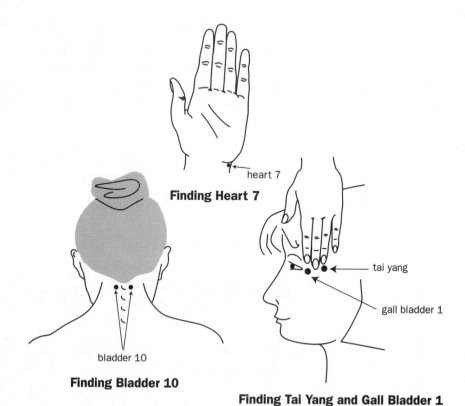

Finding Heart 7

Finding Bladder 10

Finding Tai Yang and Gall Bladder 1

Heart 7—on the wrist crease on the little finger side of the palm. Calm this point to calm the mind and promote blood circulation.

Liver 3—see Acupressure points for allergic reactions.

Good points to relieve headache are:

Colon 4—see Acupressure points for the digestive system.

Bladder 10—right up under the base of your skull, on either side of your spine, pressing upwards, disperse.

Tai Yang—in the depression on the upper temple, three finger widths from the end of the eyebrow (third finger finds the spot), disperse.

Gall bladder 1—at the outer corner of the eye, in the slight depression just outside the orbital ridge of the lower temple, disperse.

Herbs, oils and yoga for PMS

There are many herbs that you might find useful at this time. Some of these are sold as tablets or teas, already formulated for PMS. The herbal remedy of choice is *Chaste Tree* (see Irregular cycles and hormonal imbalance section). If you are making this remedy yourself, the berries are the part from which you should make an infusion.

A more comprehensive formula might include a liver drainage and detoxifying herb to help remove waste oestrogen, and various herbs to address specific symptoms, such as fluid retention and anxiety.

- Hormone-balancing herbs—*Chaste Tree, Sarsaparilla, False Unicorn Root, Bladderwrack, Dong Quai, Squaw Vine, Wild Yam, Fenugreek, Peony.*
- Liver herbs—*Dandelion Root, St Mary's Thistle.*
- Diuretic herbs—*Dandelion Leaf, Juniper Berries, Uva Ursi (Bearberry), Parsley, Horseradish, Buchu.*
- Nervine herbs—(for anxiety and irritability) *Vervain, Chamomile, Skullcap, Valerian.*
- Nervine herbs—(for sleeplessness) *Passiflora, Hops, Chamomile.*
- Herbs for depression and fatigue—*Damiana, Oats, Gotu Kola, Ginseng.*
- Herbs for headaches—*Fringetree, Wood Betony, Valerian, Skullcap.*
- Herbs for nausea—*Ginger, Black Horehound, Wild Yam.*
- Herbs for sore breasts—*Blue Flag, Poke Root, Thuja.*
- Herbs for pelvic congestion—(see Dysmenorrhoea).

Essential oils
Ylang Ylang is particularly effective for easing PMS, as are *Clary Sage* and *Neroli*. Use them combined (two drops of *Ylang Ylang* for every drop of *Clary Sage* and *Neroli*), in the bath or in an oil burner.

Yoga for PMS
Use the same poses as for hormone imbalance.

You may well be able to manage your PMS with a combination of some of these self-help suggestions, or you may need, or prefer, to seek professional help from a natural health practitioner.

Discharges and infections
Vaginal discharges can be due to thrush, which is Candida, or yeast, infestation. This can be caused by:

- Hot weather
- Tight trousers
- Synthetic underwear
- Constant douching
- Intercourse (semen is alkaline)
- Vaginal deodorants
- Antibiotics
- Oral contraceptives
- A lack of acidity in the vagina (normal pH 5.5) will inhibit the action of the 'good' bacteria needed to maintain vaginal health.

You may experience intense itching, burning, and a white discharge that smells yeasty. There is not usually an offensive odour, but it is different from your normal smell.

If the discharge is profuse, yellow-green, slightly foamy, smells bad (fishy) and causes itching and soreness, it may be caused by the protozoan organism—trichomonas. If it doesn't itch, isn't sore, but smells offensive, and is grey in colour, it may be a bacterial infection such as gardnerella. Trichomonas or bacterial infections may respond to herbal douches, and internal herbal medicine. For further information on genito-urinary infections see Chapter 10.

Characteristics of discharge from vaginal infections

Condition	Smell	Colour	pH	Consistency	Effect
Candida albicans	Yeasty	White	4	Curdy, thick	Itching, burning
Trichomonas	Bad (fishy)	yellow-green	5–6	Foamy, profuse	Itching, soreness
Gardnerella	Bad (fishy)	Grey	5–6	Foamy, profuse	Itching, soreness

Herbs and other supplements for vaginal discharge

Golden Seal, Echinacea, Picrorrhiza, Wild Indigo, Uva Ursi, Sage, Thyme and *Myrrh* can be taken internally, and *Pau D'Arco* is specific for Candida. These stimulate your immune system and help fight bacterial and fungal infections. Citrus extracts can be very helpful in controlling bacterial, fungal and protozoan (trichomonas) infections. Other herbs that we have previously mentioned, such as *Astragalus*, the two varieties of *Ginseng,* and mushrooms such as *Reiishi* are useful for building immunity in the long term in those individuals who have an obviously depleted immune system. Don't forget the hugely important role that all the nutrients play here, especially the anti-oxidants *Vitamins A, C, E* and *zinc*. *Vitamin C* can be taken to bowel tolerance (see Chapter 4).

Acidophilus and *Bifidus* powders or capsules will help to replenish the healthy, yeast-gobbling bacteria that you need when the yeast (thrush) has got out of control.

Garlic is another good immune stimulant. It is strongly antibacterial and antifungal, can be taken internally in large doses and can even be inserted into the vagina. A garlic oil capsule, or a clove, carefully peeled so that it isn't nicked, wrapped in gauze with a tail you can pull on, and dipped in vegetable oil, can be inserted as a pessary (change every eight hours), or you can douche with the following herbs:

Golden Seal (antibacterial)
Uva Ursi (disinfectant)
Witch Hazel (astringent to repel pathogens)
Calendula (antibacterial and antifungal).

Glycerine makes a good base for a douche, and you can add a few drops of *Tea-tree oil* for the strong antifungal and antibacterial properties. Use equal parts of all the herbs and glycerine, and always add white vinegar to help re-acidify the vagina.

Intercourse should be avoided, as it spreads the infection back and forth between partners (you should both be treated), or make sure you use condoms. Semen is alkaline, and will encourage infections. If your partner needs treatment, he can use the same herbs and treatments as you. Instead of douching, he can dunk.

Try this recipe:
Mix four drops of *Tea-tree oil* (a strong antifungal and antiseptic agent), plus two tablespoons of *white vinegar* (to re-acidify) in 1 litre of warm (purified) water. Don't use the vinegar if you have any cuts or abrasions. You can douche, bathe (in a sitz-bath, basin or bath) or soak a tampon in the mixture, depending on whether the infection is internal or external. *Never leave a tampon in place for longer than eight hours, or you could suffer Toxic Shock Syndrome.* The amount of solution required will vary according to the method used (you obviously don't need as much to dunk your tampon in as you do to sit in). Keep the proportions the same.

How to douche:

A douche has a rubber bulb attached to a plastic nozzle and can be bought from a chemist. To douche, suck up the solution by squeezing the bulb, then squirt it into your vagina. Sitting in an (empty) bath allows you to raise your hips and keep the solution in the vagina for two to three minutes. *Never douche if you are pregnant or have given birth in the last ten weeks.* Use two or three times a day, depending on the severity of the condition, until the symptoms have subsided and have stayed that way for several days, otherwise they will reappear.

Creams and lotions containing *Tea-tree oil* will soothe external itching and irritation. Tea-tree pessaries, if available, will help the internal symptoms. *Acidophilus yoghurt* (live culture) from health food outlets can also work well. It should be taken internally and/or used locally, and will also help to kill pathogens and re-acidify the vagina (see next section).

Preventive measures for avoiding vaginal infections

- Avoid recurrent use of antibiotics. Use *Acidophilus* and *Bifidus* lactobacilli after each course, to re-establish the healthy bacteria.
- Avoid taking the contraceptive pill.
- Treat your partner at the same time as yourself to avoid re-infection.
- Don't use soap, vaginal deodorants or bath preparations. Ask your pharmacist for a soap alternative.
- Don't use detergents to wash underwear (for alternatives, see Chapter 3).
- Eat wisely, and include yoghurt in your diet.
- Avoid tight trousers, synthetic underwear and pantyhose.
- Wipe from front to back (from the vagina to the anus).
- Keep your vagina acid (measure this with a pH stick available from your chemist), and douche with white vinegar or yoghurt.

Seek advice

If the condition does not respond, you should have a diagnosis carried out by a health practitioner. And, if you are having recurrent Candida infections, you will need to investigate the possibility that you are suffering from Candida systemically (in the gut). This is covered more fully in Chapter 11.

Other possible causes of discharge are:

- A retained tampon.
- Vaginal deodorants and spermicides.
- Cervical erosion.
- Infections such as chlamydia or gonorrhoea, which will need professional treatment.

A damaged cervix may respond to *Vitamin E oil* or the juice from an *Aloe Vera* plant, which you can dab on with a cotton swab. An infected cervix may respond to douches or *Garlic*. We look at more treatments for infections and other problems of the cervix later in this chapter.

Genito-urinary infections

As well as the more common infections listed in the previous section, there are other genito-urinary infections, which can affect either male or female partner, which may be sub-clinical, or cause no symptoms in the adult, but have a disastrous effect on the embryo and/or the pregnancy. The pathogens involved in these infections can cause the release of endotoxins, which lead to the release of inflammatory prostaglandins. These initiate premature contractions and weaken the amniotic membranes, which in turn leads to a miscarriage.

In Chapter 10, we look at these in greater detail, and in Chapter 9 we discuss their diagnosis, but here we want to give some further remedies that may help to deal with these, sometimes quite stubborn, infections.

Internal remedies

In the previous section on vaginal discharge we looked at herbs, mushrooms and nutrients that you can use to boost your immune system, and Chapter 4 will give you more information. The herbs *St John's Wort* and *Thuja* can be helpful for some viral infections and *Pau D'Arco* may be effective for ureaplasma. Anti-oxidant dosages will need to be raised at these times, and you can also use herbal antibacterials and immune stimulants.

An excellent internal remedy is *Citrus Seed extract*—a natural antibiotic which is made from grapefruit seeds. This has a strong antimicrobial and anti-fungal effect, and can be taken internally at a dose of 5 to 15 drops 2 to 3 times daily. It can also be used as a douche.

Acidophilus, Bifidus, and/or *lactobacillus from whey* are also essential internal remedies, and not only for Candida (thrush). Acidophilus affects the oesophagus, stomach and small intestine, and Bifidus the large intestine, or colon. They have several helpful effects. They:

- Digest lactose (so it's OK if you're lactose intolerant even though they are milk derivatives).
- Secrete H_2O_2 (hydrogen peroxide) and inhibit growth of bacteria (such as anaerobes), chlamydia, yeasts and parasites.
- Normalise pH in intestines and vagina.
- Are resistant to antibiotics and replenish bowel flora usually depleted by these drugs.
- Help to strengthen the immune system.

The lactobacillus extracted from whey is also an immunoglobulin and antibody concentrate, which will bind to the chlamydia organism, and prevent it from proliferating, allowing the body's own immune system to inactivate it.

We suggest that you take all three of the above. There are many excellent sources of *Acidophilus* and *Bifidus*, (including live yoghurt, though this is not really sufficiently concentrated to deal with an acute infection, see Contacts and Resources for sources of lactobacilli from whey). If you are lactose intolerant, avoid the whey concentrate, though you can still take *Acidophilus* and *Bifidus*, as they will help to correct this condition. However, you may need to start on a lower dose than normally suggested, and build up to the full dose over a few weeks. Your lactose intolerance should resolve eventually (see Chapter 12). For chronic infections, you will need small daily doses, spread over a few months. For acute conditions, the bigger the doses, the quicker the results!

Bilberry and *Cranberry* juices can be effective against E-coli organisms.

In some cases it may be necessary to use antibiotics which, although we are reluctant to recommend, can be the only way to shift some very stubborn infections. If this is necessary, it is essential to use *Acidophilus* and *Bifidus* simultaneously, and to continue their use afterwards, to replenish the bowel flora.

Some people can be infected with organisms which are resistant to many types of antibiotics. These super-resistant strains have developed in response to the indiscriminate use and overprescribing of these drugs. However, we have heard of some medical practitioners who have successfully used antibiotics such as penicillin in *homoeopathic* doses, (for example, one tablet taken once or twice per week). This has, apparently, been effective in treating some chronic conditions, such as mycoplasma and ureaplasma.

Topical remedies

The douches suggested in the previous section may be helpful, or you may need to use something a little stronger. *Remember, do not douche if you are pregnant or have given birth in the last ten weeks.* The all-important first step is to ensure that the vaginal environment is acidic (the pH should be 5.5) as the vaginal lactobacilli are inhibited in too alkaline an environment. Lactobacillus Acidophilus creates acidity, and vinegar can be used as a douche (see last section). As Acidophilus also has a number of other helpful actions, including the release of hydrogen peroxide, using it as an implant is very effective. The concentration of lactobacillus in yoghurt is probably not sufficient if the infection is severe, or of long standing.

Acidophilus vaginal implant Here again, the use of a combination of the whey-based lactobacillus, Acidophilus and Bifidus is most effective. Add:
1 teaspoon Probioplex powder (not if dairy intolerant)
1 teaspoon Acidophilus/Bifidus powder
to
50 g yoghurt
and implant into the vagina at night. In the morning, douche (to rinse out) with
1 teaspoon Acidophilus/Bifidus in 300 mL purified water and vinegar (if no cuts or abrasions). Repeat for 5 to 7 days.

For more severe infections If the infection is stubborn, *Tea-tree oil* (either the recipe given in the last section or a proprietary brand of gel, cream or douche base) can be used, or you may need to try H_2O_2 (hydrogen peroxide), *iodine,* or *Citrus Seed extract.*

Iodine (povidone-iodine) is often effective against chlamydia and mycoplasma, and can be used as a pessary. Insert one *Isodine* pessary (available from pharmacies), twice daily for one week. Follow this with the Acidophilus implant. The iodine rarely causes irritation or sensitivity.

A 1 per cent solution of hydrogen peroxide (H_2O_2) (available from your pharmacy) can be used as a douche, twice daily, for 4 to 5 days. Remember that the Acidophilus will also cause the release of H_2O_2.

Citrus Seed extract can also be used as a douche, by adding 1 to 3 drops per each 200 mL of (purified) water. Douche once daily for a week, or more often if required. Do not use undiluted and if irritation occurs discontinue use immediately.

As the infections you are trying to eliminate are often 'hidden' in the woman, that is, they are inside the cervix, douching will be more effective mid-cycle, when the mucus is thin, and may allow penetration into the cervix. The cervix is also open at this time (and also at menstruation). For affected men, as in the last section, dunking can replace douching, with the remedies remaining the same.

Summary of general guidelines
for GUI treatment

- Increase your immunity with herbs such as *Echinacea, Pau D'Arco* and *Picrorrhiza,* (or *Astragalus* and *Ginseng* for long-term conditions), nutrients (especially anti-oxidants such as *Vitamin C*, with *bioflavonoids*, and *zinc*, mushrooms, such as *Reiishi*, and *Garlic*.
- Take herbal antibiotic remedies internally. Useful herbs include *Golden Seal, Wild Indigo, Myrrh, Thyme, Uva Ursi, Sage, Citrus Seed extract, Bilberry* and *Cranberry* juice, or antiviral herbs, such as *St John's Wort* and *Thuja*.
- Use *Acidophilus* and *Bifidus* and whey-based lactobacilli as an implant, as well as internally.
- If necessary, use oral antibiotic therapy, but always accompanied (during, and for a week after, treatment) by Acidophilus and Bifidus taken internally.
- If necessary, use *Citrus Seed extract, Tea-tree, H_2O_2* or *iodine* topically. Remember to use mid-cycle.

- Avoid unprotected sex until the condition is cleared in *both* partners.
- Always re-acidify, using *Acidophilus* and/or *vinegar.*
- Always establish, through repeat pathology tests, that the infection has been successfully treated in both partners before ceasing treatment or attempting conception.

Herpes

Herpes blisters usually occur on the external genitalia, but occasionally on the buttocks and thighs, or inside the vagina. The risk from herpes infection is greatest to pregnant women since the chance of miscarriage increases if they contract the disease while pregnant. If there is an active outbreak around the time of birth, delivery by Caesarean section is necessary to avoid the newborn suffering possible brain damage, blindness, or death.

It is impossible to completely eliminate the herpes virus from the body, but a lot can be done to keep it dormant and treat the blisters.

Dormancy

To keep it dormant, you need to boost your immune system by:

- (Surprise, surprise) eating properly, eating more fish, though avoiding nuts which are high in arginine (especially almonds and peanuts).
- Dealing with your stress levels, and PMS.
- Cutting out smoking, alcohol, chocolate and drugs.
- Using anti-oxidants *zinc, manganese, magnesium, Vitamins A, B1, B6, E* and *C (with bioflavonoids).*
- Taking amino acid *L-lysine* (1,200 mg daily), and avoiding *arginine. Lysine*-rich foods include halibut, salmon and turkey.
- Taking *Evening primrose oil,* lots of raw seeds, fish, fish oils and cold-pressed vegetable oils.
- Taking *Echinacea, St John's Wort, Lemon Balm* and other herbal immune stimulants, such as *Reiishi* and *Shiitake* mushrooms.
- Taking *Garlic.*

Lesions

To treat lesions, use:

* *Garlic* capsules, taken *before* the lesions develop. At the first sign of tingling, take twelve capsules immediately, and then three every four hours for three days.
* *Ice* applied to the site at first appearance of symptoms.
* The homoeopathic remedy *Rhus Tox* 3–6 × potency, five to ten drops as lesions start to develop.
* *Calendula* or *Witch Hazel* extract, or ointment, applied topically.
* *Aloe vera* applied topically.
* Herbal ointment of *Solanum Nigrum.*

If you are sexually active during an outbreak, cover the blister with a sticking plaster.

Genital warts

Medical treatment for warts (or Human Papilloma Virus, HPV) is harsh. Freezing or acid-burning treatments can leave scar tissue. Laser, electrical and chemical treatments are not without problems, and may not be successful in the long term. Holistic treatment includes dietary and stress control approaches, with the accent on improving the immune system.

Thuja (pronounced 'Thoo-yah') is the wonder herb for all wart virus complaints. Taken internally, it can be extremely effective, especially given the support of immune-stimulant herbs such as *Echinacea* and *St John's Wort.* Thuja can also be used homoeopathically, although classical homoeopaths will want to treat the whole person and not just the symptoms. *Thuja must not be taken if you are pregnant.*

Tea-tree oil, Citricidal, or the fresh juice of the plant *Greater Celandine* applied topically, with the support of *Thuja* ointment, can complete the cure. Of course this should be done before conception (see previous sections on vaginal discharges and GUIs).

Hypnotherapy can also be very effective. 'Magic' or suggestion has traditionally been used for eliminating all forms of warts, using 'spells' which involve tying a string around them, or 'telling' them to go away.

Cervical dysplasia, damage or infection
Dysplasia

If a pap smear shows abnormalities, treatment should be started as soon as possible, since once you are pregnant it is better not to treat the cervix, especially with douches.

There are three degrees of severity, CIN (cervical intrepithelial neoplasia) 1, 2 or 3.

CIN 1 refers to mild dysplasia, which may not deteriorate further, with a majority of sufferers experiencing remission without any treatment.

CIN 2 involves more advanced changes, though 20 per cent of cases recover naturally.

CIN 3 involves changes to the full covering layer of the cervix. This is still not a cancerous condition, but definitely needs treatment.

Exposure to herpes and genital warts can predispose the cervix to dysplasia. Nutrient deficiencies, oral contraceptive use and cigarette smoking also increase the level of risk to CIN 1, 2 or 3, and of this condition progressing to cancer. A colposcopy allows a closer view of the cells of the cervix through a special microscope, and is normally used to confirm the diagnosis.

Natural remedies are to be preferred, as medical treatment of this condition can be quite harsh, involving cauterisation, freezing, or removal of part of the cervix (cone biopsy). However, frequent checks on progress should be made by your medical practitioner. To assist recovery:

- Avoid multiple sexual partners.
- Use natural contraception (see Chapter 7) or barrier methods until you are ready to conceive, rather than the pill.
- Stop smoking (as if you haven't already!).
- Increase all nutrients, especially *Vitamin C, beta-carotene* and *folic acid*. Research shows a typical sufferer ingests less than 30 mg Vitamin C daily, and is deficient in beta-carotene, and that this can increase the chance of cervical dysplasia by 300 per cent. *Folic acid* taken in the dose range of 10 mg daily over three months (always in conjunction with the other *B-complex vitamins*), can heal quite severe cases of dysplasia.

- You can also use the herbal remedies, internal and topical, suggested in the sections on vaginal infections, and warts (if this is part of the problem), or as follows for cervical dysplasia.

Soak a tampon in a mixture of:
Sweet almond oil 60 mL
Wheat germ (or Vitamin E) oil 20 mL
Essential oil of Thuja (if you can get it) *10 drops*
Essential oil of Cypress 10 drops

Insert the tampon in the vagina, up against the cervix, every night and *remove in the morning*.

Infections
To treat infections, the remedies suggested for vaginal discharges due to infections are relevant here.

Damage
If the cervix has been damaged, for example through medical treatment for dysplasia, or by previous infection, it may not be able to produce sufficient wet, or fertile mucus to enable the sperm to survive in the female reproductive tract. This is quite common after a cervical cone biopsy for precancerous conditions, when the mucus-producing crypts may be damaged, or removed.

If the cervix is sufficiently damaged, it will become incompetent and have to be sewn together during a pregnancy to avoid losing the foetus. Therefore, a course of treatment should always be undertaken as soon as possible after the damage occurs. Natural medicine can sometimes reverse scarring damage to tissue. You can try a course of treatment internally, including the herbs:

Golden Seal   Calendula   False Unicorn Root

and *Vitamins A, C, E* and *B-complex* with extra *folic acid,* and *zinc, selenium, calcium* and *magnesium* in adequate doses. The douche described in the section on Candida (thrush) can be helpful, as can *Vitamin E oil* or *Aloe Vera juice* (direct from the leaf) applied directly to the cervix.

'Hostile' mucus production

Even an undamaged cervix may not produce healthy mucus. 'Hostile' mucus is the main reason for mutual fertility problems (when the sperm do not survive in the female reproductive tract). Apart from cervical damage, there are four main reasons why mucus may be hostile: It may be of poor quality (lack of ferning) or insufficient quantity; it may be too acidic; it may contain sperm antibodies; or it may be toxic.

To increase fertile mucus production

If the mucus is too dense, the sperm cannot penetrate it (see Chapter 7). If only sticky, infertile mucus is produced, this is usually a result of a hormone imbalance (particularly insufficient oestrogen). Apart from developing good eating and exercise habits, you can use hormone-balancing and ovarian tonic herbs, plus mucous membrane tonics to improve the quality of mucus.

Hormone balancers—*False Unicorn Root, Dong Quai, Black Cohosh, Peony* and *Saw Palmetto.*

Mucous membrane tonics—*Golden Seal* and *Bayberry.*

Phyto-oestrogenic herbs can also help (see Irregularity and hormone balance section), if given in the pre-ovulatory phase of the cycle.

Calcium, magnesium, zinc and the celloid, or tissue salt, *potassium chloride* are essential nutrients for the fertility (wetness and stretchiness) of the mucus. Thyroid disorders can also adversely affect mucus.

Medically, oestrogen can be given.

Acidic mucus

If the mucus is too acidic, the sperm are immobilised. This can be detected by a post-coital test, which examines the mucus after intercourse to see if sperm are surviving and swimming well (see Chapter 14).

This condition is usually responsive to dietary remedies. You need to avoid eating too many *acid-producing* foods (not to be confused with foods that *are* acidic, such as tomatoes, pineapples, grapefruit, oranges and lemons, which become alkaline once digested).

Acid-forming foods—Meat, fish, eggs, all animal products, sugar, coffee and tea, alcohol, grains and seeds, plums, prunes and cranberries.

Alkali-forming foods—Nuts (especially almonds and hazelnuts), all fruit (especially cherries, though see above), all vegetables (especially alfalfa and red clover sprouts), cider vinegar.

You will get greater benefit from vegetables if you juice them, though of course you will still need to eat whole vegetables for their fibre content. A good juice base is carrot and celery, beetroot is excellent, and you can add whatever else you have available. *Alfalfa* and *Red Clover* sprouts are strong alkali-forming agents, and both these herbs can also be taken as teas or herbal extracts. Fish is less acid-forming than meat.

Until your mucus is no longer acidic, you should continue to eat a balanced diet using foods from both groups, but with the emphasis on the alkali-forming foods, especially vegetables and vegetable juices. You can test acidity with pH sticks (available from your chemist), or have a test carried out by a pathology laboratory. Your vagina should be slightly acidic (pH 5.5), although your mucus should not. The celloid sodium phosphate is a specific remedy.

Chemical douches and lubricants may also kill sperm, as can saliva. The only safe lubricant to use, if you are trying to conceive, is raw egg white. This should bring a note of hilarity into your conception attempt, just in case it has become too clinical!

Sperm antibodies

If the mucus contains sperm antibodies, the sperm are also immobilised. This is a result of the woman's body (it can happen in the man's body, too) reacting to the sperm as to an allergenic substance— an invading pathogen, from which it needs to protect itself. High toxin levels (such as lead) in the sperm may contribute to this reaction.

Medical treatment for this condition involves taking immuno-suppressive or antihistamine drugs, which have many undesirable side-effects, or, more commonly, by direct referral to an IVF program.

Natural medicine attempts to re-educate the woman's immune system, and ensure that her cervical mucus is not a channel for toxic-waste elimination. Detoxification of the male is also necessary to prevent the woman's body rejecting the toxic sperm but, of course, your preconception care will automatically include detoxification procedures. A condom should be used (for up to six months) to allow the body's reaction to subside, and the immune system treated with diet, supplements and herbal or homoeopathic medicine, while the detoxification program is followed.

Herbs which improve appropriate immune response and reduce sensitivity and allergic reactions have been detailed in the section on the immune system. The *Reiishi mushroom* is specific for reducing an overproduction of antibodies.

Sperm antibodies

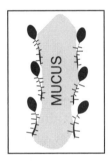 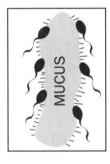 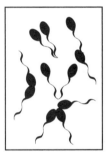

Sperm antibodies in the male cause the tails of the sperm to stick to the cervical mucus

Sperm antibodies in the female cause the heads of the sperm to stick to the cervical mucus

Sperm antibodies cause the sperm to stick together (agglutination) head to head, head to tail and tail to tail

While you are following these treatments, you can learn to recognise signs of fertility by charting symptoms such as cervical mucus changes and basal body temperature readings (see Chapters 7 and 13). This will help you to ensure that the condom is removed *only at the moment of your conception attempt.* This prevents your body having time to produce antibodies and build up sensitivity again. This treatment has the added benefit of making sure that you start your pregnancy with a healthy immune system, so you will be less likely to suffer allergies during your pregnancy, which can be transmitted to the baby.

Toxic mucus

If your mucus is toxic, it may kill or immobilise sperm. Since the mucus is a channel for detoxification, these processes must be completed well before conception is attempted.

Diagnosis and treatment

To diagnose the exact nature, and cause, of any problems with cervical mucus, and to put into effect relevant remedies, you should consult a health practitioner, and refer (with him or her) to this section and to Chapter 14, section on 'Non-invasive tests'.. Medically, the answer to mutual fertility problems is to use IVF procedures. Luckily, much can be done using natural remedies, and in many cases the situation can be resolved without recourse to such programs.

Breast lumps

Not all breast lumps are cancerous, although if you do find one it is important to have it investigated by a health practitioner. You may find you have a tendency to 'benign' lumpiness in the post-ovulatory phase. This is called fibrocystic breast disease, although there is some doubt about whether it really is a disease. Cysts filled with fluid develop in the breasts, causing lumps, pain and swelling.

Fibroadenomas are lumps that do not fluctuate with the menstrual period. They can be removed surgically, although there is a great deal that you can do before resorting to this. X-rays and surgery are contraindicated during pregnancy, even though these problems are often exacerbated at this time.

Professional supervision is recommended, although there is much that you can do to help yourself.

Useful supplements

- *Vitamin B-complex* (especially *B1, B3* and *B6*), *C* and *E, selenium, zinc, manganese, calcium* and *magnesium*. Remember, you need a prescription for selenium.
- *Garlic* supplements with *allicin* and *selenium* (high dose, 500 mg garlic three times daily with food).
- *Evening primrose oil.*

Useful herbs

- Diuretic herbs (see PMS section this chapter) may help temporarily.
- Liver herbs may be useful to help eliminate excess oestrogen, (which exacerbates the problem), and to deal with fats. Try *St Mary's Thistle* or *Dandelion Root.*
- *Violet Leaves, Blue Flag* and *Poke Root.* Take care with *Poke Root,* it can be toxic, and the dosage is critical. *Do not take during pregnancy.* (In fact, don't take anything in pregnancy that is not absolutely necessary, and that has not been shown to be completely safe.) *Poke Root (Phytolacca Decandra)* is also very useful as an ointment, as is *St John's Wort,* and bruised, wet or steamed *cabbage leaves* make a good poultice.
- Massaging the breasts can also help.
- Avoid alcohol, coffee, saturated fats, dairy foods, refined carbohydrates, salt and cigarettes because they may all be part of the problem. Make sure that all chickens are organically fed and free-range, in this way you avoid ingesting artificial hormones. Try to find organically fed meats, and remember to trim off all the fat.

Endometriosis

This is a condition in which the uterine lining (endometrium) breaks off and enters the abdominal cavity, where it grows in an abnormal situation, such as attached to the Fallopian tubes, the ovaries or behind the uterus. Blood-filled cysts may form on the ovaries. Since this migrating tissue is part of the endometrium, it builds up each month and then bleeds as usual, although the blood is unable to leave the body with the menstrual flow.

This condition usually causes pain which may worsen before, during or after menstruation. It may not be the bleeding which causes the pain, but a chemical reaction in the endometrial 'implants' that irritates the lining of the pelvis. There may also be lower backache, pain on intercourse, or, sometimes, no symptoms at all.

In severe cases, the scarring, distortion of tissue, or formation of adhesions where the endometrium has attached, can cause infertility. Endometriosis can also lead to infertility in less severe cases, where the reasons are not so obvious, though these may be to do with an effect on the sperm. Altogether, 40 per cent of women suffering from this condition will have fertility problems, and 30 per cent of female infertility is due to it. The cause of the disease is not clear, though hormone imbalance, inflammation and immunological dysfunction are all contributing factors.

Medically, it is diagnosed by laparoscopy, and treated with drugs which suppress ovulation (and menstruation), or with laser surgery. Some of the drugs used are based on male hormones, and can increase male characteristics.

We know of at least one case, when conception occurred within a short period of the use of these drugs, where the female offspring subsequently developed a severe case of hirsutism (facial and body hair) to the point of needing a full face and upper body waxing at the start of each day; as well as deepening of the voice. Fortunately for this young woman, treatment with natural remedies such as herbs and nutrients has brought about a significant reduction in her testosterone levels. Of course, whether her unfortunate condition can definitely be attributed to the effects of the drugs given to her mother cannot be confirmed without further generational studies, but we believe that her case provides a very strong argument for avoiding all drugs in the months before conception!

In fact, surveys show that although drugs may reduce the occurrence of endometriosis (in the short term though not necessarily in the long term, since they do not deal with the root cause of the disease), they do not improve the pregnancy rate, since the problems of scarring and adhesions, which are already affecting the reproductive system, are not treated. Laser surgery is required to remove as many adhesions as possible, although some of these, as well as any severe scarring, may not be amenable to medical treatment.

Natural remedies for endometriosis can be very successful, and though treatment may be rather prolonged to reach a complete remission, symptoms are often alleviated soon after initiating treatment. As well as natural medicines, yoga can be very helpful. If you suffer from endometriosis, please seek professional help.

Herbal treatment

This focuses on several areas:
- Hormone-balancing herbs—to reduce excessive oestrogen. This can include phyto-oestrogens which can be most effective (not

in excessive amounts). *Chaste Tree, Sarsaparilla, Wild Yam, Fenugreek, False Unicorn Root, Peony.*

- Alterative and lymphatic drainage herbs—to reduce congestion and toxicity. *Calendula, Poke Root* (remember previous warnings), *Cleavers, Thuja, Red Clover, Burdock.*
- Liver herbs—to detoxify and reduce blood fat levels. *Dandelion Root, St Mary's Thistle, Burdock, Bupleurum, Globe Artichoke, Salvia, Schisandra.*
- Anti-inflammatory herbs—*Wild Yam, Liquorice, Rehmannia, Feverfew, White Dead Nettle.*
- Immuno-suppressive and anti-allergic herbs—To deal with any allergic or auto-immune factors. *Hemidesmus, Albizzia, Baical Skullcap, Siberian Ginseng, Astragalus, Rehmannia.*
- Herbs to protect against infection—*Golden Seal, Echinacea, Wild Indigo, Garlic.*
- Uterine 'tonic' herbs—*Blue Cohosh, Dong Quai, True Unicorn Root.*
- Astringent herbs to reduce bleeding—*Shepherd's Purse, Beth Root, Ladies' Mantle, Cranesbill, Periwinkle, White Dead Nettle, Raspberry.*
- Pain-relieving herbs—*Pulsatilla, Cramp Bark, Wild Yam, Black Haw, Motherwort, Peony.*

Important supplements

Supplements that are particularly useful include:

- *Zinc*—for immune function, tissue repair, hormone balance and detoxification (dosage 20 to 60 mg daily according to Zinc Tally, see Chapter 9).
- *Vitamin A*—for immune function, tissue repair and detoxification (10,000 iu or 6 mg beta-carotene daily).
- *Vitamin E*—for immune function, hormone balance, circulation, detoxification, as a pain (prostaglandin) inhibitor, anti-inflammatory and for scar tissue (1,000 to 2,000 iu daily).
- *Vitamin C*—(*with bioflavonoids*) for immune function, detoxification and tissue repair (to bowel tolerance).
- *Evening primrose oil*—as a hormone balancer and anti-inflammatory (high doses here—6,000 mg daily).

- *MaxEPA*—for more essential fatty acids (also high doses—4,000 mg daily)
- *Garlic*—to reduce infection, congestion and blood lipids.
- *Celloids*—*sodium sulphate* and *sodium phosphate* (to help liver drainage), *iron phosphate* (to reduce inflammation), *potassium chloride* (for endocrine, glandular health and lymphatic drainage), *magnesium phosphate* (for pain).

Dietary recommendations

Foods containing saturated fats, especially dairy foods, may aggravate the situation. Endometriosis sufferers frequently eat excessive amounts of cheese (made from cow's milk).

Avoid animal products which contain saturated fats and eat foods containing the helpful essential fatty acids (fish, olive oil).

Other remedies

- Systemic Candida often accompanies endometriosis, and treatment for this condition is an important part of full recovery.
- Castor oil packs on the abdomen, of two hours duration, three times weekly, can be an effective remedy. However, this is a difficult condition for self-help, and it is usually best to seek professional advice, while taking all possible precautions yourself.
- Pregnancy is often offered as a cure when the disease is mild, as the nine-month period free of ovulation and menstruation can allow healing to occur. However, if the underlying cause is not dealt with there may be a recurrence. Other treatments (including the herbal ones outlined above) would need to be concluded before conception. Indeed, the medical drugs used would make conception impossible.
- Many practitioners in clinical practice find that endometriosis seems to be more common in women who have a history of sexual abuse, and this could be an important consideration in treatment. Therapy such as counselling or hypnotherapy may be useful, and the flower essences may have a role to play (see Chapter 6).
- Yoga (see Irregularity and hormonal balance section) has been found to be particularly helpful in resolving endometriosis.

Pelvic inflammatory disease (PID)

This is an infection or inflammation of the pelvic organs, including the Fallopian tubes (when it is also called salpingitis) and of the ovaries and uterus. The infection responsible may be of the genito-urinary type (GUI) such as chlamydia or gonorrhoea, or may be caused by an IUD, dilation and curettage (D and C), termination or a pelvic operation. PID can be exacerbated by systemic Candida. If the cause of this condition is GUI, or if Candida is present, it is also necessary for your partner to be treated.

Diagnosis is normally confirmed through laparoscopy, but may be achieved through symptom analysis. However, the main problem is that you may be asymptomatic (without symptoms) until the condition is well advanced, when scarring or adhesions to the tubes may already be such as to cause infertility, or ectopic pregnancy. The increase in white cell production in a woman with PID can kill sperm in her reproductive tract.

Symptoms

If symptoms are experienced they may include:

- Feeling unwell, loss of appetite, nausea, vomiting, chills.
- Severe lower abdominal pain, usually on both sides, aggravated by movement or sexual activity.
- Abnormal, possibly offensive, vaginal discharge.
- Irregular vaginal bleeding.
- Raised temperature and fever.
- Tender uterus.
- Pelvic swelling.
- Worsening of all symptoms after menstruation.
- Pain starting pre-menstrually, and occurring at other times during the cycle.

About 2 per cent of sexually active women are affected each year, and of these, after one attack, 14 per cent will be infertile; after two attacks, 40 per cent will be infertile; and after three attacks, 80 per cent will be infertile. Another subsequent risk is ectopic pregnancy.

Medical treatment of PID is with antibiotics. If you decide on this course you must remember to use *Acidophilus* and *Bifidus* to replace normal bacterial flora, and to prevent Candida infection.

Natural remedies

- Anti-inflammatory, immune-stimulant and antiviral herbs, including *Echinacea, Astragalus, Calendula, Golden Seal, Wild Indigo, Wild Yam, Feverfew, Poke Root* (do not use this herb if attempting conception or if you are pregnant) and *Thuja* are recommended (the same ruling applies).
- Increase your body's resistance to infection through maintaining good nutrition. *Vitamin C* (5 g or more, with *bioflavonoids*), *Garlic* (two capsules, three times daily), *zinc* (50 mg or more), *Vitamin A* (10,000 iu or *beta-carotene* 6 mg), *selenium* (100 to 200 mcg), *Vitamin E* (500 to 1,000 iu) plus general supplements, including *Evening primrose oil*, will all help, when taken daily.
- Saturated fats should be avoided.
- Systemic Candida must also be treated if suspected.

If the cause of PID is genito-urinary infection (see section in this chapter and Chapter 10), your partner should be checked, and treated, if necessary, to avoid re-infection. Avoid tampons, douching and having intercourse while your cervix is open (that is, during your period and at mid-cycle) or until you are both declared free of infection. All treatment, medical or natural, should be carried out by a health professional, as antibiotics may be necessary to avoid scarring on the Fallopian tubes, which can result from prolonged infection.

Blocked Fallopian tubes

Your Fallopian tubes may be blocked either by adhesions or by scarring. This may be caused by conditions such as endometriosis, appendicitis, peritonitis (inflammation of the membrane lining the abdominal cavity) or by infection, such as in PID. An accurate diagnosis and relevant treatment will be best achieved with professional help.

Scarring may be reduced by the use of *zinc, magnesium, selenium* and *Vitamins A* and *E*. Herbs such as *Calendula* and *Golden Seal* and the tissue salts *potassium chloride* and *silica* can also be effective. Medically, there is the possibility of microsurgery, though this does not have a high rate of success.

Tubes may also be blocked with mucus. This is a common reaction to allergenic foods. Foods to avoid are the common allergens such as dairy produce (from cow's milk and related products), wheat, yeast and eggs. You may have other allergies which may also contribute to this problem.

Herbs such as *Garlic, Fenugreek, Golden Seal, Golden Rod* and *Horseradish* can help to clear the congestion. The tissue salt *potassium chloride* is also beneficial. If your tubes remain blocked, assisted reproduction technology, such as IVF, may be necessary, although sometimes the passage of dye during laparoscopy or hysterosalpingogram (see Chapter 14) may clear the blockage.

Even if the tubes are not blocked, there may be a problem with the transport of the sperm or fertilised egg. This is dependent on the cilia, which may become damaged, and be unable to perform their task effectively. *Zinc, magnesium, selenium* and *Vitamin A* will help.

The tubes also assist the movement of eggs and sperm through the pulsating action of their walls. This action is hormonally controlled, and will benefit from general remedies for hormonal health. The same action has recently been recognised as occurring in the uterus, and helps the sperm on their upward journey. As one medical practitioner noted 'sperm are not salmon—they can't swim upstream!'

Adhesions

These may result from infection, from pelvic surgery, or from an acute condition such as a burst appendix. Adhesions can cause dysmenorrhoea, and if they are on the ovaries, can affect ovarian function. Adhesions may also block the Fallopian tubes, or obstruct implantation of the embryo, if they are inside the uterus, thus leading to infertility. If there are adhesions in your bowel you may suffer disruption to digestion and pain.

Medically adhesions can be treated by cutting, but this involves (further) surgery which will have its own risks.

- *Silica, zinc* and *Vitamins A* and *E* can help to soften adhesions if they are not too severe.
- *Selenium, calcium* and *magnesium* are also important nutrients.
- Lymphatic drainage herbs such as *Calendula* and *Cleavers* can help, and the homoeopathic remedy *Mustard seeds* (3 × potency) has been known to correct even severe cases.

It's best to consult a health professional for effective treatment.

Uterine fibroids

Fibroids are non-malignant tumours of the muscle wall of the uterus. Over one-third of women over the age of 35 will have one or more fibroid. They do not necessarily cause symptoms, but can result in heavy bleeding, painful periods, backache and swelling.

They start off tiny, grow past pea-size, golf-ball size, and may end up resembling a tennis ball or grapefruit. They are sensitive to oestrogen, which causes them to grow, sometimes to enormous sizes. This means that pregnancy and oral contraceptives will accelerate growth, although they will usually shrink after menopause, unless hormone replacement therapy is given. They have been known to weigh as much as nine kilos. If the fibroids grow outward, they can be felt as lumps, if inward, they can restrict the passage of sperm, or the implantation of the fertilised ovum.

Fibroids can be removed by surgery. The uterus can be reconstructed (myomectomy) or in severe cases, hysterectomy can be performed. They are sometimes treated medically with *Lucrin,* a drug that suppresses ovarian function, and therefore the release of oestrogen, which causes fibroid growth.

Naturopathically, they are treated with herbal medicine, homoeopathy or acupuncture, together with a very strict diet. This means eating lots of fresh vegetables and avoiding fats, dairy products and foods containing synthetic oestrogens, such as meat from animals or birds which have been hormonally treated. Phyto-oestrogenic foods, in moderation, will be helpful as they reduce excessive oestrogen. *Alfalfa* and *soya* products such as *soya milk* and *tofu* are important although they must not be taken in excess. See the Irregularity and hormonal balance section.

Herbs and supplements

- Important nutrients—are *magnesium, zinc* and *Evening primrose oil,* and these should be taken in reasonably high doses, along with the full range of supporting vitamins and minerals. Celloid or tissue salt *potassium chloride* is also supportive, as is *sodium sulphate* for liver function.
- Liver herbs—are important to eliminate excess oestrogen and to deal with fat. Try *St Mary's Thistle* and *Dandelion Root.*

- Hormone-balancing herbs—such as *Damiana, False Unicorn Root, Dong Quai* and especially *Chaste Tree, Wild Yam, Peony* and *Fenugreek* are useful.
- Traditional herbal remedies—include *Thuja, Poke Root* (remember the warnings about these two herbs), *Blue Flag, Red Clover, Turmeric, Bayberry* and *Violet Leaves*.
- Lymphatic drainage herbs—such as *Calendula, Cleavers*.
- Astringent herbs—to shrink the tissue: *Ladies' Mantle, Sarsaparilla, Raspberry, Cranesbill, Periwinkle* and if there is excessive bleeding add *Shepherd's Purse* and *Beth Root.*

Treatment may need to be lengthy, especially for large fibroids, and may not always be successful. However many cases respond quickly and reduction can be substantial, and often complete. Fibroids are not a common cause of infertility problems, and if the symptoms are not severe, do not present a great threat. However, since they grow during pregnancy, and can press on the foetus, it is best to attempt treatment before conception. Professional help should be sought.

Retroverted uterus

Don't worry! 20 per cent of women have a uterus which is tipped back. It is not a cause of fertility or reproductive problems.

Ovarian cysts

These are fluid containing swellings in the ovary which are usually only a few centimetres in diameter. Occasionally, the cysts become cancerous or grow larger. They can also be caused by endometriosis (when they are filled with blood). If they twist, rupture or bleed, they can cause severe pain. More frequently, a follicle in the ovary can develop into a type of small, relatively harmless, thin-walled cyst. This causes few, if any, of the symptoms of the full-grown version, and tends to disappear spontaneously. Diagnosis is through palpation, ultrasound or laparoscopy.

You may experience no symptoms, or suffer, among other things, swelling or intermittent pain especially during menstruation, ovulation and sexual intercourse. The small, non-malignant cysts may persist for years without symptoms, whereas malignant cysts grow rapidly and can spread. Thyroid dysfunction has been associated with ovarian cystic disease.

Benign and small cysts aren't really a problem, but they can be treated. *Vitamins E* and *B-complex* are needed and herbal medicines are very effective, although the treatment may need to continue for some months, and should be supervised by a health professional.

Herbal remedies

- Anti-cystic herbs—*Thuja, Poke Root, Red Clover, Violet Leaves, Blue Flag.*
- Lymphatic drainage herbs—*Calendula, Cleavers.*
- Circulatory stimulants—*Ginger, Prickly Ash, Cayenne.*
- Organ remedies—*Chaste Tree, False Unicorn Root, Golden Seal.*
- Anti-congestive remedies—*Garlic, Fenugreek.*
- Liver drainage remedies—*St Mary's Thistle, Dandelion Root.*

A good herbal formula on which to base individual treatment is *Poke Root* (take great care with this herb—it can be toxic if the low, safe dosage is exceeded), *Calendula, Thuja, Fenugreek, Golden Seal, Ginger* and *False Unicorn Root. This formula must not be used while attempting to conceive.* Conception will have to wait until treatment is concluded.

Foods to avoid include dairy produce, fats and any toxic additives.

Larger cysts may respond to similar treatment, but attention may need to be directed to an associated underlying condition. If the cyst does not respond, and is large enough to impair ovarian function, it can be surgically drained or removed.

Polycystic ovarian syndrome (PCOS)

In this condition, there are multiple follicular cysts on the ovaries, which may show as enlarged in ultrasound or during laparoscopy. Multiple follicles start to grow, and, in the more severe conditions, none ripen sufficiently to release an egg. There is often, therefore, irregularity or an inability to ovulate. This can be confirmed through temperature readings or blood tests to show progesterone levels. 35 per cent of female infertility, and 40 per cent of amenorrhoea, is due to PCO syndrome.

The syndrome is caused by an abnormality in the pituitary or hypothalamus or an imbalance between the ovarian and adrenal hormones. There is often excessive production of male hormones, and symptoms can include hirsutism (facial hair), acne and obesity.

Blood tests will often show raised testosterone levels, and raised LH (luteinising hormone) as the pituitary attempts to 'wake up' the resistant ovaries. Sufferers of PCO syndrome often have normal levels of oestrogen, and this may bring increased risk of uterine and breast cancers, due to the lack of ovulation, which leaves the oestrogen unopposed by progesterone.

Medical treatment is with ovarian stimulatory drugs such as clomiphene citrate (Clomid) which can trigger ovulation through stimulating FSH release from the pituitary gland. However, this does not treat the cause of the disease, and may in fact exacerbate the problem, as many follicles are stimulated simultaneously, and normal hormonal balance may be further disrupted. An oversensitive response to these ovarian stimulant drugs can actually induce a polycystic condition.

Natural treatments are similar to those outlined for ovarian cysts, with emphasis on detoxification of the whole system. Hormone-balancing herbs, such as *Chaste Tree,* can be useful, as they bring down testosterone levels, though this herb should *not* be used if LH levels are also high (which they often are). *Black Cohosh* will help to lower LH, as may *Bugleweed* or *Hops.* Increasing oestrogen levels, through the use of *False Unicorn Root, Dong Quai* and again *Black Cohosh,* as well as the phyto-oestrogens can be useful, though it's important to avoid any sources of synthetic oestrogens or steroids. Two herbs that have proven very effective are *Liquorice* to reduce androgens and *Peony* to stimulate female hormone levels.

Treatments for normal pancreatic function can help, as increased insulin can also be a contributing factor. *Zinc, magnesium, chromium* and *vanadium* are important nutrients here. Weight reduction is also critical as sufferers are frequently obese.

Treatment with natural remedies is often successful, with the ovaries reverting to normal size and function. Though this type of treatment can be prolonged, it has an advantage over drug therapy in that the condition is often completely resolved. Acupuncture and herbs combine most successfully for treatment of polycystic ovaries, although professional help is required.

Before we finish looking at female reproductive health, we would like to re-emphasise the importance of our pet topic, *nutrition!* All of the remedies included here for reproductive health will only be truly effective if you follow our advice in Chapter 1.

MALE FERTILITY

At last! You men must have wondered if we'd forgotten all about
you! Well, babies have fathers too—and this is where we look at any
reproductive problems that you might have which will hinder your
quest for healthy offspring. Male fertility problems are generally
acknowledged as being as prevalent as those affecting the female,
and although studies give varying figures, the causes of a couple's
infertility are approximately assessed as:

30 per cent female fertility problems
30 per cent male fertility problems
20 per cent mutual problems
20 per cent unexplained problems.

Male fertility is less complex and therefore much more easily
assessed than female. It may be helpful, if you are planning to
conceive a child soon, to have a semen analysis performed. This test,
though perhaps a little embarrassing for some, is not surgically
intrusive or painful and has no possible side-effects, unlike the tests
that need to be carried out to assess female fertility (see Chapter 14).

The other difference between tests for male and female fertility
is that, as the only factor in real need of assessment is the viability
of the sperm, (which are readily available), the results are much more
conclusive. After allowing for periodic fluctuation by having more
than one test, for the effects of prior abstinence (by varying this from
one to five days) and for the effects of stress associated with the test
which can prevent the sperm being added to the semen, a clear
picture of the viability of the sperm can emerge.

This will tell you whether you have sufficient numbers of sperm
per millilitre of semen (count), whether they move well (motility)
and in the right direction (progressive motility), and whether or not
they are deformed (morphology). It will also tell you if the volume
and viscosity of the semen is adequate, and if pH levels are appropriate (not too acidic).

It will not tell you, however, whether your sperm contain too
many toxins or insufficient nutrients to form a really healthy embryo.
Although medically speaking a sample may actually be considered
viable, there may be indications that the conception resulting from
these sperm will be less than optimally healthy. This is why it's so

important to follow the advice in the rest of this book. Toxicity and nutrient status are not measured in a semen analysis, but poor motility or lots of abnormally shaped sperm will give an indication that these factors are of concern, and need particular attention.

Other possible causes of fertility problems for the male are:

- *Hormonal imbalance*—e.g. excessive prolactin or raised LH and FSH, which can cause damage to the testes, other malfunctions of the pituitary or hypothalamus glands or inadequate testosterone.
- *Damage to testicles*—from drugs, surgery or radiation or from TB, mumps or gonorrhoea.
- *Effect of certain drugs*—antibiotics, steroids, beta-blockers, calcium channel blockers and ACE inhibitors.
- *Blocked tubes*—see previous section for females.
- *Excessive heat.*
- *Antibody production*—see previous section for females.
- *Undescended testicles*—(surgery is possible).
- *Varicocele* (varicose veins) *in the testicles*—(surgery is possible, though often not effective).
- *Infection*—of prostate or seminal vesicles.
- *Abnormal penile erection* or ejaculation—usually a stress or emotional reaction.
- *Stress*—especially through its effect on the adrenal glands.
- *Nutrient deficiencies* and high toxin levels.
- *Excessive exercise*—though you do need enough.

Sperm *morphology*, as well as count and motility are all adversely affected by cigarette smoking, alcohol and other mutagenic agents such as chemicals, drugs, environmental toxins and nutrient deficiencies. Adverse effects may be exerted directly or through reduction in nutrient status.

So—it's a squeaky clean life you need to live if you want to have healthy sperm!

Heat is very damaging to sperm which is why the testes hang in the scrotum, outside the body cavity, where it is too hot for them. Pressure is also bad news. Consequently, saunas, hot baths, tight trousers or underpants, and wetsuits are all potential sources of problems, as is sitting on anything hot, such as an engine, or even

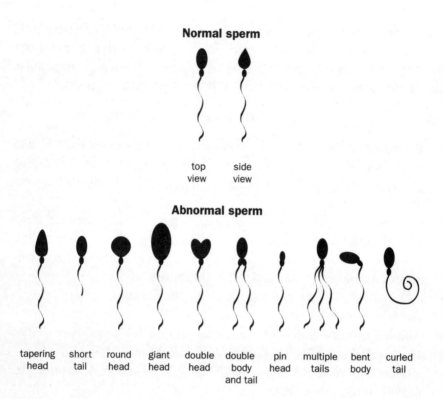

Normal sperm

top view   side view

Abnormal sperm

tapering head   short tail   round head   giant head   double head   double body and tail   pin head   multiple tails   bent body   curled tail

just sitting for prolonged periods in a warm or hot environment—so wear loose trousers and boxer shorts. If necessary, you can even dunk the testicles in cold water to cool them down—do this for a few minutes, several times a day!

Remember—it takes approximately three months for sperm to mature—so you need a *minimum of four months preconception care*, since the sperm now being ejaculated began their formation in the health conditions which prevailed three months previously. This also means that there's no point repeating your semen analysis at intervals of less than this, and expecting to see much change.

Remedies for improving male fertility
Nutrition

Remember—all the advice in this book refers to *both* prospective parents! All attempts to improve the health and numbers of sperm will be compromised if you are nutrient deficient.

Above all—enjoy your food! If this means making lots of changes, find an affirmation that you can use to help you feel good about making positive choices. As we have said, a good diet is essential, but so are your supplements. *Anti-oxidants* are of particular value, and, in fact, in a healthy and fertile man, seminal and prostatic fluids are high in these, especially *zinc* and *selenium*.

Oxidative activity has been shown to have an extremely deleterious effect on sperm. One effect of reduced levels of anti-oxidants is that the sperm will become hyperactive while still in the male reproductive tract. They are not supposed to get this excited until they make contact with the female's cervical mucus, and this 'premature excitation' can result in them becoming exhausted before they have reached their goal!

Other helpful supplements

Bee Pollen has a reputation for being a fertility booster for men, and also *octacosanol*, a substance that is found in wheat-germ oil, also high in *Vitamin E*. These can be obtained from your health food shop.

The following amino acids are needed for sperm production and motility, and healthy testes. *Arginine* (specific for count, but not if there is a history of herpes)—2–4 g, 3 × daily; *Carnitine* (specific for motility and count and morphology)—600–1200 mg, 3 × daily; *Histidine* (specific for motility)—300–600 mg, 3 × daily, between meals with water.

See also the nutrients suggested in Chapter 1, but note that requirements for *Calcium*, *Magnesium* and *Vitamin B6* will be lower than the doses suggested in Chapter 1, because men need less of these than women: *Calcium* 400 mg; *Magnesium* 200 mg; *Vitamin* B6 50 mg daily.

Helpful herbs and remedies

Herbal remedies are extremely effective in resolving male fertility problems, especially when they are combined with nutritional supplementation, exercise, detoxification and stress control. We will look at some specific examples in the following sections, along with some helpful techniques which can be used prior to the conception attempt.

Acupressure points for male fertility

There are several points which are useful to increase male fertility. *(These points should not be used on a pregnant female.)*

Conception vessel 6—On a vertical line, two finger widths (second finger locates the point) below the navel. Tonify this point.

Conception vessel 4—On the same line, four finger widths (fourth finger touches the spot) below the navel. Tonify this point.

Conception vessel 2—On the same line, at the crest of the pubis. Tonify.

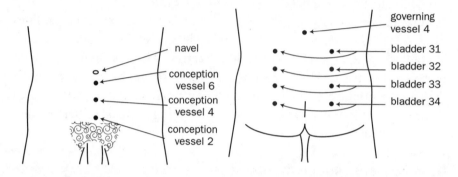

Finding Conception Vessel 2, 4 and 6

Finding Governing Vessel 4 and Bladder 31, 32, 33 and 34

Bladder 31, 32, 33 and 34—Along each side of the sacrum to the tip of the coccyx. These four points run down either side of the spine, parallel to the four fused vertebrae of the sacrum. The points are three finger widths on each side of the backbone. Tonify.

Governing vessel 4—Between the third and fourth lumbar vertebrae. Tonify.

Hormonal imbalance

See the previous section on female fertility for ideas on lowering raised prolactin, LH and FSH. Testosterone levels can be raised with the use of many herbs, and most of our clients find this results in increased vigour, body hair, sexual appetite and a deeper voice, all symptoms of increased male sex hormone levels, and traditional signs of virility.

Herbs which are effective include:

Panax Ginseng   *Oat Seed*   *Sarsaparilla*
Ginkgo   *Gotu Kola*   *Damiana*

Low sperm count

Good nutrition and stress reduction will make a huge difference to sperm production. As we have already suggested, stress at the time of ejaculation can result in little or no sperm being added to the semen. Stress may also have more long-term effects, especially through its action on nutrient levels and on adrenal function. Herbal remedies are valuable adjuncts to your attempts to reduce stress in your life, and if this is an important consideration for you, the *oats seeds*, used for low sperm count, can be replaced by a fresh tincture of *green oats*. Other helpful herbs for stressed male adrenals are *Witharia*, *Schisandra* and *Liquorice*. If treatment for the prostate is indicated, you can add these herbs to your mix: *Saw Palmetto* and *Pygeum*.

A dysfunctional hypothalamus can also be part of the problem (see 'Female Reproductive Health' earlier this chapter). Herbs for lymphatic congestion such as *Cleavers* and *Calendula* and the celloid or tissue salt, *potassium chloride,* may be helpful to clear congestion and toxicity.

Abstaining from sex for 3 to 5 days prior to the act of intercourse, which is timed to occur just before ovulation is due (see Chapter 7), will normally result in a higher sperm count. This can be clarified, if necessary, by doing two or more semen analyses after different intervals of abstinence. Abstinence for more than five days can be counterproductive, as the available sperm will be too old.

Abstinence, as a way of boosting sperm count, can be improved upon by using techniques that form part of the Tantric Yoga tradition. This is a form of yoga that uses the sexual act as a meditative practice, and encourages certain levels of control over ejaculation. The Tantric pump technique was developed in response to oriental philosophy which teaches that semen is a concentrated and valuable essence of fluids and energy, to be nurtured and not indiscriminately wasted. This is reflected in the Monty Python jingle, which was intended as a satire on Roman Catholic attitudes to contraception.

> *Every sperm is sacred,*
> *Every sperm is great,*
> *If a sperm gets wasted,*
> *God gets quite irate!*

This has a further meaning, these days, given the recent use of the word 'wasted' to mean stoned or intoxicated! Normally, Western medical attitudes to frequency of ejaculation are that it has no effect on the health of the individual. However, the Tantric pump, which is sometimes referred to as 'sensual sex,' although intended to be used to preserve the man's health and 'life-force', can also be used to increase sperm count.

Sensual sex can be practised in the five-day period of abstinence prior to your conception attempt and also at other times. It involves intimate contact, with extensive and prolonged foreplay but no ejaculation. When the urge for orgasm becomes too strong for comfort, sexual contact is ceased until the penis is flaccid. You can try a cold shower, or a run around the block, or a game of Scrabble! Then, sensual contact is resumed.

The idea is that the erotic stimulation, coupled with the gaining and losing of erection, acts, over a period of time, as a 'pump' to increase sexual energy and sperm quantity and quality.

Obviously, this technique should only be used by those who have sufficient control, or the period of abstinence will be interrupted.

The same idea is behind the suggestion that at the conception attempt itself, foreplay should be extensive, raising the sexual energy, and providing for another possible boost to the numbers of sperm in the semen.

Your sperm count may also be higher at times which correspond with a fertility biorhythm, the lunar cycle. We talk more about this cycle and its effect on fertility in Chapters 7 and 13, when we look at timing for contraception and conception, but it's worth noting that there may be a boost to sperm count occurring once a lunar month, when the moon phase which was present at the time of the man's birth recurs.

There is substantial evidence that this biorhythm, which starts at the moment of birth, seems to have a peaking effect on female fertility once a lunar month, but there is only anecdotal evidence that it causes an increase in sperm count. We have carried out semen analyses at 'peak' times, and half-way between two peaks (at a trough) and found that in a reasonable proportion of cases the count is considerably higher (sometimes up to tenfold) at the biorhythm peaks. A study of a (small) sample of men in England returned similar findings.

In cases where the sperm count is low, it may be worth attempting conception at this peak time. As this may not coincide with a fertile time in the woman, some manipulation of her cycle may be necessary. Whether this is desirable, and how to achieve it, is discussed further in Chapter 7.

Low levels of motility

Thorough detoxification and good nutrition are important to help remedy this problem, and avoidance of drugs, radiation and chemicals is mandatory. The main herbs to use are those mentioned in Chapter 4 which focus on the liver and lymphatic drainage. *Zinc* and *Vitamin C* are particularly important, and an extra herb to add to those already mentioned is *Astragalus.* Another helpful supplement is *Co-enzyme Q10* which will also help to raise the sperm count. You also need to check for infections.

High levels of abnormal sperm

High levels of abnormal sperm are an even surer indication of poor nutrition and high toxicity and studies show they are related to an increased rate of miscarriage. A hair analysis will give more specific indications of both (see Chapter 9). The anti-oxidants, such as *zinc, Vitamins A, C* and *E* and *selenium* will all be required in substantial doses, as well as all the detoxification herbs and remedies previously indicated.

Too much ejaculate

You might suspect that a low volume would be a problem, and in fact this may indicate low fluid intake (drink more water) or a general lack of reproductive health (use the supplements and herbs already suggested). However, if the volume of ejaculate is too high it may 'dilute' the viable sperm.

The 'split ejaculate' is a good way of getting around this problem. In this technique, only the first and healthiest gush of the ejaculate is deposited in the vagina, the penis being withdrawn before the ejaculation is complete. The healthy sperm may have a better chance if unhindered by their less healthy brothers. This may also increase the chances of a healthy conception. *Black Willow* herb may be helpful in reducing semen volume.

Semen viscosity

If your semen has been diagnosed as being too thick, you may need to drink more water. Mucus solvent herbs such as *Fenugreek, Golden Rod, Golden Seal* and *Garlic* may also be of assistance.

Acidity of the semen

If the pH is too low (acidic) it can cause the sperm to be immobilised. This is usually a result of general systemic acidity, and should respond to a more alkali-forming diet. This consists of a high intake of vegetables (especially vegetable juices), fruit (except plums, prunes and cranberries) and nuts (especially almonds and hazelnuts) and a low intake of animal foods, including meat, fish (though this is less acid-forming than meat), eggs and dairy produce, sugar, coffee and tea, grains and seeds.

Good bases for vegetables juices are *beetroot, carrot* and *celery*, and *Alfalfa* and *Red Clover* are both specific for increasing alkalinity. *Fresh cherries* are the most effective fruit, and the celloid or tissue salt *sodium phosphate* is also a specific remedy.

Genito-urinary infections

The white cells generated in the presence of GUIs damage sperm and testes through the effect of free radicals. This means that anti-oxidant therapy is of supreme importance. See 'Female Reproductive Health' (this chapter) and Chapter 10.

Medical treatment of male infertility

This can be done with hormonal drugs, if testosterone is low, or surgery for varicocele. Otherwise IVF procedures, where sperm is treated and micro-injected, are used to bypass the problem.

Varicocele surgery, when it is successful, can improve all aspects of sperm health. It also, in some cases, seems to reduce heat in the scrotum, which may be part of the problem. In men with varicoceles, there is often nutrient loss and oxidant damage to the sperm, so anti-oxidants are particularly helpful.

Remember—Diet, exercise and losing excess or gaining extra weight are as important for the prospective father as for the mother. Supplementing, abstaining from all drugs, taking care with environmental, domestic and industrial pollution, managing stress levels as well as all the other advice in this book can and should be applied to both of you!

9

SOME HELPFUL
DIAGNOSTIC TESTS

ONE OF THE MOST important diagnostic tests which
should be performed well in advance of any pregnancy
is a *hair trace mineral analysis*. Other tests include
blood pressure, blood tests, Zinc Tally and
semen analysis.

HAIR TRACE MINERAL ANALYSIS

This test is used to determine levels of essential minerals as well as
those of toxic metals.

At least four months before you plan to conceive, both of you
should send a sample of your hair to a laboratory for analysis. Details
can be found in Contacts and Resources. This is what you need to
do: send only recent hair growth for analysis. To do this you must
cut the hair *from close to the roots*. This should provide fresh,
chemically untreated hair which will provide the best results. Hair
should be taken in small snippets from the back part (occiput region)
of the scalp. The nape of the neck is a good place from which to
take the sample, and its removal can be easily concealed.

Use stainless steel scissors only. Thinning scissors may be used
if hair is very short. The sample should be no more than 3.75 cm

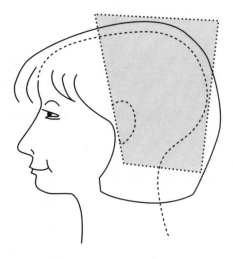

Occiput region of scalp

long. Cut off the old growth (excess) hair. Ideally the sample should weigh about 0.5 g. This is about one heaped tablespoonful of hair.

In this chapter you will find a sample request form for hair trace mineral analysis. You will need to photocopy a separate form for each of you and after checking cost details with the laboratory, you can send your hair samples away for analysis. Two copies of each result will be returned to you within three to four weeks. One copy is for you and the second is for your health practitioner. Each copy will include basic information about the test, as well as specific recommendations about diet and supplementation.

Why hair analysis?

In the preceding chapters we have explained how important it is for both of you to have adequate levels of all the essential minerals before conception. As you now know, it is equally important that both of you are free from a burden of any of the toxic metals before your child is conceived. It has been shown conclusively by investigators in many countries, including the Foresight research team in the United Kingdom, that hair trace mineral analysis gives a reliable overall picture of an individual's essential mineral status as well as an accurate indication of any toxic metal contamination. Hair is now used as the tissue of choice by the NSW Environmental Protection Authority to determine toxic metal exposure.

What is hair analysis?

The metabolic rate of hair is very high in its growing phase. Hair is in fact the second most metabolically active tissue. During its growth, hair is exposed to the internal environment of the body including exposure to extracellular fluids such as circulating blood and lymph. Then, as the hair reaches the surface, the outer layers harden, and lock in the accumulated metabolic products. Hair element levels therefore provide vital information about the metabolic activity which occurred in the body during the period of hair growth.

Put a little more simply, it gives us information about levels of exposure to essential minerals and toxic metals over the previous six to eight weeks as opposed to blood levels which are related to the supply of elements in the preceding hours or days only. Furthermore, since the composition of blood is extremely complex, and whole blood, serum, erythrocytes and leucocytes will each exhibit different concentrations of trace elements, and since nutrients present in blood are not always available to tissues, hair appears to give a much more useful assessment of element status, and is particularly useful in assessing exposure to the toxic or heavy metals. There are some other advantages in using hair as a biological sample. Hair is an inert substance and does not undergo any changes or biological break-down, samples can be collected quickly, easily and non-invasively, and, finally, the concentrations of most trace elements are high in hair compared to other body tissues.

Patterns which may appear

In the past, the usefulness of hair trace mineral analysis as a diag-nostic tool has been debated. It now appears that much of the debate was due to practitioners using the results of this test inappropriately. Hair trace mineral analysis reveals typical patterns which should always be considered in light of the patient's individual history. Practitioners should also consider the ratios of one mineral to another. The reasons for this should be apparent from our earlier discussion of zinc and copper which are antagonistic minerals. You will remember that low zinc levels, which may be caused by a number of factors including the use of oral contraceptives, IUDs and inorganic iron supplements, will lead to inversely high copper levels.

To consider the level of each essential trace mineral on an individual basis may not give a reliable picture of *nutrient status*, although individual levels (both high and low) of toxic or heavy metals do accurately reflect body burden. In some instances, zinc for example, a high reading may in fact indicate that you are suffering from a deficiency, due to slow hair growth. Therefore, while it is possible for you to send your own hair sample for analysis, and we give you all the appropriate information right here, we also strongly recommend that you consult a practitioner who has experience in interpreting the results. You should also remember that if, for example, both you and your partner exhibit very similar patterns for toxic metals, this may give you a clue as to the source of any environmental contamination.

Some of the typical patterns which emerge in hair trace mineral analyses are summarised below.

Multiple deficiencies/toxicity

- *Scattered low essential minerals* right across the chart—this pattern is due to a *poor diet*, or one which is high in white flour and sugar-containing products. As you have already learned, a diet which is high in these products will also be low in essential nutrients and, as well, the minerals and vitamins needed for the metabolism of the refined products will be leached from body stores leading to generally depleted nutrient levels.

  This pattern, reflecting oversupply/undernutrition, can be improved by removing nutrient-low foods from the diet and replacing them with nutrient-dense ones such as fresh fruit and vegetables, whole grains, legumes, and high quality protein. Supplementation should consist of a combination of all essential vitamins, minerals, amino and fatty acids.

- *Low potassium and sodium*, indicating adrenal stress, *together with low minerals* across the range—this pattern shows *malabsorption of essential minerals*. If your hair trace mineral analysis indicates that you are suffering from a malabsorption condition, it means that food, and therefore essential nutrients, are poorly absorbed from your gastrointestinal tract. This, of course, means insufficient nutrients for ensuring the optimum health of sperm or ova, and if this condition is untreated in the mother, it will seriously compromise the supply of nutrients available to the developing foetus.

Malabsorption can be due to a variety of conditions, which include lack of hydrochloric acid in the stomach (hypochlor-hydria). It may also be the result of allergies or infections, chronic Candida, nutritional deficiencies, a high body burden of any of the toxic metals, irritable bowel syndrome, Crohn's disease, coeliac condition or colitis.

If your hair trace mineral analysis indicates a pattern of this type, it is advisable that you seek the help of a practitioner. You will probably need to undergo further testing to determine the reasons for this malabsorption, and, after appropriate treatment, you will need to take steps to improve your nutritional status. You will find more information about the diagnosis and treatment of allergy and Candida in subsequent chapters.

- *High potassium and sodium*, showing kidney irritation by toxic metals, occurs typically with *high heavy metal contamination.*

As we have already described, the heavy metals such as lead, mercury, cadmium and aluminium, have been implicated in many adverse effects on reproductive and foetal health. If by hair trace mineral analysis, either of you is shown to have a high body burden of any of the heavy metals, you must take steps not only to locate and remove the source of the contamination, but to reduce the toxic burden to acceptable levels before you make any attempt to commence a pregnancy.

In earlier chapters we looked at ways of reducing levels of toxic metals. These include supplementation with *ascorbic acid (Vitamin C)*, as well as with the *B-complex vitamins*. Supplementation with *garlic* as well as specific antagonistic minerals such as *calcium* for lead, *selenium* for mercury and *zinc* for cadmium is also useful. There are some foods which you should eat regularly if your toxic levels are found to be high. These include garlic, onions, peas and other legumes. Apples stewed with the pips (for pectin) can also help to reduce high toxic levels (see Chapter 4).

If your hair trace mineral analysis shows a body burden of any of the toxic metals, your health practitioner may wish to consider additional testing of sweat or blood. However, you should remember that blood testing alone appears to be of limited use, since your body's homeostatic mechanism will keep blood levels of heavy metals relatively low, by removing them from the circulation and concentrating them in other body organs. For example, lead becomes concentrated in the bones, cadmium in the liver and kidneys, and both become highly concentrated in the placenta.

Deficiency of a single essential mineral

A hair trace mineral analysis of this type usually reflects a particular lifestyle condition. We have given a few examples of single mineral deficiencies and their possible meanings.

- *Low calcium* often indicates an undiagnosed cow's milk allergy. In Chapter 12 you will find out how you can determine if you are allergic to dairy foods, and also what foods you should eat as an alternative source of calcium. This pattern may also reflect a lack of oestrogen or magnesium or Vitamins A, D and C.
- *Low zinc* may be due to use of oral contraceptives, IUDs or to other lifestyle factors such as smoking, drinking, injury or stress. Since zinc is intimately involved in many aspects of reproduction, strenuous efforts must be made to remove the offending causative factor and to restore adequate zinc status before a pregnancy commences.
- *Low manganese* may be due to organophosphate use. This may occur if you are involved in farming, gardening or mothproofing activities. A test for xenobiotic overload (pesticides) may also be necessary if low levels of manganese are revealed by hair trace mineral analysis.
- *Low chromium and cobalt* may indicate heavy consumption of alcohol or sugar. These nutrient-poor foods must be replaced with nutrient-dense ones, and appropriate supplementation taken to restore chromium and cobalt levels. Low cobalt alone may occur in vegetarians. Low chromium means impaired glucose tolerance, which can have serious effects on foetal growth.
- *Low selenium* on hair trace mineral analysis appears commonly in Australia since selenium levels in the soil are very low. (New Zealand's soil is even more selenium-depleted than Australia's and has in fact the lowest levels of selenium in the world.) Low selenium levels have been said to be implicated in allergies

affecting the lungs, in immune incompetence and cardiovascular disease. Selenium supplements are available only on prescription as selenium can be toxic in excess.

- *Low iron* may be due to a vegetarian diet or excessive menstrual bleeding.
- *Low potassium* may be due to the use of diuretics or too much salt.
- *Low sodium* is not usually a problem but may be due to caffeine, weight loss or gastrointestinal disturbances.
- *High calcium levels, relative to potassium* a pattern of this type may indicate hypothyroidism. Confirmation of an underactive thyroid gland must be obtained by other diagnostic tests.

Checking your progress

If your initial hair trace mineral analysis shows that treatment is necessary for the restoration of essential mineral levels, a further analysis must be carried out to check the effectiveness of the treatment and supplementation program after 60, but before 90 days. You should not make any attempt to commence a pregnancy until this re-test has shown that your essential minerals are at adequate levels. Remember that these must be so for *at least four months prior to conception*. This may mean a frustrating delay for some and is, of course, one reason why we recommend that whenever possible you allow yourselves more than the minimum period of four months to prepare for a pregnancy.

Sometimes, if the level of heavy metal contamination is very high and of long standing, treatment to reduce toxic levels may take some time. This is particularly true if the contamination is due to lead which will continue to be pulled from its storage sites in bone. As we have already discussed, treatment to reduce a high body burden of mercury may involve the removal of amalgam fillings and replacement with an alternative compound. This may be time-consuming too, and needs to be completed well before conception, as initially levels of mercury in the body will rise due to release of the filling material. It may even be preferable to leave the amalgam fillings in place if you feel that a long wait may be too much to bear. In this case, detoxification procedures are particularly important.

Once again, you should have further hair trace mineral analyses performed to check your progress. You must be prepared to wait until the toxic body burden of both partners is at acceptably low levels, and has been so for at least four months, before you make any attempt to conceive, because, as you have seen, the ill effects of commencing a pregnancy with even a moderate burden of any of these substances can be quite severe.

Whether low essential mineral or high toxic metal levels, or both, are the problem, we strongly recommend that you seek the help of a practitioner who is familiar with the interpretation of hair trace mineral analysis charts and who can order the necessary supplementation and additional treatment.

Hair Trace Mineral Analysis Request

CLIENT DETAILS

Surname   Given Name

Address

Postcode   Telephone

Sex   Age

Height   Weight

Race   Occupation

Nature of problem (answer is optional).

HAIR SAMPLE DETAILS

Date of sample

Any previous report? YES/NO   If YES, date?

Location of sample NAPE/OTHER

Natural hair colour

Hair preparations (colour*, bleach, perm etc.)

* If colour is used, a sample of pubic hair should also be
  included so that laboratory may verify levels of lead.

Shampoo

Referred by

Address

Town/Suburb   Postcode

Telephone   Signature

Send results to REFERRER/DIRECT TO CLIENT

OTHER DIAGNOSTIC TESTS

Some of the following tests are ordered routinely once a pregnancy is confirmed. However, we believe that it makes better sense to have these performed some months beforehand. In this way any undiagnosed medical conditions are far less likely to jeopardise your baby's early development. If, for example, your iron stores are found to be inadequate or if you are found to be suffering from a genito-urinary infection, the necessary course of treatment can be completed well before you become pregnant.

There are some tests which we believe should be undertaken by everyone, both male and female, and we have marked these clearly. There are others which should only be performed if your previous health or history indicates the need for such investigation. If infertility problems are part of your reproductive history, you will find that we have divided these tests into non-invasive and invasive procedures, and you will find them listed fully in Chapter 14.

We have also listed a number of alternative tests which may be available to you depending on the training of your practitioner. The fact that we list them here does not necessarily mean that you must seek out a practitioner who can perform them. Rather we have listed them alongside those which are more orthodox, for the information of those of you who are in the care of a complementary or holistic health-care provider.

A general practitioner will be able to perform most of the standard diagnostic tests and will refer you to an appropriate specialist for others which may be necessary. A complementary health practitioner will need to refer you to a doctor who can order the necessary pathology.

Tests for all women

Blood pressure

This measurement is important as high blood pressure is a condition which may produce few adverse symptoms and, for that reason, it may frequently go undetected. If you are found to be suffering from elevated blood pressure, this does not necessarily mean a lifetime of antihypertensive drugs. There are several measures which may be sufficient to reduce your blood pressure to within normal limits, and these should be tried first. These measures include:

- Losing excess weight
- Undertaking regular exercise
- Reducing stress levels
- Giving up alcohol
- Reducing the amount of salt in your diet
- Taking herbs such as *Hawthorn, Lime Flowers*
- Taking nutrients such as fish oil (*EPA*), *Vitamins E, C* and *B6*, *zinc*, as well as *calcium* and *magnesium* (taken in the ratio of 2:1).

Blood pressure readings are always taken once a woman realises that she is pregnant. However we recommend that you have this reading done in advance of a pregnancy, since it is advisable to have your blood pressure well within the normal range before you conceive. High blood pressure can put enormous stress on the kidneys and heart, and toxaemia (eclampsia) of pregnancy can threaten the life of both you and your baby.

Thyroid and ovulation status

You can perform a simple test at home to indicate whether you are ovulating. If you are using Natural Fertility Management you will already be familiar with this method of taking your temperature. Buy an ovulation or fertility thermometer which has large, easy-to-read markings, and then take your temperature every morning on waking. Do this before you get out of bed by placing the thermometer under your tongue and leaving it there for two minutes. At ovulation your basal temperature will normally rise and will remain elevated for the remainder of your menstrual cycle. If your temperature remains the same for the whole cycle, you should seek your health practitioner's advice. A small number of women who ovulate do not show the typical temperature rise, but your doctor will be able to order more comprehensive testing to assess ovulatory function.

If your chart shows temperatures which are excessively low (frequently right off the graph), then you may be suffering from hypothyroidism. Once again your doctor will order further testing.

Blood tests

A full blood count should be performed. This will show if there are any abnormalities of red or white cells. For example, a deficiency of red blood cells can indicate an anaemia, and proliferation of white blood cells is the body's response to infection. Your eosinophil (a particular type of white cell) count will be raised if illness is due to allergy. It is also sensible for your blood group and Rh factor to be determined at this time.

Your serum ferritin level, which indicates the amount of iron stored by your body, should be assessed. It is important that this level is *tested well before conception.* This amount of stored iron should be in the range of 55 to 65 mcg per litre if you are to have sufficient iron stores for the pregnancy. We want to emphasise that if you are anaemic at the commencement of your pregnancy there are irreversible changes which will occur no matter how much your iron levels may subsequently be supplemented. We would also like to emphasise that only 40 per cent of women have iron stores which are within the appropriate range before they conceive. Remember, supplementation with iron, which must be organic and chelated, is not necessary unless the need is proven.

A full blood test will also indicate whether you are suffering from an infection called toxoplasmosis. Toxoplasmosis is a teratogenic disease (one which can cause birth defects) which is carried by cats and may be contracted from handling cat litter or infected meat. Medically, there is no specific remedy for toxoplasmosis, but herbal medicine makes use of antivirals and immune stimulants to treat this condition.

Your rubella (German measles) status will also be indicated by a full blood count. Since rubella is another teratogenic disease, you may choose to be immunised if your immunity is below acceptable levels; you must then wait at least four months before attempting to conceive. However, if you feel that immunisation puts foreign substances into your body which you would rather avoid, you may choose to strengthen your immune system by other methods.

A blood test may indicate the presence of genito-urinary infection(s) which must be treated before you attempt to conceive, but do remember that a negative blood test for GUI is not definitive. Other tests (see below) will give you better information about the presence of such infection(s).

A blood test can indicate thyroid function if your doctor considers that there is any possibility that this is abnormal. However, this test may not always be reliable.

Your doctor may also ask for blood levels of Vitamin B6, zinc, copper and lead to be tested. As we have already explained, blood levels, particularly of heavy metals, may not always accurately reflect the true body burden, so, ideally, these results should be regarded in conjunction with those of a hair trace mineral analysis or other assessment for nutrients such as Vitamin B6.

Blood may also be analysed to indicate liver function. This may be a useful test if you have been over-indulging, or if other symptoms such as liver tenderness, headache, nausea, or gastrointestinal disturbances such as bloating, are present.

Urine analysis

Your urine should be tested for sugar and protein. The presence of either of these substances in your urine can indicate that you are suffering from conditions which could seriously compromise the outcome of your pregnancy. Excess sugar (glucose) may indicate that you are suffering from a pre-diabetic or diabetic state, and the presence of albumin may indicate high blood pressure (called toxaemia or pre-eclampsia) during pregnancy. Your doctor can carry out a urine analysis in the surgery using a simple dip stick method.

Pap smear

A general internal examination and pap smear should be performed.

Colposcopy for genito-urinary infection

Since blood and urine tests may not always give evidence of genito-urinary infection, we recommend that females have a colposcopy examination. This is similar to a smear but involves a small microscope-type device being inserted into the vagina. This appears to be the most reliable way to test for all types of sexually transmitted disease or genito-urinary infection. Your general practitioner will need to refer you to an obstetrician or gynaecologist who has the appropriate equipment to perform this test. If a colposcope is not available, a swab must be taken from high inside the cervix.

Zinc Tally (or Zinc Challenge)

Many researchers feel that zinc deficiency is widespread in the general population. In fact, a recent study carried out by the CSIRO showed that the levels of zinc and magnesium were marginal or below the RDA in the diets of 67 per cent of Australian men and 85 per cent of women. Zinc Tally is an easy way to test for adequate zinc status. This is a proprietary solution of Zinc Sulphate which may be purchased from any pharmacy or from your natural health practitioner. To test, you put 5 mL of the solution into your mouth and swish it about.

If your zinc status is adequate, you should experience a *strong unpleasant* taste, promptly!

If your zinc status is marginal, you will experience a *dry mineral, sweet* or *furry* taste.

If this is the case, you should supplement with tablets of zinc chelate.

If you experience *little* or *no* taste, then you need to take 25 mL of the Zinc Tally solution twice daily until the taste sensation which you experience is strong and prompt. Once this is so, you can revert to the normal recommended dose of zinc (chelate) in tablet form.

It is strongly recommended that both prospective parents do this simple test.

Dental check-up

For reasons already mentioned, we recommend a full dental check-up for both prospective parents well in advance of any intended pregnancy. Any X-rays should be completed *at least four months before conception* and any fillings should be completed using an alternative to amalgam. *Do not attempt to have your mercury-containing amalgam fillings replaced at this stage, as four months may not be long enough to eliminate residual mercury.*

Tests for all men
Blood Pressure
Zinc Tally or Zinc Challenge
Dental Check-up
Blood Count—may indicate presence of genito-urinary infection, but we recommend also
Urine
Urethral Smear

Semen sample

It is strongly recommended that a full semen analysis is carried out. This will include a sperm count and will also assess motility, morphology, pH and volume—in other words the test will look at both the quality as well as the quantity of the sperm. Many doctors are concerned only with a viable level of forward, progressive sperm to achieve conception. We feel that if the motility and morphology are poor, then the health of all sperm is compromised and treatment is essential before any attempt is made to conceive. Treatment to improve motility and morphology will include detoxification, herbs and nutritional supplements. A pH which is too acidic or too alkaline can be corrected through diet. If the volume of ejaculate is too high, then the technique of 'split ejaculate' can be tried. This involves depositing only the first gush of semen (the healthiest fraction) in the vagina before the penis is withdrawn.

It is preferable to have 2 to 3 semen samples analysed to give an accurate picture, since some factors can vary. The samples should always be taken under similar conditions, that is, after the same number of days abstinence (preferably 3 to 5) and delivered to the laboratory within the same length of time (preferably within 2 hours and not collected in a condom containing spermicide). Then 2 to 3 full semen analyses should be repeated after implementing diet and lifestyle changes and appropriate supplementation, and after three months have passed, during which time fresh, hopefully healthy sperm have been manufactured. No attempt should be made to conceive until the quality of the sperm is assessed as suitable.

We want to emphasise that, if possible, all prospective fathers should have this test performed. Of course, it is mandatory if there have been any suspected fertility problems at all. We are well aware that masturbating into a specimen jar is probably not anyone's idea of fun, and that the stress of the ordeal may in fact affect the count, but we feel that any inconvenience/embarrassment which you may experience is relatively minor and actually pales into insignificance when compared to some of the investigations which may be recommended for your partner if infertility is a problem. This is also a fairly definitive test, since the only factor involved in male fertility is the production of adequate numbers of healthy sperm.

Tests if previous history indicates the need
Stool samples

If your doctor considers that there is a possiblity of infestation in either you or your partner, he/she may order a stool analysis to check for threadworm or tapeworm. If your or your partner's hair trace mineral analysis shows below normal levels right across the chart, this indicates a possible malabsorption problem. In this case your doctor may order further testing or screening for coeliac disease.

Drinking water analysis

We have already recommended the use of a water filter for all prospective parents. However, in some areas you may suspect that your water has higher than average levels of heavy metals or pesticides. For example if, after filtering, the water turns white dinnerware blue, then heavy copper contamination may be a problem. Contact your local water authority for details of available analyses. In city areas, if you filter your water, it is probably unnecessary to have a water analysis carried out.

If you use rainwater collected on your property, it may be necessary to ensure that there is no local airborne pollution which could be dissolved in the water, and that the roof it is collected from is not made from toxic metals such as aluminium. You should also be aware that galvanised storage tanks may contribute to high zinc levels in the drinking water—this may be reflected in a very high zinc reading on your hair trace mineral analysis.

Some complementary tests

Some of the following diagnostic tests may be unfamiliar to many GPs but they are tests which have been recently developed, and are now used in many clinics in Europe and the United States. They are specifically designed to detect sub-clinical conditions—in other words, to detect conditions which produce only vague symptoms, in that window between optimum health and frank pathology states. These tests may be recommended if your health or energy levels seem to be chronically below par.

Clot retraction test (CRT or HLB)

By close examination of the clot retraction patterns in blood samples, acute or chronic conditions can be differentiated and an indication of your general metabolic state may be given. This test may also indicate specific organ function, hormone imbalance, physical and psychological stress and allergies.

Live blood analysis

Blood is drawn from a capillary in your finger and examined immediately—the examination is therefore of active, motile cells. This test is usually ordered in conjunction with CRT to ascertain health status and body function. Live blood analysis can also show the presence and activity of systemic *Candida albicans*.

Testing for allergies and sensitivities

There are numerous diagnostic tests such as ALCAT, cytotoxic or IgE-mediated, which may be offered to ascertain which foods or other substances you may be sensitive or allergic to. In our experience, none of these tests can be considered to be 100 per cent accurate in assessing allergens, nor can they be considered 100 per cent accurate in eliminating those substances to which you do not react.

Part of the problem with these diagnostic tests is that the manner of testing is frequently very different from the manner in which your body handles the test substance (that is, the test is done in vitro not in vivo). This problem may be compounded by the absence, or presence, of other stressors (we will talk more about this in Chapter 12). If your practitioner orders any of these tests for allergy, you should be prepared to accept the results with a certain degree of caution, and remember that the most reliable test for food allergy is certainly an elimination diet with subsequent food challenge.

ALCAT or cytotoxic testing may also be used to determine sensitivities to commonly used domestic, agricultural or industrial chemicals.

Lymphocyte viability test

A lymphocyte viability test can give an indication of whether you have a healthy or compromised immune system and can also be used to monitor the effects of dental procedures on your immune system.

Biocompatibility

Your immune response to a number of dental materials can be assessed using this test.

Urine challenge test for mercury

This test may be performed if it is suspected that your symptoms of ill-health may be due to chronic mercury toxicity, or if your hair trace mineral analysis chart shows a high body burden of mercury.

Urinary indicans test

This test, which can be performed in the clinic, measures the level of *E. coli* in your bowel. If an overgrowth of this organism is indicated, then you have a highly toxic system. This test does not measure the overgrowth of other organisms such as Candida.

Sweat test for zinc levels

This test is regarded as the most accurate assessment of zinc status. It involves the passive collection of sweat, but unfortunately you may have difficulty in finding a laboratory who is able to perform it. Hopefully, this situation will change in the near future!

Iris diagnosis (iridology)

Your health practitioner may be trained in iridology or iris diagnosis. In the hands of an experienced practitioner, this method of diagnosis is able to give a fairly accurate picture of your overall health and can also give clues to some of the factors which may be contributing to any ill-health.

Muscle testing (applied kinesiology)

The availability of this test will depend on the training of your health practitioner. It is useful for detecting allergies or sensitivities, or for Sherlock Holmes type investigations. That is, muscle testing can give an idea of which organ or system is under stress, or diseased, or what foods or conditions you may be sensitive to.

Urine screen for heavy metals

A test kit is available to detect the presence of heavy metals in urine. Although this test gives limited information on degree of contamination and with which metal(s), it is useful as a first screening test.

10

CLEARING
GENITO-URINARY
INFECTIONS

INFECTIONS OF THIS type are due to a variety of
organisms but it is important that you do not dismiss
the significance of these conditions even though some
cause few, if any, symptoms. *The presence of one or
more of these infections has the potential to
adversely affect fertility, foetal health and the health
of the newborn.*

THE TERM SEXUALLY TRANSMITTED disease (STD) may actually
be more familiar to you than genito-urinary infection (GUI). However,
we prefer referring to these infections as those of the genito-urinary
type. This name not only avoids the stigma of the more familiar name,
but is in fact more correct, as not all of the infections which we are
about to discuss are sexually transmitted, and many of them may be
present in couples who are in a stable, long-term relationship with no
history of extra-marital or extra-partnership affairs.

INCREASES IN INFECTIONS

The prevalence of this group of infections has increased dramatically
in recent years. There is no doubt that changed attitudes to sexual
relationships before, during or outside marriage are a major factor

in the proliferation of infections of this type, but other factors, such as compromised immunity due to poor nutrition, lifestyle factors and environmental pollution, are also partly responsible.

Where once these infections were due largely to gonococcal organisms (those responsible for causing syphilis and gonorrhoea) a host of other types of organisms are now found to be responsible for most cases of genito-urinary infection. These may include bacterial, viral, mycoplasmal and fungal pathogens.

However, the single factor which makes all of them so problematic is the ease with which they can avoid detection! The infection site may be hidden well inside the cervix and may therefore not be detected by a routine pap smear or vaginal swab. Similarly, blood or urine samples from male sufferers may not show any signs of infection, and a swab should be taken from the urethra.

The infections may also be sub-clinical (without apparent symptoms) in the adult, but have devastating effects on the viability of a pregnancy and the foetus. They cause few symptoms because the majority of the pathogens involved are not very powerful inducing agents. This means that the immune system does not respond strongly (there is no high temperature, etc.) but the inflammatory response may cause obstruction of the tubes which can lead to infertility, and the level of white cells in the woman can kill the sperm. In his book, *The Fertility Solution* American obstetrician and gynaecologist Dr A. Toth states that, *in his opinion, at least 50 per cent of infertility cases are caused by common genito-urinary infections!*

TYPES OF INFECTIONS

Bacteria

Chlamydia trachomatis is the most common of the offending pathogens and is reputed to be the cause of up to 60 per cent of genito-urinary infection in both males and females. Initial infection with chlamydia produces far less severe symptoms than gonorrhoea and its presence may therefore go undetected until further problems arise. It has been estimated that as many as 70 per cent of female sufferers are asymptomatic (without symptoms) and as many as 50 per cent of males. This fact makes *chlamydia trachomatis* a very insidious infection indeed!

Initially in females, the organism infects the cervix causing cervicitis, it then spreads to the endometrium causing endometritis (this is an inflammation of the endometrium and should not be confused with endometriosis) and, finally, if undetected or untreated, may spread to the Fallopian tubes causing acute salpingitis and/or pelvic inflammatory disease (PID). The damage which may be done to the Fallopian tubes is the most common cause of female infertility.

Alternatively, chlamydia may not be present in the cervix, but may lie dormant in the Fallopian tubes. It can become active during pregnancy, or as a result of investigations to assess tubal function.

Chlamydial infection has been found to be responsible for miscarriage, ectopic pregnancy (one which occurs in the tubes), premature birth, infant mortality, and many clinical infections in the newborn and older infant.

In males, chlamydial infection has been shown to be directly responsible for inflammation of both the epididymis and urethra.

Viruses

The two viruses which have been shown to be most commonly associated with compromised reproductive and infant health are *cytomegalovirus* and *herpes virus hominis*. As well, cervical lesions which have been caused by recurring viral infections form a focus for persistent cervicitis or recurrent thrush.

Infection with cytomegalovirus during pregnancy carries a one in five chance of severe and permanent brain damage in the foetus. Infection with genital and cervical herpes is also extremely common. If the mother suffers a primary attack at the time of delivery this can result in damage to the central nervous system, eyes, skin or liver of the newborn. If the mother suffers a recurrent attack close to the time of the birth, it is usually considered necessary to deliver her baby by Caesarean section.

Mycoplasmas

Mycoplasmas are the smallest organisms which are capable of life outside a cell. Infection with these organisms, *mycoplasma hominis* and *ureaplasma urealyticum* being the most common, can result in a considerably higher incidence of infertility, spontaneous abortion, prematurity and neonatal morbidity. Infection with these organisms can be extremely stubborn and may be resistant to antibiotic treatment (see Chapter 8, section on 'GUIs' for details of treatment recommended in stubborn cases).

Other infections

Other infectious agents, which are frequently sexually transmitted, have also been found to cause serious complications such as infertility. Serious diseases, such as AIDS or Hepatitis, will normally be screened during any fertility investigations. Treatment for these diseases lies outside the scope of this book. We have already discussed infection with *Candida albicans* (for more information see Chapter 11 and for treatment see Chapter 8, section on 'Discharges and Infections'), but include below a comprehensive list of those pathogens which have been implicated in the full range of compromised reproductive outcomes and ill health in the neonate.

Organisms commonly causing GUI

B. streptococcus   *Haem influenza*
Candida albicans   *Herpes virus hominis*
Chlamydia trachomatis   *Klebsiella*
Cytomegalovirus   *Staph aureus*
E. coli   *Strep milleri*
Enterococcus   *Ureaplasma urealyticum*
Gardnerella

Symptoms of infection

Female   Male
Unusual vaginal discharge (smell, colour)   Discharge
Vaginal irritation or itching   Irritation/itching
Urinary frequency   Urinary frequency
Abdominal pain

It would be simple if the absence of the foregoing symptoms also indicated the absence of genito-urinary infection. However, we would like to emphasise that the majority of sufferers of genito-urinary infections may remain symptom-free, which is why it is so important that screening for these infections is carried out well before any attempt is made to conceive.

We have listed below some risk factors, which may be more helpful for you than a list of symptoms.

Risk factors

Female	Male
Early sexual activity	Early sexual activity
Promiscuous sexual activity (several partners)	Promiscuous sexual activity (several partners)
Oral contraceptive use	Poor immune function
IUD use	Candida infection
Poor immune function	Gonorrhoeal infection
Candida infection	
Gonorrhoeal infection	

Conditions indicating possible GUI

We would also like to list some medical conditions which may indicate that you are suffering from infection of this type, as this too may be more useful information for you than a list of possible (or non-existent) symptoms.

Female	Male
Recurrent thrush	Urethritis
Cervicitis	Epididymitis
Cervical dysplasia	Infertility
Endometritis (which is an inflammation of the endometrium and should not be confused with endometriosis)	High level of deformed sperm
Salpingitis (infection of the Fallopian tubes)	
Pelvic Inflammatory Disease	
Infertility	
Ectopic pregnancy (risk may increase by factor of 7 to 10 after one period of inflammation)	
Miscarriage	
Premature rupture of membranes	
Premature birth	

Perhaps you have given birth to a child who exhibited physical or mental ill health which may have been due to infection of the genito-urinary type.

Newborn/infant

Conjunctivitis
Otitis media (inflammation of the middle ear)
Gastroenteritis
Pneumonitis
Congenital defects (physical/mental)

WHO SHOULD BE TESTED FOR GUI?

As we have already stated, lack of well-defined symptoms is not a clear indicator of freedom from genito-urinary infection. Unfortunately, these infections may also be present in couples who are completely faithful to one another, and some infections are transmitted by means other than sexual intercourse. Screening would also be a much simpler affair if blood or urine sampling always showed the presence of infection. However, this is not the case and the combination of all these factors probably accounts for the high incidence of undetected genito-urinary infection in the general population. Recent screening at an infertility clinic in London detected 69 per cent of couples suffering from one or more of these infections. Therefore, knowing the very high incidence of these infections and the damage which they can cause, we recommend that all couples contemplating pregnancy undergo testing for GUI.

It is also important to realise that although you may have already had many tests for infection (for example, during IVF procedures), due to the extensive list of offending organisms, and due to the fact that they are often missed during a routine vaginal swab/pap smear, because the infection is inside the cervix, it may be necessary to carry out further testing. We have treated many cases where couples are confident that they have been tested for every organism possible and we have still found one or more genito-urinary infections to be present!

A full check for the organisms that commonly cause GUIs will involve the following tests:

Females	Males
Blood	Blood
Urine	Urine
Pap Smear	Urethral Smear
Colposcopy (or if this is not available, an intra-cervical smear should be taken from inside the cervix).	Semen analysis

In Chapter 8, section on 'GUIs' we give a list of alternative treatments which are available if either you or your partner, or more frequently both of you, are found to be infected with one or more of these organisms. However, antibiotics are often called for since a quick resolution of the infection is usually required. Remember it is important to maintain abstinence from sexual intercourse, or to use condoms, until absence of infection(s) is indicated in both partners.

11

THE CANDIDA FACTOR

THIS CONDITION IS MORE correctly termed 'chronic Candidiasis', or 'systemic *Candida albicans*,' it is also commonly called 'thrush', but we will refer to it simply as 'Candida' which we feel is less cumbersome. There are two main reasons why this condition needs to be resolved before conception. (1) *Candida can seriously affect fertility and reproductive health*; and (2) *Candida can worsen significantly during pregnancy due to hormonal activity, and may cause considerable ill health in the mother and adversely affect the child.*

ARE YOU SUFFERING FROM CANDIDA?

At the outset we want to emphasise that it is possible for either one, or both, partners to suffer from Candida, and that it does not simply refer to *'vaginal thrush'*.

The following questionnaire is based on one taken from Peter de Ruyter's excellent book *Coping with Candida*. The questions below will give you some idea of possible symptoms, and your score will indicate whether indeed there is a likelihood of a Candida infestation in your system. We want to emphasise that the answers to the questions must refer to the present, and past symptoms should *not* be included!

The Candida questionnaire

Symptom level	Score
Occasional or mild	1 point
Frequent or moderately severe	2 points
Constant or disabling/very severe	3 points

Symptoms	Score
Abdominal bloating	_____
A lot of wind	_____
Belching	_____
Abdominal pain/colic	_____
Irritable bowel syndrome	_____
Bowel motions that are alternately too loose and then too firm	_____
Indigestion/heartburn	_____
Coated tongue	_____
Bad breath	_____
Metallic taste in mouth	_____
Lethargic/tired/fatigued/feeling drained	_____
Easily depressed for no reason	_____
Feelings of 'can't cope'	_____
Anxiety spells for no reason	_____
Frequent mood swings	_____
Irritability	_____
Unable to make decisions/concentrate	_____
Poor memory	_____
Feeling spacey/disconnected from your body	_____
Insomnia	_____
Hyperactivity	_____
Dizzy spells	_____
Spots before the eyes	_____
Blurry vision	_____
Tinnitus (ringing in the ears)	_____
Cold sweats	_____
Rapid heartbeat	_____
Headaches	_____
Migraines	_____
General muscle aches for no apparent reason	_____
Muscles feel weak and paralysed	_____

Joint aches _____
Weakness and trembling _____
Numbness/tingling in limbs _____
Cold hands/feet _____
Chronically congested/blocked nose _____
Nasal/throat catarrh (mucus) _____
Post nasal drip _____
Chronic colds/flu _____
Chronic bronchitis/cough _____
Chronic ear infections _____
Chronically sore throat _____
Sinusitis _____
Hayfever _____
Asthma (resistant to treatment) _____
Allergies to yeast/mould _____
Allergies to foods/environmental substances _____
Very sensitive to odours (perfumes, cigarette smoke, car
   fumes, household chemicals, airborne pollutants) _____
Hypoglycaemia _____
Cravings for sugar/sweet foods/fruit/fruit juice _____
Cravings for alcohol _____
Easily adversely affected by alcohol _____
Cravings for bread _____
Cravings for certain cheeses _____
Sudden hunger _____
Itchy eyes _____
Itchy ears _____
Itchy nose _____
Itchy anus _____
Itchy scalp _____
General body feels itchy _____
Scaly scalp/dandruff _____
Eczema (resistant to treatment) _____
Psoriasis _____
Tinea of feet/groin/fingers/nails _____
Chronic acne _____
Hives _____
Skin rashes _____

Dry scaly skin   _____

Scaly skin behind ears/in eyebrows/on eyelids/either side
of nose   _____

Very dry mouth/lips   _____

Cracked corners of mouth   _____

Gums that bleed easily on brushing   _____

Gums that feel tender/sensitive/sore   _____

Mouth ulcers   _____

Oral thrush   _____

Chronic vaginal thrush (resistant to treatment)   _____

Vaginal itching/burning   _____

Cystitis (bladder infection) especially in females
(resistant to treatment)   _____

Premenstrual tension (PMT)   _____

Menstrual problems (sore breasts/fluid retention/painful
or heavy periods/irregular periods)   _____

Endometriosis/PID   _____

Infertile (for no apparent reason)   _____

Loss of libido (sexual desire)   _____

Discomfort during sex   _____

Impotent (unable to be sexually aroused in males)   _____

Chronic urethritis in males (resistant to treatment)   _____

Prostatitis (resistant to treatment)   _____

Urgency to urinate for no apparent reason   _____

Bedwetting   _____

Bad body/foot odour   _____

Hypothyroidism   _____

Use of antibiotics (especially for acne), now or in past
five years   _____

Use of cortisone (or other immuno-suppressive)
tablets/sprays/creams, now or in past five years   _____

Use of the oral contraceptive pill, now or in past five years   _____

Use of hormone replacement (HRT) for menopause, now
or in past five years   _____

Do damp, mouldy places make you feel worse?   _____

Do you live in a damp, mouldy home? (YES = 3 points)   _____

Have you had several, debilitating pregnancies, one after
the other, in the past few years? (YES = 3 points)   _____

How you score

Females

- Less than 79 points indicates possible Candida
- Between 79 and 158 points indicates probable Candida
- Between 158 and 240 points indicates almost certain Candida

Males

- Less than 72 points indicates unlikely but possible Candida
- Between 72 and 144 points indicates probable Candida
- Between 144 and 219 points indicates almost certain Candida

If you score highly on this questionnaire you may wish to confirm a diagnosis of Candida by other methods. The most reliable test is the Live Blood Analysis (see Chapter 9). It is also possible to have a conventional blood test for Candida antibodies. This will be performed in a pathology laboratory at the request of a medical doctor. It may also be helpful for you to learn a little more about this condition.

WHAT EXACTLY IS CANDIDA?

Candida albicans, normally a benign yeast organism, present in the gut of all healthy people, can, in some circumstances, mutate to a fungal form which proliferates and causes an invasive overgrowth in the gut. Candida commonly occurs if you have been given long-term or recurrent antibiotic therapy, if you have used the oral contraceptive pill or have taken cortisone or other immuno-suppressive drugs. It is more likely to be a problem:

- If you have had persistent infection with the Epstein-Barr virus (glandular fever) or cytomegalovirus, which can exhaust the immune system.
- If you have a high level of sugar in the blood resulting from diabetes or excessive sugar consumption.
- If you are deficient in biotin, a B-complex vitamin.
- If you have a hypothyroid condition.
- If your liver is sluggish.
- If your immune system is depressed due to excessive stress.

In many instances, Candida occurs together with other infections, particularly those of the genito-urinary type.

Unfortunately, some members of the medical profession are wary, to say the least, of a diagnosis of Candida. However, holistic and natural therapists have realised for some time that Candida is a significant contributing factor in a vast range of different disorders. You can see from the list of symptoms that Candida may manifest as a very wide variety of both physical and mental conditions. The fact that Candida may be implicated in so many different complaints is perhaps the reason that a diagnosis is sometimes controversial. However, Foresight studies have found that infection with the Candida organism is implicated in the full range of compromised reproductive outcomes, which include subfertility or infertility, miscarriages, premature births and compromised health in the newborn. It also occurs commonly in endometriosis sufferers.

The Candida infection, per se, may not be totally responsible for all of the reproductive problems which have been observed. They may be contributed to, in part, by the underlying factors which predisposed the sufferer to chronic Candida in the first place, or to those conditions which are exacerbated by the overgrowth of the organism.

For example, poor nutritional intake, oral contraceptive use, stress, smoking, drinking and subsequent inadequate levels of zinc and other nutrients, can lead to compromised immunity. If your immune function is inadequate, the yeast may mutate and proliferate, and you will be more likely to suffer from other concurrent infections and allergies.

Overgrowth of the Candida organism in the gut appears to make the gut wall porous, allowing poorly digested food particles to be absorbed. This results in malabsorption (or poor absorption) of nutrients, and absorption of poorly digested food may also cause intolerances or sensitivities. Both malabsorption and food intolerances will exacerbate nutritional deficiencies.

Furthermore, toxic by-products are released when the yeast is killed (die-off) and these substances also, can contribute to a range of adverse symptoms. Finally, as we have already mentioned, pregnancy itself can predispose you to Candida, or can cause the pre-existing condition to worsen.

The chronic Candida sufferer must frequently resort to drug use to control both the physical and mental symptoms of this condition. These drugs may lead to further nutritional imbalances or they may have adverse effects on the developing embryo.

You can see that if you suffer from chronic Candida you are caught in an extremely vicious circle indeed. It is therefore absolutely essential that if you suspect that any of your ill health is due to this condition, that it is diagnosed, and properly treated, well before conception, and that it is kept under control throughout your pregnancy. Since chronic Candida is definitely an indication that something much more fundamental is amiss, the underlying problems must also be identified and treated appropriately.

WHAT CAN I DO?

From what we have said it should be clear that the treatment of chronic Candida will involve you in a several-pronged attack on your condition. The treatment is best carried out in the care of a practitioner, but there is lots that you can do for yourself. Treatment will aim to do several things:

Restore your nutritional status
See Chapter 1.

Strengthen your immune system
- Specific nutrients, especially *anti-oxidants, Coenzyme Q–10, Kelp, Vitamins A, C , E* and *B-complex, biotin, zinc, selenium, magnesium, EFAs (Evening primrose oil* and fish oils—*MaxEPA* or cold-pressed olive oil).
- Herbs such as *Pau D'Arco, Echinacea, Astragalus, Siberian Ginseng.*
- The amino acid *Arginine* (but not if suffering from herpes or schizophrenia).
- Stabilised oxygen.

Avoid allergens
You can give your immune system a rest and a chance to recover by avoiding any substances you are allergic to. Refer to Chapter 12 for information on what to do in this regard.

Avoid other stressors

These include oral contraceptives, antibiotics, corticosteroids, etc.

Starve the yeast

The anti-Candida diet which excludes refined carbohydrates (which act as food for the organism) and all products containing yeast will have to be strictly adhered to. This means that you must avoid:

- alcoholic and fermented beverages
- foods containing yeast, to which you may be allergic (e.g. breads)
- products containing white flour, such as pastry, cake, bread, breadcrumbs and pasta
- white rice (although whole grains may be eaten)
- all sugars (including honey) and foods containing sugar (including dried fruit)
- malt products including milk drinks, cereals and sweets
- tea (including commercial herb teas) and coffee
- cow's milk/dairy products (although live sugar-free yoghurt may be eaten)
- pickles/relishes
- soy sauce
- vinegar and vinegar-containing foods such as mayonnaise and salad dressing
- peanuts/peanut butter and pistachios (which usually contain mould)
- fungi (such as mushrooms), except Shitake and Reiishi which may be useful
- fermented foods (such as miso)
- mouldy foods and left-overs
- processed and smoked meats
- animal foods containing antibiotics or hormones
- antibiotics, especially the broad spectrum ones such as ampicillin and amoxicillin
- food additives
- packaged or processed foods
- melons—watermelon, honeydew and especially rockmelon (contains mould)
- B-complex vitamins unless labelled yeast-free and sugar-free

Even fruit and fruit juices may need to be eliminated initially, as fructose can contribute to yeast growth. Dried fruit is high in sugar and should definitely be avoided.

This may be a difficult diet to follow at first since some of the foods which the yeast likes best are those which you will crave, although the anti-Candida diet is little more than the standard, healthy preconception diet. However, once the overgrowth of Candida is under some sort of control, you will notice an unpleasant return of symptoms if you stray at all from the dietary guidelines.

Kill the yeast

Supplements and herbs such as *Garlic, Caprylic acid* (derived from coconut), *Citrus seed extract* and *Probioplex* (derived from whey) are all helpful (see Chapter 8, section on 'Discharges and Infections' and 'GUIs').

Some authorities feel that it is not possible to treat the overgrowth by dietary and lifestyle modification alone, and recommend the use of the anti-yeast preparations *nystatin* (Mycostatin, Nilstat) or *amphotericin* (Fungilin-oral). While drug use during pregnancy must certainly be kept to an absolute minimum, nystatin (which acts locally and is quite non-toxic), can be used, and seems preferable to allowing the yeast to proliferate. We suggest that you use natural remedies as a first preference, and stress that two other pharmaceutical antifungals—*griseofulvin, Ketoconazole* and related antifungals should definitely be avoided.

Reline your gut

- Nutrients, see Chapter 1.
- Bitter tonic herbs such as *Golden Seal, Agrimony, Gentian, St Mary's Thistle*, which all restore normal digestive function.
- *Acidophilus/Bifidus* which restore the friendly bacteria in the gut which control levels of Candida.
- *Digestive enzymes* and *hydrochloric acid* to restore gastric activity.

Detoxify

Liver herbs are of primary importance (see Chapter 4).

Treat the symptoms

This should be done using appropriate natural remedies, which can be prescribed by your natural health practitioner.

Usually you will need to stay on the full anti-Candida diet for at least one month, but perhaps for as many as three months. You may then need to introduce a Rotation Diet (see Chapter 12). You can use muscle testing (see Chapter 9) to ascertain when to re-introduce foods such as fruit. After the initial die-off and exacerbation of symptoms, you will see a great improvement in all symptoms and experience a general feeling of well-being.

We also recommend that you read further and recommend Peter de Ruyter's book (see Suggested Reading) which contains lots of recipes to make it easier for you to adhere to the diet.

12

ARE YOU ALLERGIC?

THERE ARE TWO MAIN reasons why these
conditions need to be detected and treated
before conception:
(1) *They have the potential to adversely affect
fertility (of either partner) as well as
your general reproductive health.*
(2) *They may be transmitted to your child.*

ARE YOU SUFFERING FROM
ALLERGIES/INTOLERANCES?

We are extremely grateful to Phillip Alexander for permission to
reproduce Classic Allergy Symptoms from his book *It Could Be
Allergy and It Can Be Cured*. You can consider yourself a strong
candidate for allergy if you have one or more of the symptoms
mentioned below and have been unable to get rid of them with
standard treatments. Most people have a combination of symptoms
and some people have as many as a dozen. If, after reading this list,
you think that you could be suffering from an allergy, we strongly
recommend that you read Phillip's book, which deals with the subject
of allergy and intolerance in far greater detail than we are able to
here. We would like to stress that this is not really a self-help area,

but one which is definitely best tackled with the help of a health practitioner who has experience in the field of clinical ecology.

Classic allergy symptoms

- *Headaches*—various kinds, including migraine.
- *Eye conditions*—conjunctivitis, eye pain, periods of blurred vision, sensitivity to light, teary eyes, temporary refractive changes.
- *Ear conditions*—hearing loss, infections, inflammation, Ménière's syndrome, noises in the ear, repeated ear trouble.
- *Cardiovascular*—angina, high blood pressure, irregular heartbeat, low blood pressure, rapid pulse.
- *Gastrointestinal*—constipation, diarrhoea, gall bladder pains, gas, gastric ulcer, gastrointestinal bleeding, heartburn, haemorrhoids, indigestion, mucus colitis, nausea, nervous stomach, pains or cramps, spastic colon, vomiting.
- *Respiratory*—asthma, chronic rhinitis, coughing, frequent colds, hayfever, mouth breathing, nosebleeds, post-nasal discharge, sinusitis, stuffy nose, wheezing.
- *Urological*—bed wetting, frequent night urination, frequent urination, painful or difficult urination.
- *Musculo-skeletal*—arthritis, joint pains, muscle cramps, muscle pains and aches, muscle spasms, muscle weakness.
- *Skin*—hot and flushed for no apparent reason, excessive perspiration, itchiness, red patches, dryness, flakiness, dandruff, acne, hives, eczema, dermatitis, boils, psoriasis, blushing, black rings under eyes, sensitivity to sunlight, small white spots on face, legs and body.
- *Mental and behavioural*—anxiety, delusions, depression, dizzy spells, drowsiness, epilepsy, floating sensations, general fatigue, hallucination, hyperactivity, insomnia, irritability, learning disorders, minimal brain dysfunction, nervousness, periods of confusion, phobias, poor concentration, poor memory, poor muscle coordination, restlessness, schizophrenia, falling asleep at inappropriate times, sleeping too little or too much, chronic fatigue syndrome, unsteadiness.
- *Miscellaneous*—abnormal body odour, diabetes, excessive sweating, hypoglycaemia, general weakness, night sweating, overweight, underweight, virus infections, bad breath.

So many symptoms?

The fact that all of the foregoing physical and mental conditions may be due wholly or in part to allergies or intolerances to foods, chemicals or other environmental agents may surprise some of you. You might wonder what causes the body to react in inappropriate ways to substances present in your food or in your immediate surroundings. However, it is estimated that at least 20 per cent of the population is seriously affected by these types of conditions and a much larger percentage is believed to be moderately afflicted, if we include those individuals who suffer from minor allergic reactions such as itching, sneezing or hayfever. Phillip Alexander believes that this number may actually be close to 60 per cent.

The reason that so many people are affected by these conditions is undoubtedly due to the way in which the chemical contamination of the food supply and of the general environment has increased during the last 200 years. Or, to put it more simply, many individuals have simply been unable to adapt to the vastly increased load of allergens or stressors with which their bodies have to deal.

Here we will briefly discuss some of the mechanisms of allergy or intolerance, and will also outline what you need to do if you suffer from these conditions. It is impossible in one chapter to fully cover this very complex topic, so we have listed some further books in Suggested Reading. If you suspect that your ill health may be due to allergy or intolerance we recommend that you read at least one of these titles for a more complete understanding of the subject.

Essentially, the holistic approach to the treatment of these conditions involves improving your overall health (a healthy gut lining, competent immune system, etc.) so that you can in fact tolerate exposure to the offending substances. Even though it is usually necessary to identify the offenders, and although avoidance of these will be necessary initially, this most definitely does not mean that you will have to live the rest of your life eating only pears and lamb chops!

Why do you have an allergy?

Your allergies or intolerances may have been passed to you if your mother suffered from allergic reactions during her pregnancy, or they may have begun in infancy when you reacted to certain allergenic foods or chemicals transmitted to you during breastfeeding. Alternatively, these conditions may have begun with the too-early introduction of cow's milk products or solid food to a digestive system which was still immature and meant to receive only breast milk. The list of symptoms which you may have suffered as an infant and which may have been due to these adverse reactions to food or chemicals could have included: colic, prolonged crying spells, nappy rash, eczema, diarrhoea, constipation, colds, runny nose, coughs and ear infections.

The acute phase of these allergies or intolerances may have disappeared as you matured, or as your body learned to adapt to the offending substance or substances. You may have then become relatively symptom-free.

At a later date, which may be days, months or even years afterwards, following a stressful period such as an illness, or simply if you fail to maintain good health, exposure to the offending food or chemical may again trigger a reaction.

In some instances the conditions may not have resolved themselves as you grew and matured. You may have continued to suffer from ear infections, asthma or constant sneezing for example, or you may have suffered from a variety of different symptoms which were never diagnosed as being due to allergy or intolerance. As a toddler you may have suffered from tantrums, you may have touched everything in sight in a mad haphazard fashion, you may have felt no sense of danger or you may have suffered from nightmares.

As you grew older you may have had frequent headaches, unexplained joint and muscle pain or you may have continued to wet your bed. You may have developed 'glue ear'. Some of the symptoms may have been neurological—you might have been clumsy, had difficulty completing a task, had a reading problem, you may have had trouble with mathematical processes, or you may have been disruptive at school or at home.

If you were sensitive to foods or chemicals as a child then you are probably an adult with similar sensitivities, but as an adult you may exhibit a different set of symptoms. Since your immune or other affected system has been under stress all your life, you may become increasingly less well as the years go by and the number of substances which make you unwell may increase in number. Alternatively, as we have already explained, you may be relatively free of symptoms for many years until a period of ill health or extreme or constant stress triggers an allergic or intolerant reaction.

Through the years, your symptoms of allergy or intolerance may be inconsistent or unpredictable and for this reason you and your health practitioner may fail to recognise the real cause of your condition. We now know that there is a threshold level of stressors, below which symptoms fail to appear, but if your body is affected by a combination of stressors which exceed this threshold, (and we will talk more about the various factors which may cause this to happen) then you will exhibit symptoms. In other words, if you have previously recognised, or on reading this now recognise, that you may be exhibiting allergic or intolerant symptoms, you should be able to identify the offending substances, and if you avoid them, be able to restore yourself to better health by giving your body the opportunity to rest and recover.

We should say at the outset that the study of allergy/intolerance or 'clinical ecology' as it is more correctly called, is relatively new and the findings are not always as cut and dried as some orthodox practitioners would like. Results from various tests may vary just as your symptoms may vary, so before we get to the 'What do I do if I am allergic/intolerant?' question, we would like to explain some of the actual mechanisms of allergies, intolerances or sensitivities in a little more detail.

Mechanisms of allergy

Food intolerance

We have used the words 'food intolerance' as opposed to the more commonly used term of 'food allergy'. The term 'allergy' properly denotes an immune response. In a true *allergic reaction* an 'allergen', which is the substance to which an individual is sensitive, triggers a reaction as the immune system tries to deal with what it perceives as a foreign invader. A true allergy will produce severe and acute symptoms which may require hospitalisation. While some reactions to foods may be true allergies, many others are not.

In these others, *incompletely digested particles of food* can be absorbed through the gut wall. They can set up an inflammatory reaction at an organ site. The site which is affected will depend on your biochemical make-up, and the symptoms which you display will depend on the site at which the inflammation occurs. For example, if the brain is affected you may exhibit psychological or neurological symptoms, if the gastrointestinal tract is affected you may suffer from diarrhoea or stomach cramps, if the lungs are affected then you may have asthma, if it is the skin then you may develop hives or eczema, and so on. However, you may not always exhibit the same symptoms, and they may change over the years.

This leaky gut wall may be due to the too-early introduction of solid food or to nutritional deficiencies which cause the lining of the intestine to break down and become porous. An overgrowth of *Candida albicans* has been implicated in causing incompletely digested food to pass through the gut wall, leading to these sorts of reactions.

Metabolic problems can also increase sensitivity to a wide range of foods.

Chemical sensitivity

Chemical sensitivities may be due to food additives or naturally occurring food chemicals. The mechanism of the sensitivity reaction is not always completely understood. Researchers have found, for example, that sensitivities which were previously thought to be due to the gluten fraction of wheat are in fact due to the chemicals with which the wheat has been sprayed. This simply means that if you appear unable to tolerate products of any kind which contain wheat, you may be able to tolerate those made with wheat which has not been chemically treated at the seed stage, and which has been organically grown.

Salicylates which are naturally occurring substances, similar in chemical composition to aspirin, may also be a trigger for sensitivity reactions. Salicylates are found in many fruits and vegetables, as well as in nuts, and concentrations are particularly high in spices and herbs. They are also found in cola drinks, tea, coffee, peppermint tea and fruit juices. Packaged or canned foods may also contain significant amounts.

Foods containing *vaso-active amines* are another cause of intolerance and these substances are of particular concern for those suffering from irritable bowel syndrome.

Artificial additives such as preservatives and colourings are also implicated in many instances of sensitivity or intolerance. Researchers have found that tartrazine (a commonly used red/orange colouring agent) causes an increase in the urinary excretion of zinc, particularly in hyperactive children. Since zinc is intimately involved in brain function, this loss can lead to a variety of behaviour or learning problems. This finding provides solid scientific evidence for the use of the controversial Feingold diet. This diet for hyperactive children involves the avoidance of all colouring and salicylate-containing products, and, despite its many clinical successes, has been criticised for its lack of scientific basis.

Common offending foods

- dairy products and beef
- wheat/rye/oats/maize (corn)
- hen's eggs and chicken meat
- chocolate/tea/coffee
- cane and beet sugar
- colourings and preservatives
- yeast
- pork
- peanuts
- citrus fruits
- alcohol
- salicylate-containing foods
- vaso-amine-containing foods

Airborne pollutants

In other instances, you may be adversely affected by airborne pollutants such as cleaning or household solvents, chemicals, dustmites, or pollen. If you suspect that these substances may be the trigger for your reactions or ill health there are a number of provocation tests which experienced practitioners can use to identify offending substances. You can then take the necessary steps to avoid these wherever possible.

In many instances allergies or intolerances will be due to a *combination* of foods, chemicals and airborne pollutants.

Identifying allergenic substances
Why?

If you have been adversely affected by various foods or environmental agents for most of your life, you may wonder why we recommend identifying and avoiding them now. Obviously those conditions which may be due to food or chemical intolerance such as eczema, asthma, migraine, epilepsy, insomnia, gastrointestinal disturbances, neuroses or psychoses all cause episodes of ill health and stress. Ill health and stress can severely compromise your nutritional status. Furthermore, medication which may be necessary to control or alleviate symptoms may not only be best avoided in pregnancy, but may lead to malabsorption of essential nutrients. To sum up—your general health and consequently the health of sperm and ova, as well as the health of the developing foetus, may be seriously affected if these conditions are left untreated.

It is also recognised that if you suffer from untreated allergies or sensitivities, then you are likely to have children who suffer from similar allergies or intolerances. In fact, if both you and your partner are allergic or intolerant there is about a 60 per cent chance that you will have an allergic child. This is particularly true if you suffer from allergic reactions during pregnancy.

How?

In Chapter 9, we listed some of the ways in which your health practitioner may determine which substances are the offending ones. You can also, in simple cases, identify the offenders for yourself.

If you suspect that your health problems may be due to food intolerance, keep a diary in which you keep a scrupulous list of everything you eat. You should also take note of any other relevant factors, for example: were you sick, were you unduly tired, were you exposed to any other stressors? Ask yourself which food it is that you like best. If you are exhibiting symptoms of food intolerance it may mean that you will actually crave the offending food. If there is something which you feel you could not live without, removal of that food from your diet may cause initial worsening, followed by a reduction, in symptoms.

There will be instances when the offending foods may not be easily identified, and then you can try the 'lamb and pears diet' or a 'modified exclusion diet'. These are both reliable methods (we think the best methods) for the detection of food sensitivity, but this detection and treatment is best undertaken with the help of a practitioner who has experience in this field.

In fact, whether you can easily identify the offending food or not, we recommend that you *seek help from a trained health practitioner*. If you have to avoid any one or a number of major food groups, you can very easily become vitamin or mineral deficient, and it is important that you seek professional advice to ensure that you continue to receive appropriate nutrition while on the exclusion diet. If exclusion diets are undertaken without supervision, or if they are followed for prolonged periods, existing problems may be exacerbated, simply because large numbers of essential nutrients are missing from your diet. New intolerances may also arise if the number of foods eaten is extremely limited. Concurrent nutritional support/supplementation is essential to give the gut lining a chance to regenerate, to strengthen the immune system and to improve your general nutritional status.

It is definitely not the ultimate aim for you to continue on a restricted diet forever—the aim of naturopathic treatments is for you to regain robust immune and digestive systems that can tolerate a wide and comprehensive range of foods. We all know of people who can't eat this and that and have a considerably restricted lifestyle. Most people should be able to resolve their intolerances, allergies and sensitivities and resume normal, healthy eating habits.

Other contributing factors

As we have already said, you may encounter some sceptics who doubt that food can affect your physical or mental health. The reason for this doubt probably stems from the difficulty of reproducing consistent results. In other words, there will be times when you will exhibit no symptoms at all, or perhaps you will not always exhibit the same symptoms. In fact, the symptoms will depend on the total load of stressors which are affecting you at any particular time. These stressors may be psychological, they may be environmental, or they may be other problem foods. We have listed below some additional factors which might contribute to the condition of food intolerance:

- Pollutants in water (pesticides, flocculants).
- Naturally occurring chemicals in food, such as salicylates or artificially added chemicals (preservatives, colourings).
- Compromised nutritional status, particularly zinc deficiency.

- Stress of any sort (remember that positive as well as negative events can be regarded as a stress).
- Airborne pollutants (chemical sprays, agricultural and industrial pollution, low cloud cover, high pollen levels, strong winds blowing off the land, animal fur or feathers).
- High body burden of any of the toxic metals, especially lead, but also copper, aluminium, mercury and cadmium.
- Subtle world (fluorescent lights, television, noise and colours).

Therefore, if you are to properly treat your food intolerance, you must reduce the total load of stressors on your system. To put it another way, if you find that you are suffering from food (or chemical) sensitivity, you can greatly reduce the severity of your symptoms and sometimes see them completely disappear, simply by making changes to your diet and lifestyle, which is really what we have recommended in all the preceding chapters.

Exclusion diets for detecting food intolerance
Lamb and Pears Diet
Yes, we know, we know, but we did say that you won't have to live on it forever!! This is an extremely successful diet for identifying offending foods, but should not be followed for longer than seven days.

- Eat only lamb and peeled pears
- Drink only bottled spring water

You may grill, roast or casserole your lamb with pear slices. In the original lamb and pears diet, lamb offal is allowed, however we prefer that you avoid this due to reasons already mentioned. If seven days on this one seems like more than you could possibly bear, you may like to try the following diet.

Modified exclusion diet
Remember, use organically grown/fed produce wherever possible.

Food	Avoid	Eat only
Meat	Beef, pork, bacon, sausages, delicatessen meats	Lamb, rabbit, turkey, game. Use only lean cuts/cook plainly.

Food	Avoid	Eat only
Fish	Shellfish, smoked fish	White fish
Vegetables	Potatoes, onions, sweet corn, soya beans	Lettuce, celery, spinach, leeks, peas, lentils, all beans (not green or broad), brussel sprouts, cabbage.

If you suffer from gastrointestinal symptoms, avoid beans, lentils, brussel sprouts, cabbage.

Fruit	Avoid tomatoes and all fruits except those in opposite column	Bananas, mangoes, papaya, peeled pears, pomegranates
Cereals	'Big grasses'— wheat oats, barley, rye, corn	Rice, tapioca, sago, millet, buckwheat, rice flour, rice cakes
Cooking oil	Corn, soya, vegetable oils, and nut, especially peanut	Olive, sunflower, safflower, linseed oils
Dairy products	Cheese, milk, butter, yoghurt and some margarines from cow's milk. Also goat's, sheep and soya products, and eggs and chicken	
Drinks	Tea, coffee (instant, ground or decaf.), fruit squashes, orange and grapefruit juices, alcohol, unfiltered water.	Herbal teas, bottled, filtered water
Other	Chocolate, sugar, honey, herbs, spices, yeast, preservatives and all additives	Sea salt

Some tips about exclusion diets

- Your allergic symptoms may be worse if you are exposed to lots of other stressors (see above) or if you are suffering from numerous nutrient deficiencies.
- Exclusion diets are only useful for identifying offending foods— they should not be considered as treatment.
- Your symptoms may worsen initially on the diet.
- If sensitivity to certain foods is indeed the problem, you should experience an improvement, or complete disappearance of symptoms, while on the exclusion diet.
- Improvement may take some time Sometimes it may take weeks.
- If your symptoms disappear when you are on the diet, you need to find out what foods were causing them.
- To identify the offending foods, re-introduce them *only one at a time*. The speed of the reaction to the offending food will vary from minutes to hours to days.
- Re-introduce foods singly, at one or two day intervals, and in normal-size portions.
- When re-introducing foods, choose those least likely to be problematic initially, and leave more commonly allergenic foods (see above) till last.
- If you suffer a reaction, wait until this settles down before introducing another food.
- Take two teaspoonsful of sodium bicarbonate in a glass of water if the reaction is severe.

The pulse test

You may also be able to track down offending foods by using the pulse test which, although not 100 per cent reliable, has been found by many practitioners to be useful. To perform it, you must take your resting pulse rate before eating a particular food. *This should be measured in beats per minute.* (See Chapter 5 for how to take your pulse.) Perform this measurement when you are relaxed and sitting quietly, then perform the test again at intervals of 10, 20, 40 and 60 minutes after eating the food. If your pulse is elevated or decreased by more than 10 beats per minute, you can consider that the particular food is causing a stress response. Be aware, however, that the absence of an altered pulse rate does not mean that the food is not a problem one. Sometimes symptoms will occur without alteration in pulse rate and vice versa. You must also be careful to rule out a raised pulse rate which is due to emotional factors, or to increased physical activity.

Nutrients/herbs for concurrent use

You will find the full range of nutritional supplements helpful to boost your immune and digestive system. As well, herbal medicine can be used to make a several-pronged attack on the problem of allergy/intolerance.

For different organ systems

- Gut—Bitter tonics: *Golden Seal, Gentian, Agrimony, Dandelion Root*
- Liver—*St Mary's Thistle, Globe Artichoke, Barberry, Bupleurum*
- Immune system—*Echinacea, Astragalus, Siberian* and *Korean Ginseng, Reiishi, Hemidesmus*
- and for allergic reaction—*Albizzia, Baical Skullcap*

For symptoms

- Respiratory—*Elecampane, Gindelia, Horehound*
- Sinus/congestion—*Garlic, Horseradish, Golden Rod*
- Skin problems—*Calendula, Burdock, Cleavers*
- Nervous disorders—*Oats, Vervain, Valerian*
- Mental confusion—*Ginkgo, Rosemary, Schisandra*
- Inflammatory conditions—*Liquorice, Wild Yam, Black Cohosh, Rehmannia*

Once you have identified the offending food(s)

Once your immune system is no longer constantly under stress, and once the tissue of your gut lining has been given a chance to regenerate, you should be able to tolerate the previously offending foods. We recommend that, initially, you eat them only in small quantities and on a rotating (every four to seven day) basis. This is important for you to remember, since it is believed by many researchers in this field, that the foetus which is exposed to small quantities of previously problem foods will be less likely to develop intolerances than the foetus from which these substances are totally excluded.

If allergies or sensitivities appear to be a problem for either partner, ample time (which may be significantly *more than four months before conception*) must be allowed for their detection and appropriate treatment.

What if I am allergic to dairy products?

Once you are pregnant, you may be advised to drink cow's milk or eat dairy foods to ensure that sufficient calcium is available for the formation of your baby's strong bones and teeth. If, however, like a significant proportion of the population, you suffer from an allergy or an intolerance to dairy products, that problem should be identified well before conception, and you should not revert to heavy consumption of these products during pregnancy for the sake of your baby. If you need to avoid cow's milk products, then it means that you will have to obtain your calcium from other dietary sources. These include legumes, green leafy vegetables, eggs, fish with the bones (such as salmon and sardines) and tahini (sesame seed) paste and goat's milk.

You can of course also use calcium supplements, but remember to add magnesium (calcium: magnesium in the ratio of 2:1) which is required, as is Vitamin D, for the proper absorption of calcium.

Lactose intolerance, a major cause of dairy allergies or sensitivities, can be effectively treated by the use of *Acidophilus* which, although a milk derivative, digests lactose. Starting slowly, on a low dose of *half to one teaspoonful 2 to 3 times daily*, and doubling the dose at weekly intervals for the first few weeks, you should be able to tolerate milk and related products after 2 to 3 months.

It is probably also worth remembering that the majority of the world's population does not eat dairy foods and that a diet which is high in processed food, in red meat, in protein or in fat increases your body's needs for calcium, as does the consumption of alcohol, caffeine and excess sugar and salt. Conversely, weight-bearing exercise such as walking, running and cycling will keep calcium in the bones, maintaining your bone density, and reducing your need for calcium from dietary sources.

PART THREE

Time to conceive

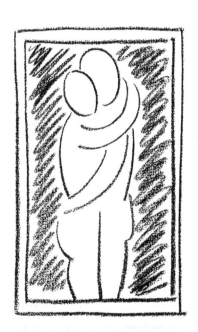

13

CONCEIVING CONSCIOUSLY

TO CONCEIVE CONSCIOUSLY AND optimistically, and
to be aware of and loving toward your child from the
very beginning, can provide the *best possible
environment* for healthy emotional growth, and your
experience will also be a profoundly joyful one.

SO, NOW, AFTER ALL that, you've prepared yourself for conception,
and you're ready to go! Everything that you have done so far should
make you supremely confident that you will easily conceive a beautiful, bright, healthy baby. The timing techniques we discussed in
Chapter 7 can now be reversed to achieve a conception, and with all
the preparation you have done, this should, for most of you, happen
easily.

However, most of you will have spent your sexually active lives
actively avoiding conception. Unless you have suffered from a fertility problem, the number of times in your fertile life that conception
is actually sought are few and far between. In addition, most women,
or couples, are usually unaware if they have conceived until several
weeks later, and cannot then confidently assess which sexual act
resulted in the conception.

But once you are aware of how to accurately identify your fertile
times this information can be used to predict confidently that on a

particular day, your love-making will also become baby-making. In this way you can *consciously* conceive, embracing all the consequences of your act of love, and welcoming your child into the physical world from the very beginning. So—confident that you have provided an optimally healthy physical environment for your child— you can do the same on an emotional and psychological level.

If you have made sure that you are reproductively healthy, and you have learnt to identify your fertile and ovulation days, you can then be reasonably confident that intercourse will result in conception and, indeed, accurate timing of intercourse can sometimes be all that is required to overcome a fertility problem. However, timing for conception is a little more complex than simply reversing the directions for contraception. You need to be aware that the sperm can live for 3 to 5 days and the egg is only viable for 12 to 24 hours. This makes optimum timing quite a precise exercise. Consider the following 'romance'.

The romance of the egg and the sperm

The healthy, well-nourished egg is released from the ovary, and is caught by the waving arms of the tiny filaments (fimbriae) around the end of the Fallopian tube. This tube is about as wide as a hairbrush bristle, and about 10 cm long. The egg itself is even smaller than the dot at the end of this exclamation mark! You think that's incredible? Well, to the sperm, the egg is a giant. 25 million sperm could fit on this full stop.

As far as sperm are concerned, we always talk in millions. *Normal* sperm counts range from 30 to 60 million per millilitre of seminal fluid, which will result in a healthy male depositing 280 to 400 million sperm in the vagina during one ejaculation. This may seem like an enormous number when only one is needed to fertilise the egg, but sperm face many hazards on their journey. They move along by lashing their tails, and are enabled to do this by a substance found in the female reproductive tract. It takes them roughly an hour of vigorous tail-lashing to complete the 18 cm marathon trip from the cervix (neck of the uterus) to the place in the Fallopian tubes (the ampulla) where, hopefully, the egg is waiting.

While the egg waits, a constituent of the fluid that surrounds it is sending out 'love letters'—messages to the sperm, alerting them to its presence and triggering their swim in the right direction. It's possible that these messages are selective, attracting the highly motile and vigorous sperm, rather than the very young or old, which might be less viable. The signals may also chivvy the sperm on from their resting places along the way.

On this journey, many of the sperm will be immobilised by the acidity in the vagina before they reach the relative safety of the alkaline cervix. Then many get lost in the uterus, simply swimming around and around until they die, never finding the two exits to the Fallopian tubes, in one of which the egg is waiting.

Many which do find one of the tube entrances will choose the wrong one (pick a tube—any tube!) An egg is normally released by one ovary in each cyle, usually alternately. So—what starts off like the crowd at a fun run, thins out just as rapidly.

The egg will wait for Mr Right for 12 to 24 hours, and then, if he hasn't arrived, will give up and die (broken-hearted—or just tired of waiting?) The sperm live longer, up to 3 to 5 days. Although they take 10 to 11 weeks to be produced, once released into the vaginal tract, 5 days is the most they can survive. However, it is extremely unlikely that such a geriatric sperm could hobble its way to the egg, and win this very competitive race.

In fact, sperm life reduces by one-third each day, and 16 to 18 hours is an average life span. The number of sperm also drops each day, and falls below a viable level within 3 days. Three days is, therefore, normally considered to be the maximum viable life span of the sperm.

Before the lucky, one-in-a-zillion sperm can penetrate the egg, it has to be 'capacitated'. This may sound like a scary initiation rite, but is in fact when hormonal secretions in the female cause the release of two enzymes from the sperm, making the way clear for the final breakthrough by enabling the sperm to burrow through the egg's two outer coatings.

Then the fertilised egg is majestically wafted down the rest of the tube, aided by the tube's rhythmic contractions and by the little cilia or hair-like projections that line it. This slow and stately progress takes about a week, after which the egg reaches the uterus, and implants in the endometrium. From that moment on, everything moves very quickly. The moral of the story is:

Timing is critical

If you have spent some months preparing for the big event, and if you want to be sure that you know which sexual act results in conception, then you need to know exactly when to 'do it'.

As we have discussed, adequate amounts of the right type of mucus are necessary to:

- Protect the sperm from the acidity in the vagina, and
- Nourish and guide them up into the cervix and the uterus.

Because this mucus is usually present before your mid-cycle ovulation and may perhaps be triggered by a spontaneous ovulation (see section on the lunar cycle in Chapter 7), the sperm can be ready and waiting for the egg as it comes down the Fallopian tube. This is much more likely to result in conception than having the egg wait for the sperm. The egg is an impatient lady, and won't wait long. So, if ovulation occurred in the morning, and intercourse took place that evening, the egg might already be dead.

Also, we aren't that good (yet) at telling precisely when ovulation occurs, so it is vital to know in advance that *ovulation is about to take place*. Information that tells you that ovulation has already taken place, such as that given by basal temperature readings, will be useless if there is any chance that it occurred up to, or more than, 12 hours previously, or if there is no opportunity for intercourse in the next 12 hours.

Baby snatching

There is another timing factor to take into consideration to ensure a healthy conception. *Ageing sperm and ova are potentially defective.* Therefore, you need to use your timing techniques to make sure that the romance between the egg and the sperm is a story of young love! Two scenarios to avoid are:

- A single sexual act several days prior to ovulation, which is likely to furnish the ovum with ageing and potentially defective sperm.
- A single sexual act just after ovulation, which creates a higher risk of the sperm meeting an ageing and potentially defective egg.

Frequent intercourse during the peak fertile time, until ovulation is over, ensures that fresh sperm meet a fresh egg. So, having waited until the right moment to start, you then keep going until you are sure that you have ovulated, with the optimum frequency being every other day. This ensures that live, fresh sperm are waiting all along the Fallopian tubes, ready for contact with the egg as it descends.

Conception at mid-cycle

Obviously, the best way to tell that you are about to ovulate, is through your mucus observations. Hopefully, you will be getting good at these by the time you plan to conceive. Another advantage of spending a few months learning about symptom observation is that, after the birth of your baby, you will already be an expert in natural contraception. Breastfeeding is not the easiest time to practise natural birth control if you are a novice.

Once fertile mucus has been detected, there is a good chance that sperm deposited in the vagina will be ready and waiting for the egg when it is released. However, you can improve upon this procedure.

By using a combination of temperature and mucus observations over several cycles, it is possible to come to a fairly precise understanding of exactly where ovulation falls in your mucus pattern.

Using the day at the beginning of the temperature rise as the most likely day for ovulation to have taken place, you can learn if there is a regular mucus pattern preceding this day. There usually is. You may find that you usually ovulate on the third day of wet mucus, or usually the fifth, or the second day of 'spinn', following three to four days of wetness.

Personal repeating patterns are uncovered in this way, and other symptoms, such as ovulation pains (called *'mittelschmerz'*, which means *'pain in the middle'*) can help to confirm this. The lymph node in your groin will also swell, on the side from which you are ovulating, at approximately the same time. You cannot expect to pinpoint ovulation to the exact day, but you *can* expect, through the cycles spent in preconception care, to refine your understanding considerably.

The day before ovulation is the most important day for you to have intercourse! Then you can be sure that fresh, vigorous sperm are ready and waiting for the egg, since the front-runners are the healthiest, while the less viable sperm trail along behind, and take longer to complete the journey. This optimum day for intercourse should be identified through observing your mucus pattern over several cycles.

Preceding this, you should have spent several days building the sperm count. Several days (3 to 5) of abstinence (no ejaculation) can help to build a high count of healthy sperm.

Ejaculation results in loss, not only of sperm, but of large amounts of essential nutrients, such as zinc and selenium. A period of abstinence which is longer than 3 to 5 days can, however, be counter-productive, as the sperm may age before ejaculation. In Chapter 8, in the section on 'Male Fertility', we looked at how you can use ancient yogic practices to improve sperm count even further.

Once you have reached the day in your mucus pattern that you consider usually precedes the day of ovulation, intercourse can start—provided this is not later than day 17 of your cycle, as this may cause problems in the pregnancy (see Chapter 7). It should then continue, with the optimum frequency being at least every other day, until you are confident you have finished ovulating.

The sperm should be deposited high in the vagina, near the cervix (penetration from the rear is most successful). After ejaculation, the penis should be left in the vagina until it is flaccid, to prevent 'pulling' the semen out. The woman should then lie down for a few minutes, to make sure that the semen remains in the appropriate place. You should avoid lubricants as they may interfere with sperm motility—even saliva can be spermicidal. If a lubricant is necessary, you can try raw egg white, which should bring a few laughs!

If your mucus pattern changes suddenly, and you suspect that ovulation has occurred, and that you have missed your chance, don't just go ahead and have intercourse anyway. Wait for the next cycle and avoid the possibility of fertilising an ageing egg.

Temperature readings obviously do not, by themselves, give you this warning of ovulation. However, they are an essential part of the process of refining your understanding of the significance of your unique mucus pattern.

You may also be interested to attempt conception at your lunar fertile time.

Conception on the 'lunar' cycle

As we have said before, there may be another cycle influencing your fertility, the biorhythmic lunar cycle. Research and clinical experience shows that women conceive at this time of peak fertility, whether or not it coincides with the mid-cycle ovulation. In Francesca's book *Natural Fertility* there is an attempt to give possible explanations for this, but, although many questions remain unanswered, conceptions do occur! Sometimes these happen at exceedingly unlikely times, such as when the lunar peak coincides with menstruation. This is also possible in short cycles, when fertile mucus may be starting to build even through bleeding.

Most surveys have found that fertility is increased if the mid-cycle ovulation occurs at the lunar peak, and, in fact, that this is a common occurrence. If these peaks do not coincide for you (see Chapter 7 on how to achieve this) then you may still choose to attempt conception at this time of seemingly heightened susceptibility to a 'spontaneous' ovulation. If using this time to attempt conception, intercourse should be frequent within the peak 24 hours, as it is the sexual stimulation which may trigger the release of the egg.

These times need to be charted for you in advance, and these calculations form part of the Natural Fertility Management kits that you can order from us (see Contacts and Resources for details). The kits for conception teach you how to plan for, and time, your conception attempt, to make the best possible use of your fertility.

Preparation for your conception attempt

In the few days preceding a conception attempt, there are several things that you can do to create a more supportive environment, and make the experience more joyful, and more likely to succeed. There are many ideas in Chapter 6 for stress relief and positive thinking, including visualisations that you can adapt for this time.

You may be using abstinence to build sperm count. This ensures that there is a vigorous, healthy, first swarm of sperm that reaches the egg just in time for fertilisation to occur. But abstinence may be stressful, and stress hinders conception (see Chapter 6). Therefore it might be helpful to use this time to offer emotional support in other physical ways. Plenty of cuddles, sexual activity that does not involve ejaculation, or massage can be great ways to lead up to this auspicious event. Massage each other's feet, hands, backs, necks, shoulders and heads. Even a novice can do remarkable things with touch. As part of the actual foreplay, a peristaltic massage (of the tummy, with strokes from the chest to the groin, or in clockwise circles, and done in time with the breathing rhythm), can be excellent for reducing abdominal tensions. Take it in turns.

You might like to create a special atmosphere, with candles, flowers, fragrances, or whatever you enjoy most. This child's conception is as important as its birth.

When you have conceived

You can be confident you have conceived if your body-at-rest temperature has been elevated for more than 20 days. You can then confirm this with a pregnancy test.

Your pregnancy will last nine lunar months (265.5 days) from the date of conception, which, of course, you have identified. During this time there will be more that you can do to support the health of yourself and your child, with continuing good nutrition an essential part of pregnancy care.

14

SOME THOUGHTS
ON INFERTILITY

A COUPLE IS DIAGNOSED as infertile if they have
been unsuccessful in conceiving after a year of trying. It
is estimated that between 10 and 15 per cent of couples
are presently in that situation, which means that about
one couple in every six is experiencing some difficulty
conceiving, and this rate is significantly higher than it
was just 30 years ago. However, where once infertile
couples simply resigned themselves to their
childlessness or adopted a child, the increasing
incidence of infertility has seen millions of dollars
poured into medical technology in an attempt
to solve the problem.

CAUSES OF INFERTILITY

The medical causes of infertility are many and varied and include
irregular ovulation, disorders of the Fallopian tubes, endometriosis,
and hostile mucus in women, and undescended testes, varicocele (a
varicose vein in the testicle), as well as low sperm count and poor
sperm motility (sperm quality) in the male. As well, of course, there
are always those cheerless terms, 'idiopathic infertility' or 'infertility
of unexplained origin', which give those on whom they are pinned,
not even the cold comfort of a medical diagnosis.

Causes of infertility in women
Disorders of Fallopian tubes
  —30 per cent
Disorders of ovulation
  —20 per cent
Endometriosis—15 per cent
Disorders of mucus—10 per cent
Other mechanical causes (e.g.
  fibroids)—5 per cent

Causes of infertility in men
Disorders of sperm (quantity
  and quality)—50 per cent
Disorders of sexual intercourse
  —30 per cent

20 per cent of infertility in both men and women is unexplained

Furthermore, the Fertility Clinic at the Royal Women's Hospital in Sydney provides the following figures which show clearly (and dispel popular misconceptions) that the male is just as likely to have infertility problems as the female:

Female problems	30 per cent
Male factors	30 per cent
Mutual problems	20 per cent
Unexplained origin	20 per cent

But many of the conditions which are given as causes of infertility are merely symptoms of something much more fundamental that is amiss. Infertility is not a disease in itself—it is a condition arising from certain deficiencies, and, possibly, disease states.

A generally poor nutritional status, undiagnosed genito-urinary infections, allergies, poor absorption in the gastrointestinal tract, an excessive burden of toxic metals, radiation and chemical or pesticide exposure and stress have all been shown to interfere with ovulation. Empirical studies have shown that women with endometriosis are also often zinc deficient. Zinc, as we have already seen, is essential for the proper fertility of both partners but may be squandered or lost in a variety of ways. Principle among these is the use of oral contraceptives (which ironically are frequently prescribed to reduce the symptoms and pain of endometriosis, but may only exacerbate the problem). Smoking, drinking, the consumption of caffeine, and stress, also contribute to zinc loss.

Foresight clinicians have also found that a woman will often manufacture hostile mucus if her partner's sperm are abnormal, as is the case when the male has a high body burden of lead, or an undiagnosed infection. It seems that nature may have actually developed a fail-safe mechanism to destroy defective sperm.

Smoking, drinking and social drugs have a direct and detrimental effect on healthy sperm production as we have already seen. Exposure to radiation, pesticides and other chemicals and toxic heavy metals, may also adversely affect male fertility and, of course, infections, malabsorption and allergies all contribute to poor sperm health.

FACTORS WHICH MAY CONTRIBUTE TO INFERTILITY

- General poor nutritional status, particularly zinc deficiency
- Smoking
- Drinking
- Caffeine consumption
- Residual effects of medication, including oral contraceptive pill use
- Consequences of contraception programs
- Excessive burden of any of the toxic (heavy) metals
- Radiation
- Chemical or pesticide exposure
- Stress
- Undiagnosed genito-urinary infections
- Allergies
- Dysfunctional immune systems
- Gastrointestinal malabsorption
- Some drugs and surgical treatments for infertility
- Greater age of would-be parents.

Indeed there is little doubt that the deficiencies of the average Western diet, coupled with a number of common lifestyle factors, undiagnosed medical conditions and the present cocktail of environmental pollutants are compromising reproductive health, and infertility is the most basic reproductive failure of all.

MEDICAL TREATMENT OF INFERTILITY

Despite the obvious overpopulation of the world, we have to ask serious questions about the future of a species which is losing its ability to naturally and effectively reproduce its kind. Certainly the increasing levels of infertility seem to be inextricably linked with the effects of our polluting habits, overuse of the earth's resources, and disregard for the integrity of nature, which, as by-products of the kind of society in which we live, are, in turn, the inevitable result of our population density.

Perhaps, in an evolutionary sense, Mother Nature is stepping in and halting the growth of a species which has reached plague proportions. It certainly seems that our future as a healthy race is dependent upon the recognition and correction of our careless lifestyle. Part of this recognition means that we must pay attention to the quality, not the quantity, of our children.

The future of our species does not depend on ever-increasing manipulation of the earth's resources, of human genetic material and of the reproductive processes, but on responsible personal attitudes to the health of our planet, homes, lifestyles and bodies, and, most of all, to the inheritors of it all—our children! We hope that this book clearly emphasises this message, so that by now it should be obvious that if you are experiencing difficulty conceiving, there is a great deal that you can do to remedy the situation. Often, careful attention to all of these self-help measures, many of which mean no more than assuming some responsible personal attitudes, may be sufficient to reverse your condition.

We have already referred to the 81 per cent success rate for treating infertility by natural means that was achieved by Foresight in their study. These figures are supported by our extensive clinical experience. Against these excellent results, the success rate of the medical approach of routinely prescribed drugs and surgery (which may well be necessary in some cases), with little or no regard for underlying general and reproductive health, does not fare well. We probably do not need to remind you that reproductive technology can offer at very best a 20 per cent success rate and, more accurately, only a 10 to 15 per cent chance of a 'take-home baby'. The many critics of this technology believe that such a success rate should more realistically be called an 85 per cent failure rate, and, of course, a drug with such a low success rate would never be marketed.

Statistics for Australia and New Zealand (for 1991), released in 1995, show the following:

GIFT	25.2 per cent pregnant	19.5 per cent live births
IVF (to the tubes)	13 per cent clinical pregnancy	9.6 per cent live births
IVF (to the uterus)	11 per cent clinical pregnancy	7.5 per cent live births

Effect on baby's health

Babies born to couples on assisted reproduction programs have a much higher incidence of prematurity and congenital abnormalities than those born without the aid of such programs, and are more likely to die in infancy. One IVF baby in every ten is only *half* the average birth weight.

A report entitled 'Assisted Conception Australia and New Zealand 1992 and 1993', which was released by the Australian Institute of Health and Welfare (AIHW) in October 1995, gives the following figures for increased complications occurring in test-tube babies.

Category	Overall population per cent	IVF/GIFT pregnancies per cent
Mothers aged over 40	1.6	5
Miscarriages	10–15	20 approx.
Premature births	7	22–25
Multiple births	1.3	17–24
Low birth weight	6	27–34
Perinatal death rate	1.2	3.2
Major abnormalities	1.6	2.5

One mother, interviewed for an ABC 'Four Corners' program on infertility and IVF, had spent four months on the roller-coaster of neonatal intensive care after the birth of triplets who all suffered severe health problems. She was not alone—three-quarters of the Neonatal Intensive Care Unit's beds were filled by premature triplets and quadruplets—all born to mothers who had undergone treatment for infertility. Some of these babies don't survive, and some parents of those who do are left to wonder whether their child's survival was, in fact, the best thing.

Dr David Cartwright, from Brisbane Women's Hospital (also interviewed on the same 'Four Corners' program) had this to say:

> '*At any given time it is not uncommon for up to one-third of the babies in the intensive and special care nurseries to be multiple birth products,*' and
>
> '*There is an increased incidence of long-term neurological handicaps, particularly with premature babies. Some of these handicaps, such as those involving learning and co-ordination, may not be clearly obvious until the child starts school.*'

There is very little research or information available on the connection between IVF, fertility drugs and deformity, but we do know that spina bifida is five times more frequent in IVF births, and when mice are given Clomid, their babies are smaller and have an increased incidence of birth defects. Interestingly, the Clomid product information states quite clearly that there is a chance that clomiphene may cause birth defects if it is taken after you become pregnant!

Professor Les White at Sydney's Prince of Wales Hospital noticed rare cancers in babies whose mothers were treated with fertility drugs. He is not certain whether these findings are coincidental.

Effect on mother's health

There are often severe repercussions for the woman's general and reproductive health as a result of the drugs and surgical procedures used. The use of anaesthesia has the potential for serious side-effects and the surgery which is performed may well create further fertility problems.

The use of clomiphene citrate (marketed as Clomid), a fertility drug used to stimulate follicle stimulating hormone (FSH) release from the pituitary gland has been clearly linked with an increased incidence of ovarian cancer, and it has been recommended that all women considering using this (or a similar) drug should have a 'base-line' ultrasound to assess the tendency to benign or malignant tumour development. Other side-effects of this drug include 'exploding ovaries', subsequent polycystic ovarian syndrome and a host of hormone related side-effects such as nausea, gastrointestinal problems, thrush and headaches. One ironic side-effect is that Clomid thickens cervical mucus, thereby lowering fertility!

In 1989, the World Health Organisation (WHO) issued a report urging that induction of ovulation, using fertility drugs, be limited until the risks are better known. Furthermore, it said:

- These drugs should not be used for women who were naturally ovulating
- The number of cycles of use should be limited
- Drug-free IVF cycles should be aimed for wherever possible.

A senior research fellow at the University of Melbourne in the Department of Surgery, says that the long-term effects of fertility drugs are being ignored by the bioethicists. She believes that all forms of reproductive technology, including IVF, should be abolished in order to prevent continuing 'victimisation' of women during assisted pregnancies.

Problems with IVF programs

It is now acknowledged that couples doing nothing to help themselves conceive have a better chance of overcoming fertility problems than those on IVF and associated programs. Although there is a distinct lack of comprehensive scientific evaluation of IVF against either 'no treatment' or 'natural treatment', IVF is said to be 'in evolution', that is, it is experimental. In a report from the University of Western Australia and the Western Australian Health Department to the World Health Organization, the authors concluded that there was:

- A lack of standardisation in reporting the results of IVF
- Deficiencies in classifying infertility
- Inconsistencies in evaluating results, and
- Little information to compare IVF with other forms of infertility care.

We also, of course, as the providers of natural treatment for infertility, cannot comply with many of the above requirements, but the approach that we advocate does not adversely affect your physical and emotional well-being. In fact, if you follow our suggestions, the very least that can happen is that you will end up healthier!

A National Health and Medical Research Council report on the long-term effects on women from assisted conception programs concluded that:

- Some clinics provide misleading patient information which glosses over potential adverse outcomes of reproductive technologies such as IVF, and
- In many cases negative aspects of the treatment are played down with reassuring language, conveying the message that there is really nothing to worry about.

The report called for information on short-term effects such as:

- Potentially life-threatening ovarian hyperstimulation syndrome
- Higher rates of multiple and ectopic pregnancies and pregnancy loss,

and of long-term effects such as:

- The possibility of recurrent pancreatitis
- The possibility of maternal malignancy
- The possibility of psychotic reactions.

Reproductive technology puts an enormous amount of stress on both partners, although it seems that the woman usually bears a far greater burden. Not least is the feeling of disempowerment which comes from the conveyor-belt attitudes and systems which prevail in many IVF clinics, and from the lack of real information and choice offered.

We have already spoken of some of the ill-effects of stress, so it should be obvious from that point of view alone that a technologically assisted fertilisation is off to a less than ideal start. We know, however, that very few infertile couples are actually deterred by the stress involved in the procedures, but if you are aware that this alone can be a contributing factor to the success or otherwise of the techniques, then you can take steps to reduce its ill-effects by some of the methods already outlined.

Improving the success rate

In some instances, of course, the Fallopian tubes may be so damaged, or other problems may be of such long standing, that reproductive technology is the only option.

However, we firmly believe that couples who do need to use this technology, but who have cleaned up their diet, their lifestyle and their environment, and who have treated any undiagnosed medical conditions, preferably through non-invasive, natural means, will have a much better chance of an assisted fertilisation and a healthy baby than those who have not. It is significant that some prominent local IVF clinics have found that those couples who have attended fully to their preconception care at our clinic have consistently better results on assisted reproduction programs. Put simply, some sort of stress reduction, together with a much improved diet and lifestyle, the treatment of infection and removal of environmental pollutants will help to ensure that any assisted pregnancy gets off to the best possible start under any circumstances.

RESEARCH ASSOCIATED WITH REPRODUCTIVE TECHNOLOGY

Although we acknowledge the helpful role that assisted reproduction technology has in some specific fertility problems, we do feel that, apart from it being decidedly less successful, and more problematic than natural methods of fertility enhancement, there are other serious ethical, legal, social and political problems involved.

IVF clinics are funded by a huge amount of public money, as well as by extremely high payments from desperate infertile couples (and single women). The most recent figures available show that in 1991 Australian women took more than $6 million worth of drugs and hormones for infertility (most of this while on IVF programs). That's a lot of money and does not include the cost of the procedures. As well, the massive cost of postnatal care of premature, multiple or defective babies is not calculated or added when assessing the cost of IVF to the community. We feel strongly that if this money were put towards preventive health care, the results would be infinitely more successful, both in terms of increased fertility, general health and well-being and sense of empowerment for those involved.

In infertility clinics, treatment of couples occurs alongside a great deal of research aimed at improving reproductive technology. Much of this research would have read, a few years ago, like a science fiction novel! Yet, increasingly, procedures that would, until recently, have horrified us in their implications, are becoming commonplace. The result of this is that reproduction is gradually being removed from the human being (specifically the woman) to the laboratory, giving rise to a level of control that has hitherto only been hinted at in books about fearful totalitarian future societies! Genetic

manipulation gives rise to fears that fascist, sexist and racist programs could develop.

Individuals involved in this research may have the best of inten-
tions, but the technology is developing so fast, and the legal restraints
are so piecemeal, that to many of us, it seems out of control. Ad hoc
legislation arises in different countries. For example, in Britain, it is
no longer legal for a black woman to choose eggs donated by a white
woman in order to give her child a better chance in life. Similarly,
a white woman cannot choose eggs from a black donor. Also in
Britain there has been recent debate about the ethics of fielding eggs
from an unborn foetus, since the resulting child, would, in effect,
have no mother at all!

In Canada, they are considering a ban on the use of embryos in
research related to cloning and animal/human hybrids, the fertilisation of eggs from female foetuses (as in Britain), sale of
eggs/sperm/zygotes and foetal tissue, and advertising, paying for, or
acting as an intermediary for, surrogacy. In France (and perhaps soon
in Italy) it is no longer possible for post-menopausal women to
exercise their right to a child by using donated eggs and IVF
procedures coupled with massive injections of hormones. In other
countries it is illegal for *neo-morts* (newly dead women) to be kept
alive on life support systems while their wombs are used as incuba-
tors. This technique was developed in order to avoid the legal
strictures on surrogacy which refer to the surrogate mother as *she*
while a neo-mort is legally neuter. Who knows what will be next?

There is no worldwide scrutiny or control over these procedures.
It is now possible for a child to be born from an egg donor, a sperm
donor, a womb donor and to have two legal parents who are none
of these things. This child could perhaps be excused for having an
identity crisis and a confused idea of its history and heritage. Likewise, experimentation with, and (especially in cases where parents
separate) ownership of, frozen, discarded and non-viable embryos
becomes a legal and social nightmare, as does the possibility of
confusions arising with the identity and ownership of eggs, sperm
and embryos. Parents have to trust the efficiency and ethics of the
clinics, and there have been several cases where it has become
obvious, as a child is born or grows, that it does not *belong* to its
supposed parents.

BEFORE YOU OPT FOR REPRODUCTIVE TECHNOLOGY

If women and their partners choose to solve their fertility problems in the more effective natural way, they can maintain their self-respect and feel empowered. Their money is spent on themselves, on their own health and that of their children, and will not go into funding research. Even if they fail to conceive, they will be healthier, will have addressed their stress problems and have had some help and counselling in coming to terms with their infertility.

In our practice we do not necessarily see lack of conception as a failure. Couples may need support through a process of grieving for their fertility and for the children they have not been able to have, and they may need help with restoring their self-esteem as they come to terms with their infertility, but if that couple is able to go on and lead a healthy and happy life, with absolutely no doubts that they have done everything they can to resolve their problem, have a full understanding of their situation and have no feelings of guilt, remorse or resentment, then this is, in its own way, a success.

Having said all of this, we do not want you to feel that we are totally against orthodox medicine per se. This is certainly not the case, and we believe that any responsible approach to health and fertility needs to involve informed choices of the best offer from whatever source. However, we would like to feel that couples felt free to choose not to try these technological approaches, without suffering guilt and disapproval from family and friends.

We do recognise that, as well as providing effective treatment for some fertility problems, medicine has made some remarkable breakthroughs in their diagnosis. In the remainder of this chapter we have included some of the diagnostic procedures which may be helpful in determining the reasons for your infertility. We have divided these into *non-invasive* and *invasive* procedures. We strongly recommend that while you are attending to all of the measures already outlined to improve your fertility, that you choose, wherever possible, to be subjected to non-invasive procedures only.

NON-INVASIVE TESTS

In Chapter 7 we discussed in detail the temperature/mucus/symptom charts. These can reveal a great deal about any hormone/nutrient imbalances you may have and you will be able to observe these too when you practise Natural Fertility Management.

Hormone Assays

Your oestrogen level should be tested a day or two prior to ovulation when it is at its peak. The level of oestrogen will affect mucus production and ovulation. Your doctor may assume that ovulation occurs on day 14 of your menstrual cycle, but everyone is different. Charting will help you assess the best day (though mucus observations or blood tests performed by your doctor can be carried out on consecutive days to monitor hormone levels).

Your progesterone level should be tested one week after ovulation, when it should be peaking if ovulation has actually occurred. Once again, your doctor may assume that this peak will be on day 21, but it may not be so for you. Again charting will be helpful.

If there is any doubt about the regularity of your ovulation then luteinising hormone (LH) and follicle stimulating hormone (FSH) should be tested just before you ovulate.

If your oestrogen level is low and LH and FSH are high, then you may be menopausal. If your LH is high, and your FSH and oestrogen are low, you may have polycystic ovarian syndrome. If your menstrual cycles are irregular, high prolactin levels may indicate a pituitary problem (or, of course, you may be lactating). High testosterone levels may indicate that you are suffering from polycystic ovarian syndrome. High testosterone levels may simply be indicated by menstrual irregularity accompanied by obesity, acne and hirsutism. See Chapter 8, section on 'Irregular Cycles and Hormonal Imbalance' for more on how to treat all these conditions.

Post-coital Test (PCT)

This test can tell you if your infertility problem is a mutual one, and can be a useful first investigation. However, it must be carried out mid-cycle (when conception may occur) so it is important that *your preconception preparation is complete*. Intercourse at the time of ovulation is necessary and a swab (similar to a pap smear) is taken as soon as possible thereafter. This test will diagnose if the sperm survive in/penetrate the mucus, but will not tell you why not (if not), so you may then need to have a:

Sperm Cervical Mucus Contact Test (SCMCT) or Sperm Invasion Test

In this test, sperm and mucus are put together on a slide and checked against donor mucus and donor sperm and individually assessed. You can find out whether your mucus is too acidic, insufficient or of a poor quality. This may indicate a possible oestrogen or nutrient deficiency or perhaps some cervical damage.

Mucus can be 'hostile' for other reasons which include toxicity, either of the cervical mucus, or the sperm, or there may be antibodies to the sperm. Sperm antibody testing is done separately and the health of the sperm is assessed in the same way as in the semen analysis already discussed. Sperm antibodies in the male can be treated by boosting the immune system with nutrients and herbs. If the female has antibodies to her partner's sperm, condoms can be used for several months to desensitise the woman, while boosting her immune system, and while steps are taken to detoxify the male.

This test is definitely one worth knowing about, since it can be done before your preconception preparation is complete. It can highlight many problems which can be treated without resorting to more invasive procedures or to reproductive technology. However, many doctors and gynaecologists remain unaware of how these incompatibility problems can be treated by natural means, so they generally tend to go straight for assisted reproduction without ordering any prior assessment of this type.

INVASIVE TESTS

At the outset we want to say that, in our opinion, these tests should be undergone as a last resort only. If you have both exhausted every option outlined in this book, and if after a reasonable period of time there is absolutely no response whatsoever to your improved diet, environment and lifestyle, then you might consider, as an option, the procedures outlined below.

If your infertility problems are so intractable or of such long standing that these tests do become necessary, then we should emphasise that you will need to *start your preconception care all over again*, with due regard for timing of X-rays, detoxification for anaesthesia and other drugs used, and so on.

The tests listed below are not the only ones which are available. Newer ones are constantly being developed. If you are in any doubt at all about a procedure which your doctor orders for you, we suggest that you ask for a full account of exactly what is involved. We recommend that you only undergo a procedure if the outcome, or the information gained thereby, is essential to, or will substantially affect, any subsequent decisions or course of action.

Remember, too, that very few doctors who order these investigations have any knowledge whatever of natural ways of improving your fertility, and that treatment of infertility by medical means provides their livelihood. Also, they have almost certainly never undergone the procedures themselves. Their so-called 'mild discomfort' has been found by many women to be absolute agony. You should also be aware that little, if any, regard is paid to the effects the X-rays, anaesthesia, dyes and so on may have on any embryo which is conceived in the cycles immediately following these procedures.

Laparoscopy

This investigation involves a laparoscope (a small camera on the end of a filament) being inserted through your navel to view the pelvic cavity and reproductive organs. This procedure, which is done under full anaesthesia, can tell if you are suffering from adhesions, endometriosis, pelvic inflammatory disease, polycystic ovaries, fibroids, or from abnormalities of the uterus, tubes or ovaries. During this test a dye is usually sent through the Fallopian tubes from the uterus. The laparoscope determines if the dye emerges from either/both tubes. However, this merely shows if your tubes are open or closed and does not tell you if your tubal function is good. In other words it does not tell you about the condition of the cilia, nor of the tubes' ability to contract rhythmically for the adequate transport of ova and sperm.

Hysterosalpingogram

(If you can say this you can get pregnant!) In this procedure a dye is injected into your uterus and the results are observed on X-ray.

This procedure really hurts and tells you a lot less than a laparoscopy. It is debatable, of course, whether the effects of full anaesthesia or X-ray are more harmful. Although anaesthesia is generally considered to carry a greater risk, the residual effects in the body are not long lasting. On the other hand, X-rays of the lower back and abdominal region have been shown to adversely affect sperm production for up to three years, and it is reasonable to suppose that ova would be similarly affected.

Tubal Insufflation

This procedure involves the use of gas rather than dye, but gives results which are much less reliable, although it involves no X-rays and no anaesthesia.

Ultrasound

This can show if the uterus is abnormally shaped and if the ovaries are enlarged. If follicles show, then you know that ovulation has taken place, or if there are many follicles, then the ovaries are probably polycystic. We know that ultrasound affects the foetus, so we assume that it must also affect the eggs.

Dilation and curettage

This procedure is commonly ordered and is routine with most of the other procedures we have mentioned. We believe that it is rarely necessary unless your period is delayed because the endometrium is not coming away properly (not because of a delay in ovulation which is much more common). We would prefer to treat this problem with herbs, although a D and C sometimes seems to help in ways which we don't really understand.

Hysteroscopy

In this procedure a camera goes up through the cervix and into the uterus. It records the condition of the endometrium, and can see fibroids which project internally into the uterus. These are more of a problem than those that project externally because they may affect the implantation and growth of the embryo.

Endometrial biopsy

A sample of tissue is taken at approximately day 21 (or one week after ovulation) to see if the endometrium is building properly. This test will usually be unnecessary because temperature charts (or a blood test) should tell you about progesterone levels, and with good nutrition and herbs it is usually possible to deal with any problems. Clotting during a period indicates poor endometrial condition, excessive oestrogen levels or low iron status.

CONCLUSION

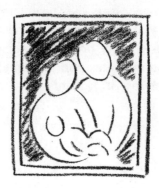

FOR THE PAST 200 years, a mechanistic view of the world and its inhabitants has prevailed. During this time we have focused our attention on the exploration and the domination of nature and on the attainment of mastery over our surroundings. We have been to the summits of high mountains and to the depths of the oceans. We have put men on the moon and sent space probes to the farthest reaches of our solar system. We have taken untold riches from the earth and turned them into housing, clothing and machines to make our lives easier. We have also used them to create weapons of destruction and a host of other products which have little intrinsic value for human-kind. We have shaped the land to produce the food we need. We have then shaped the food in the search for a bigger, more attractive or longer lasting product . . . we have conquered, plundered, changed and manipulated.

It was inevitable that we should also view ourselves and our children as machines whose workings we could further manipulate or perhaps improve upon. We have seen illness or disease, and wear or malfunction in our bodies, as isolated incidents which we could attend to in much the same way as we would attend to the repair of a flat tyre. We have embraced the science and technology which has given us organ transplants, synthetic replacements for worn parts and the drugs which can affect and alter every aspect of our being. We are now tolerating, and even encouraging, a medical and scientific

344

approach to 'better babies' which embraces genetic engineering and all its potential for fascist, racist and sexist implications.

Along with our acceptance of and reliance on this mechanistic model we have abrogated our responsibility for the well-being of the earth and for our own well-being. We have come to believe that science and technology can fill all our needs and provide the answer to all our problems and the cure for all our ills. At the same time, we have neglected or negated those aspects of our existence which cannot be measured, quantified or analysed. Our actions are now invariably the results of reasoning, logic and calculation. We no longer trust our intuition or our instincts.

But at last we are seeing a paradigm shift. Physicists, chemists, biologists and many others are starting to recognise that there is a continuum to life on earth and beyond. We are in fact rediscovering what was known by philosophers and mystics of innumerable ages past—that we are an intimate part of the earth and everything on it, and our every action will affect that whole of which we are a part. We are increasingly aware that the old Cartesian model of a single action leading to a single effect is no longer valid. Just as a tiny pebble thrown into a pond will cause ripples to go to the farthest reaches of that pond, so all the changes which we have wrought in our environment will have effects which are far-reaching and all-encompassing. 'Chaos' theory links the flap of the butterfly's wings in Peru with the tidal wave in Bangladesh.

While this switch to an holistic view of ourselves and of our world is occurring worldwide and in all fields of endeavour, nowhere is it more apparent than in our growing concern for the environment. We now generally accept that if there is to be a quality to the life of future generations, then we cannot continue to produce, consume and pollute as we do today. Recognition is at last being given to the profound effects which our tampering has had on both the macro and micro environment in which all life is created and in which it then develops and grows. In the words of Greenpeace, we are learning that we must 'step lightly' on the earth.

The validity and importance of a holistic approach is also now recognised by many health practitioners and their patients. This approach, which involves natural therapies combined with diet and lifestyle changes, means that it is the individual rather than the practitioner who is responsible for health and well-being. In the case of preconception care, two individuals assume responsibility for their own health and well-being as well as for that of their children. We believe that it is up to all of us to assume this responsibility.

We believe that if strenuous efforts are not made to do so then the numbers of future children born with a physical, mental or emotional disability, may eventually be more than the fit and well population can support. Perhaps there will come a time when couples who fail to make efforts to improve their own fertility by those methods we have outlined, will not be able to resort to reproductive technology, just as perhaps someone who continues to smoke 60 cigarettes a day will not be eligible for a heart transplant or a coronary bypass.

While this attitude may seem harsh, we firmly believe that all of us must accept responsibility for our own lives, and one of the most important aspects of those lives is our health. We should no longer expect doctors to perform endless miracles with drugs and surgery. Of course there will always be a place for crisis care intervention in medicine, but by and large preventive medicine is the medicine of the future. The health of all future children is in our hands. We must all accept the responsibility for making that absolutely sound physical, mental and emotional health.

A wise women has said that if we are to heal the earth, then first we must heal ourselves. Having 'better babies' is the first step in this healing process. Our children will live out their lives in the twenty-first century. They will encounter obstacles and challenges of which we, their parents, can only dream. If they are to overcome these obstacles, and if they are to meet the challenges head-on, it is essential that we give them all a 'better beginning', which is what Nature in her infinite wisdom intended them to have.

APPENDIX

SUCCESS RATES OF CONTRACEPTION METHODS

Ranges indicate varied results from different surveys.

Method	'Theoretical' success rate per cent	'User' success rate per cent
Pill—Combined	99.5	95–99
—Mini-pill	97–99	93–99
IUD	94–99	93–98
Condoms	97–99	80–93
Diaphragm/Cap (+ spermicide)	97–98	80–97
Spermicide (Vitamin C)	96	96
Spermicide (chemical)	85–95	75–85
Withdrawal	90	70–85
Injections (Depo-provera)	99	99
Sterilisation (male and female)	99.5–99.9	93–99.9
Natural Birth Control		
Sympto-thermal method	97–99.8	70–98
Mucus method	97–99.8	70–98
Temperature method*	93–99	75–98
Rhythm method (regular cycles)	98	60–85
Rhythm method (irregular cycles)	55	30–55
Lunar cycle (with rhythm)	98.5	97.5–98.5

*Temperature method implies abstinence in pre-ovulatory phase.

CONTACTS AND RESOURCES

We have given national contacts wherever possible. NSW contacts, when given, can usually supply you with appropriate addresses in your own state or territory. Natural health journals also contain service directories that will give many more names and addresses than we have been able to list here. All addresses and phone numbers are up to date at time of publication.

Francesca and Janette also offer the following services that can augment and update the information in this book. They are also available for conferences, community and professional seminars, media interviews, lectures and consultancy work.

THE BOOKS

These books by Francesca Naish and Janette Roberts are available through all good book stores, by mail order or through the internet. All prices are quoted in Australian dollars and include GST.

- *The Natural Way to a Better Pregnancy* by Francesca Naish and Janette Roberts, Doubleday, $25.00.
- *The Natural Way to Better Birth and Bonding* by Francesca Naish and Janette Roberts, Doubleday, $27.50.
- *Natural Fertility: The Complete Guide to Avoiding or Achieving Conception* by Francesca Naish, Sally Milner Publishing, $33.00.
- *The Lunar Cycle* by Francesca Naish, Nature & Health Books, $13.00.

For the above books, send credit card details (Visa/Mastercard/Bankcard) to: Natural Fertility Management, PO Box 786, Castlemaine Vic 3450, Australia; Ph: (61-3) 5472 4922, Fax: (61-3) 5470 5766; or email: enquiries@fertility.com.au

Please include postage costs: $10.00 for up to four books (within Australia); $25.00 for up to two books (overseas economy air).

Or order through: www.fertility.com.au or www.chakra.net

NATURAL FERTILITY MANAGEMENT

Francesca is the founder and director of Natural Fertility Management (NFM), which offers programs for:
- Natural contraception
- Conscious conception and preconception health care
- Overcoming fertility problems (male and female)
  as well as holistic health care for:
- Reproductive health (male and female)
- Pregnancy and preparation for birth
- Threatened miscarriage
- Breastfeeding
- Menopause
  You can find out more about NFM on our website: www.fertility.com.au.

Personal consultations
The Natural Fertility Management clinic offers all of the above programs and treatments at: The Jocelyn Centre, 46 Grosvenor Street, Woollahra NSW 2025, Australia; Ph: (61-2) 9369 2047, Fax: (61-2) 9369 5179.

A comprehensive range of holistic medical and natural treatments is provided by highly qualified practitioners, using natural and non-invasive therapies.

How to find a local NFM practitioner
NFM provides a referral service to NFM accredited counsellors throughout Australia, as well as in New Zealand, USA and the UK.

Send a stamped, addressed envelope to: Jane Bennett, NFM Network Co-ordinator, PO Box 786, Castlemaine VIC 3450, Australia; Ph: (61-3) 5472 4922, Fax: (61-3) 5470 5766.

Or you can contact her through our website: www.fertility.com.au, or email: enquiries@fertility.com.au

Postal and internet services
For those unable to attend personally, contraception and conception kits are also available by mail order or through the internet. The NFM kits include:
- A copy of the book *Natural Fertility: A Complete Guide to Avoiding or Achieving Conception* (or rebate on proof of purchase).
- A copy of the book *The Natural Way to Better Babies: Preconception Health Care for Prospective Parents* (for conception kits only—rebate on proof of purchase).
- An audio cassette with:
  Side 1 Instructions for contraception or conception and use of lunar cycle charts, and
  Side 2 Relaxation techniques, visualisations, and suggestions to assist the synchronisation of cycles, increase confidence and motivation, promote

reproductive health and general wellbeing, and deal with stress. In the conception kit there are also suggestions for a healthy conception, pregnancy and birth.

- Blank sympto-thermal charts for recording mucus and temperature and other observations for each menstrual cycle.
- Individual computer-calculated lunar charts showing the potentially fertile times on your personal bio-rhythmic fertility cycle for the next ten years.
- Current year Moon Calendar, showing moon phase present on each day of the year.
- Time zone calculator, to adjust times given on your personal lunar chart for different time zones.
- Attractively bound printed notes for conception or contraception, taking you through the first few months, cycle by cycle.
- Options:
  1. for conscious conception—sex selection calculations and advice;
  2. for male fertility problems—male lunar chart, male relaxation and suggestion tape;
  3. naturopathic advice for your personal situations from Francesca Naish and associates.

Orders can be placed through the website or by post: Contact Jane Bennett, NFM Network Coordinator, as above.

NFM counsellor training
Residential seminars are conducted by Francesca Naish and associates to train health professionals in NFM techniques and the *Better Babies* program of preconception health care and fertility treatments. All accredited counsellors have access to NFM kits for their patients, and professional support. You can find out more about training through the website, or by contacting the NFM Network Coordinator.

NFM and Better Babies Helpline
Francesca Naish and associates are also available for advice on all reproductive health issues, as well as those associated with fertility and contraception. Phone consultations for simple enquiries are charged by the minute. More complex problems can be addressed postally or through email. For enquiries contact the Network Coordinator. Payment for on-line, postal or telephone consultations can be made by Visa/Mastercard/Bankcard (or by cheque or money order). Individual advice for preconception health care, fertility problems or contraception can be included as part of the kits available through our postal or internet service. See above for details.

CHAKRA.NET (NATURAL PARENTING)

Jan has developed the Natural Parenting website for the chakra.net portal, a fully interactive site offering a complete range of holistic services designed to help you achieve optimum personal potential and health and wellbeing for all your family. Join on-line chats, ask questions, consult the experts on-line, find the nutritional supplements and other products that support your natural parenting choices: Website: www.chakra.net; Email: naturalparenting@chakra.net

SPA CHAKRA

Jan has developed the Chakra Baby program exclusively for Spa Chakra, which was recently voted Australia's only five-star spa. The Chakra Baby program combines a highly interactive range of educational sessions for mother, father and baby with your choice of one of the Spa's luxurious, pampering treatments. Visit the website: www.chakra.net; or contact:

Spa Chakra Sydney, 170 Victoria Street, Potts Point NSW 2011; Ph: (61-2) 9368 0888, Fax: (61-2) 9380 2950; Email: spachakra@chakra.net

Spa Chakra Melbourne, Hilton-on-the-Park, 192 Wellington Parade, East Melbourne VIC 3002, Australia. Ph: (61-3) 9412 3190; Fax: (61-3) 9412 3191; Email: spachakra.melbourne@chakra.net

FORESIGHT ASSOCIATION

Jan is the Australian representative of Foresight, The UK Association for the Promotion of Preconceptual Care. Members receive regular newsletters with updated research results. Fully referenced booklets are available, detailing the adverse effects on reproduction of the following: alcohol, tobacco, zinc deficiency, manganese deficiency, food additives, genito-urinary infections, lead and agro-chemicals. The Foresight video 'Preparing for the Healthier Baby' (running time 85 minutes) is suitable for viewing by preconception couples. Contact: Foresight, 16/133 Rowntree St, Birchgrove, NSW 2041, Australia. Ph:/Fax: (61-2) 9818 3734; Website: www.wellnesscentre.com.au; Email: janroberts@wellnesscentre.com.au

THE TUBETRAIN EXERCISE SYSTEM

Developed by Jan's business partner specifically for use in the post-natal period. Economical, portable, safe and effective – comes complete with workout video. Payment for TUBETRAIN system can be made by Visa, MasterCard or Bankcard. Contact: Tubetrain, 16/133 Rowntree Street, Birchgrove, NSW 2041, Australia. Ph: (61-2) 9818 5588, Fax: (61-2) 9818 3022; Website: www.wellnesscentre.com.au; Email: janroberts@wellnesscentre.com.au

OTHER CONTACTS AND RESOURCES

To find a doctor trained in nutritional and environmental medicine, contact:
Australian College of Nutritional and Environmental Medicine (ACNEM), 13 Hilton Street, Beaumaris VIC 3193; Ph: (61-3) 9589 6088, Fax: (61-3) 9589 5158

For names of appropriate natural health practitioners, contact:
The Australian Acupuncture and Chinese Medicine Association (AACMA), PO Box 5142, West End QLD 4101; Ph: (61-7) 3846 5866

Association of Massage Therapists (NSW), PO Box 1248, Bondi Junction NSW 2022; Ph: (61-2) 9517 9925

Association of Remedial Masseurs, 1/120 Blaxland Road, Ryde NSW 2112; Ph: (61-2) 9807 4769

Australian Association of Reflexology, PO Box 366, Cammeray NSW 2062; Ph: (61-2) 0500 502 250

Australian Homoeopathic Association NSW branch, 171 Victoria Road, Drummoyne 2047; Ph: (61-2) 9231 3322

Australian Hypnotherapists' Association, Freecall: 1800 067 557

Australian Natural Therapists Association, Freecall: 1800 817 577

Australian Osteopathic Association, PO Box 699, Turramurra NSW 2074; Ph (61-2) 9449 4799

Australian Psychological Society, 1 Grattan St Carlton 3053; Ph: (61-3) 8662 3300

Australian School of Reflexology, 25 Nords Road, Nords Wharf NSW 2281; Ph: (61-2) 4976 3881

Australian Society of Clinical Hypnotherapists, 30 Denistone Road, Eastwood NSW 2122; Ph: (61-2) 9874 2776

Australian Society of Hypnosis (members are doctors, dentists, psychiatrists, psychologists), Ph: (61-2) 9417 0091

Academy of Applied Hypnosis, 302 Pacific Hwy, Lindfield NSW 2070, Ph: (61-2) 9415 6500

Australian Traditional Medicine Society, PO Box 1027, Meadowbank NSW 2114; Ph: (61-2) 9809 6800

BKS Iyengar (Yoga) Association of Australia Inc., PO Box 159, Mosman NSW 2088; Ph: (61-2) 9948 2366

Chiropractors Association of Australia, Freecall: 1800 803 665

International Federation of Aromatherapists, PO Box 107, Burwood NSW 2134; PO Box 400, Balwyn VIC 3103; IFA National Information Line, Ph: 190 224 0125

International Yoga Teachers Association Inc., PO Box 207, St Ives NSW 2075; Ph: (61-2) 9484 2256

Natural Health Society, Suite 28/541 High Street, Penrith NSW 2750; Ph: (61-2) 4721 5068

Natural Herbalists Association of Australia, PO Box 61, Broadway NSW 2007; Ph: (61-2) 9211 6437

Reflexology Association of Australia, 22 Lagoon Street, Narrabeen NSW 2101; Ph: (61-2) 9970 6155

Reiki Network, 187a Avenue Road, Mosman NSW 2088; Ph: (61-2) 9969 1623; Freecall 1800 804 529

Shiatsu Therapy Association of Australia, 332 Carlisle Street, Balaclava VIC 3183; Ph: (61-3) 9530 0067; PO Box 47 WAverley NSW 2024; Ph: (61-2) 9314 5248

Tai Chi, the Australian Academy of, PO Box 1020, Burwood North NSW 2134; Ph: (61-2) 9797 9355

To receive an organic products directory, contact:
Heaven and Earth Systems Pty Ltd, Ph/Fax: (61-2) 9365 7668

To find a supplier of organically grown produce near you, contact:
The National Association for Sustainable Agriculture, Australia (NASAA)
    Head Office: PO Box 768, Stirling SA 5152; Ph: (61-8) 8370 8455, Fax: (61-8) 8370 8381
    New South Wales and ACT: c/- PO Box 770, North Sydney NSW 2060
    Queensland: PO Box 733, Emerald QLD 4720
    South Australia: c/- PO Box 261-7, Stirling SA 5152
    Tasmania: Post Office, Lower Longley TAS 7109
    Victoria: c/- RMB 1299, Blampied VIC 3363
    Western Australia: PO Box 8387, Stirling Street WA 6849
    The Organic Retailers & Growers Association of Australia (ORGAA), PO Box 12852, PO, Melbourne VIC 3000; Ph: (61-3) 9737 9799 or 1800 356 299

For information on genetically engineered foods, contact:
The Gene Ethics Network, PO Box 2424, Fitzroy MC VIC 3065; Ph: (61-3) 9416 2222, Fax: (61-3) 9416 0767, Email: acfgenet@peg.apc.org

To find out if drugs you need to take are safe during pregnancy, contact:
Australian Drug Evaluation Committee, PO Box 100, Woden ACT 2606;
Poisons Information Service: 13 1126 (for all states)

If you have trouble stopping smoking, contact:
Smokers' clinic, St Vincent's Hospital, 366 Victoria Street, Darlinghurst NSW 2010; Ph: (61-2) 9361 8025

If you need help overcoming an addiction to drugs or alcohol, contact:
The Jocelyn Centre, 46 Grosvenor Street NSW 2025; Ph: (61-2) 9369 2047
The Langton Centre, Nobbs Street (cnr South Dowling Street) Surry Hills NSW 2010; Ph: (61-2) 9332 8777
Alcohol and Drug Information Service, St Vincents Hospital, Victoria Street Darlinghurst, NSW 2010; Ph: (61-2) 9361 8000
Alcoholics Anonymous National Office, Joynton Avenue, Zetland NSW 2017; Ph: (61-2) 9663 1206

For information on hazards at work, contact:

Total Environment Centre, Level 2, 362 Kent St, Sydney NSW 2000; Ph: (61-2) 9299 5599

National Occupational Health & Safety Commission, 92 Parramatta Rd, Camperdown NSW 2050; Ph: (61-2) 9577 9555; Freecall: 1800 252 226

For information on safe lead removal, contact:

Environmental Protection Authority, Level 15, 59-61 Goulburn St, Sydney NSW 2000; Ph: (61-2) 9995 5000

The Lead Group, PO Box 161, Summer Hill NSW 2130; Ph: (61-2) 9716 0014; Fax: (61-2) 9716 9005; The Lead Advisory Service Aust (information and referral service on lead poisoning) Freecall: 1800 626 086

For advice on removal of dental amalgam, contact:

The Australasian Society of Oral Medicine and Toxicology (ASOMAT), Dr Robert Gammal, President, PO Box A860, Sydney South NSW 2000; Ph: (61-2) 9867 1111; Fax: (61-2) 9283 2230

For alternative pest extermination, contact:

Academic Pest Control, PO Box 714, Double Bay NSW 2028 or 12 Anderson St, West Botany NSW 2019; Ph: (61-2) 9666 8666

Systems Pest Management, PO Box 889, Epping NSW 2121; Ph: (61-2) 9869 3153 Fax: (61-2) 9869 3642

Enviropest, Freecall: 1800 048 200

For devices which can protect against electromagnetism and radiation, contact:

Integrated Functional Medicine P/L, PO Box 65, Kalorama VIC 3766; Ph: (61-3) 9761 9951, Fax: (61-3) 9761 9952

Elf Cocoon Australia, PO Box 405, Merimbula NSW 2548

Tesla's, 31 Jasper Terrace, Frankston VIC 3199; Ph: (61-4) 1899 0539

For assessment of electro-magnetic and earth energy in your home:

New directions Healing Centre, Ph: (61-2) 9415 2767

For Bach flower remedies and Australian bush flower essences, contact:

Australian Bush Flower Essences, 45 Booralie Road, Terrey Hills NSW 2084; Ph: (61-2) 9450 1388

Martin and Pleasance, 123 Dover Street, Richmond VIC 3121; Ph: (61-3) 9427 7422

To have a chart drawn by a professional astrologer, contact:

Federation of Australian Astrologers, PO Box 70, Northbridge NSW 1560

For information about full spectrum lighting, contact:

Interlight Australia, 20 Nulgarra Street, Northbridge NSW 2063; Ph: (61-2) 9958 6378

For information on paints and other house renovation products, contact:
Bio products Australia P/L, 25 Aldgate Terrace, Bridgewater SA 5153; Ph: (61-8) 8339 1923; Freecall: 1800 809 448
Planet Ark Environmental Foundation Ltd, Level 10/ 77 Pacific Hwy, North Sydney, 2060; Ph: (61-2) 9956 5500

For chelation therapy to remove heavy metal load, contact:
Omnicare, 2 Brady St, Mosman NSW 2088; Ph: (61-2) 9960 4133
Dr Ian Brighthope, Australian Detox Centre, Caulfield VIC 3162
Whole Health Medical Clinic, 31 Dunstan St, Clayton VIC 3168; Ph: (61-3) 9562 7558.

For information about water filters and water deliveries, contact:
All Clear Water Aust (61-8) 9228 8111
Aqua One Water Filters (61-7) 3890 2900
Crystal Clear Purification Systems (61-8) 8340 4344
Culligan Australia Pty Ltd (61-2) 9560 1900; 24 Hour Service Line: 1300 655 295
Neverfail Spring Water Co (61-2) 1300 300 204
The Freshly Squeezed Water Co (61-2) 9712 1022; (61-7) 3856 0988
The Pure Water Shop (61-8) 8373 2096
The Water People (61-3) 9885 0222
The Water Shop (61-2) 9956 5677
Unicorn Water Purification (61-8) 9242 1066
Water One (61-2) 9181 2983

For meditation and yoga classes, contact:
Siddha Yoga Foundation, 50 Garnet Street, Dulwich Hill NSW 2203; Ph: (61-2) 9559 5666

For ambient music and relaxation tapes, contact:
Phoenix Music, PO Box 98, Bondi NSW 2026; Ph: (61-2) 9388 0983

For DIY acupressure machines, contact:
ELF Cocoon Australia, Health and Environment Services, PO Box 405, Merimbula NSW 2548
SHP International P/L, 5/212 Glen Osmond Road, Fullarton SA 5068; Ph: (61-8) 8379 0700

For acupuncture treatments, contact:
The Jocelyn Centre, 46 Grosvenor St, Woollahra NSW 2025 Ph: (61-2) 9369 2047

For comfortable, attractive maternity & nursing underwear, swimwear and nightwear, contact:
Full Bloom Pty Ltd; Ph: 1800 068 870

For more information on hair trace mineral analysis, contact:
Interclinical Laboratories, PO Box 630, Gladesville NSW 2111; Ph: (61-2)
    9211 2200, Fax: (61-2) 9211 4409

Support groups for infertile couples include:
Access, Australia's National Fertility Network Ltd, PO Box 959, Parramatta NSW
    2124; Ph: (61-2) 9670 2380; Fax: (61-2) 9670 2608 (all states)

If you need help losing weight, contact:
Weight Watchers, Level 10, 98 Arthur Street, North Sydney NSW 2060 or PO Box
    1961 North Sydney 2059; Ph: (61-2) 9928 1300

If you have endometriosis and need support, contact:
Endometriosis Association of NSW, Hemsley House, 20 Roslyn Street, Potts Point
NSW 2011; Ph: (61-2) 9356 0450

For unbleached, chemical-free tampons and pads, contact:
Natural Fertility Management, 46 Grosvenor Street, Woollahra, NSW, 2025; Ph:
    (61-2) 9369 2047; Fax (61-2) 9369 5179
Rad Pads from: Jane Bennett, 70 Bowden Street, Castlemaine, Vic., 3450; Ph:
    (03) 5472 4922; Fax: (03) 5470 5766

You can get information on the mucus method of contraception from:
Natural Fertility Management, 46 Grosvenor Street, Woollahra, NSW, 2025; Ph:
    (61-2) 9369 2047; Fax (61-2) 9369 5179
Billings Natural Family Planning; Ph: (02) 9724 5769
Billings Family Life Centre, 27 Alexandra Parade, North Fitzroy, Vic., 3068; Free-
    call 1800 335 860
Families of Australia Foundation, cnr Belmore Road and Silver Street, Randwick,
    NSW, 2031; Ph: (02) 9399 3033

or on the sympto-thermal method from:
Australian Council of Natural Family Planning, PO Box 529, Forestville, NSW,
    2087; Ph: (02) 9452 5244

To be fitted for a diaphragm, contact your local women's health centre or FPA:
FPA Health, 328 Liverpool Road, Ashfield, NSW, 2131; Ph: (02) 9716 6099

Kits to help pinpoint day of ovulation are available from pharmacies:
Clear Plan, The Right Day, and First Response.

You can obtain a mucus microscope from:
The Jocelyn Centre, 46 Grosvenor Street, Woollahra, NSW, 2025; Ph: (02)
    9369 2047, Fax: (02) 9369 5179

You can obtain a Lady Comp or Baby Comp (computerised thermometers for timing ovulation) from:
Biotech Diagnostica Products Ltd, 29 Chantry Lane, Grimsby, South Humberside DN31 2LP, United Kingdom; Ph: (44) (0472) 356695

For more information on hair trace mineral analysis, contact:
Interclinical Laboratories, PO Box 630, Gladesville, NSW, 2111; Ph: (61-2) 9211 2200; Fax: (61-2) 9211 4409

Alternative diagnostic tests including allergy testing available from:
Australian Biologics Testing Services, 6th Floor, Fayworth House, 383 Pitt Street, Sydney, NSW, 2000; Ph: (02) 9283 0807, Fax (02) 9283 0910

Sweat analysis (available to doctors only) from:
Douglass Hanly Moir Pathology, 95 Epping Road, North Ryde, NSW, 2113; Ph: (61-2) 9855 5222

For a local source of Probioplex (lactobacillus from whey), contact:
Metagenics, PO Box 830, Hamilton, Qld, 4007; Ph: (61-7) 3260 3300, Fax: (61-7) 3260 3399; country and interstate: Freecall 1800 777 648

If you have, or suspect, an allergy and need help or support, contact:
Allergy Prevention Clinic, 1st Floor, Room 14, 370 Victoria Road, Chatswood, NSW, 2067; Ph: (61-2) 9419 7731

For advice on medical options for infertility, contact:
The Jocelyn Centre, 1/46 Grosvenor Street, Woollahra, NSW, 2025; Ph: (61-2) 9369 2047 Fax (61-2) 9369 5179

For advice on genetic engineering, contact:
The Gene Ethics Network, PO Box 2424, Fitzroy, Vic., 3065; Ph: (61-3) 9416 2222

If you have experienced pregnancy loss or the death of a child, contact:
Pen-Parents of Australia, PO Box 574, Belconnen, ACT, 2616;
Sudden Infant Death Association, Freecall 1800 651 186
SANDS (Stillbirth and Neonatal Death Support) in your state

GLOSSARY

A complete glossary would read like a medical dictionary. Terms listed here are those which are not explained in the text. If a word is not in this list, please consult the index. The definition will be found on the page which is indicated by a **bold** number.

abortifacient: a substance which can cause an abortion.

ACE inhibitor: a class of drug used in the treatment of high blood pressure.

Acidophilus: a type of bacteria present in yoghurt/used to re-establish normal bowel flora.

adrenals: glands situated above the kidneys, which are involved in stress response.

agglutination: clumping or sticking together (as of sperm).

aldosterone: a hormone secreted by the adrenals, responsible for maintaining electrolyte balance in the body.

amnionitis: inflammation of the amniotic membrane.

anaerobes: organisms that survive in the absence of oxygen.

androgen: any substance that acts as a male sex hormone.

antibodies: substances formed by the body in response to the presence of antigen/allergen.

antihypertensive: a substance used to reduce high blood pressure.

artificial insemination: an assisted conception procedure—donor sperm used in AID (artificial insemination donor), husband's in AIH (artificial insemination husband).

benzodiazepine: a class of tranquilliser (e.g. Valium, Serepax).

beta-blocker: a class of drug used to treat high blood pressure.

Bifidus: a type of bacteria present in yoghurt/used to re-establish normal bowel flora.

calcium channel blocker: a class of drug used to treat high blood pressure.

carcinogen: a substance that can cause cancer.

cardiovascular: of the heart and blood vessels.

cerebral palsy: spastic paralysis.

cervicitis: inflammation of the cervix.

cervix: the neck of the uterus, which projects into the upper part of the vagina.

coeliac condition: a sensitivity to gluten, leading to a malabsorption of fats.

colitis: inflammation of the colon (lower bowel).

congenital defect: a defect present from birth.

conjunctivitis: inflammation of the membrane covering the eyelids and front of the eye.

corticosteroid: a hormone formed by the adrenals, or a similar synthetic derivative.

Crohn's disease: inflammation of the intestines.

cystic fibrosis: a hereditary defect of various glands, including the mucous glands of bronchi.

dioxin: a toxic product released during the manufacture of organochlorines.

diuretic: a drug used to promote the flow of urine.

diverticulitis: inflammation of small pockets in the large intestine.

ectopic pregnancy: this occurs when a fertilised ovum implants in a Fallopian tube, or elsewhere outside the uterus.

embryo: from time of fertilisation to approximately two months.

endocrine gland: a ductless gland which releases a hormone directly to the bloodstream.

endometrium: the lining of the uterus, which builds each month after ovulation.

endorphins: the body's natural pain-killers, appetite suppressants, mood enhancers.

epididymis: tubes in which newly formed sperm mature.

episiotomy: a surgical cut made in the perineum to enlarge the birth outlet.

erythrocytes: red blood cells.

Fallopian tubes: a pair of tubes that collects the ovum that is shed each month and conveys it to the uterus.

foetus: an unborn infant after the embryonic stage (i.e. after approximately two months).

fungicide: a fungus-destroying substance.

gastroenteritis: inflammation of the stomach and intestines.

genetic engineering: the manipulation of genetic material in an attempt to produce superior offspring.

germ cells: sexual reproduction cells in males and females—sperm, ova.

gestation: the period between conception and birth.

GIFT: an assisted conception procedure—Gammete Intra Fallopian Transfer.

haemoglobin: the red pigment of blood, which carries oxygen from the lungs to rest of the body.

herbicide: a substance used to kill plants (notably weeds).

hirsutism: an excessive growth of hair.

holistic: in medicine, treating the whole person.

homeostasis: the process of maintaining constant conditions within the body.

hormone: a substance released by endocrine glands to regulate the function of other organs.

hydrocephalus: the enlargement of an infant's head by the accumulation of cerebrospinal fluid.

hyperemesis: severe vomiting in pregnancy.

hypoglycaemia: low sugar levels in the blood.

hypothalamus: a region of the brain.

immunosuppressive: a substance that adversely affects the function of the immune system.

in vitro: in a test tube.

in vivo: in the living body.

insecticide: a substance which kills insects.

IVF: an assisted conception procedure—In Vitro Fertilisation.

lactobacillus: a type of bacteria present in yoghurt/used to re-establish normal bowel flora.

leucocyte: a type of white blood cell.

lymphocyte: a type of white blood cell.

mastitis: fever and flu-like symptoms sometimes experienced during breastfeeding—not necessarily due to infection!

Ménière's syndrome: a disease characterised by disturbances in hearing and balance.

neonatal: of newborn babies (first four weeks of life).

neurological: of the nervous system.

nucleic acid: DNA/RNA—the stuff of genetic material.

offal/organ meats: products including kidney, heart, tongue, liver etc.

organochlorines: insecticides which break down slowly are stored in fatty tissues in living creatures and persist in the environment.

organophosphates: insecticides which break down more quickly than organochlorines.

ovary: the primary sex organ in the female.

pancreatitis: inflammation of the pancreas.

perinatal: the period shortly before, during and shortly after birth.

perineum: muscle and tissue bridge between genital organs and anus.

placenta: the organ by which an unborn infant receives nourishment from its mother.

postnatal/postpartum: after birth (as in postnatal depression).

prostatitis: inflammation of the prostate gland.

prothrombin: one of several blood clotting factors.

psychoneuroimmunology: the study of the effect of mind/emotions on immune function and general health.

pyrethroids: natural insecticides of low toxicity, although they may irritate the nose and throat.

RDA: recommended daily allowance, the dose required to prevent a frank deficiency state.

refractive: focusing (as in the eye).

scrotum: the loose bag of skin containing the testicles.

sinusitis: inflammation of the mucous membranes lining the nose.

sitz bath: a hip bath.

spermatogenesis the formation of sperm.

spermicide: a chemical used with a condom or diaphragm as a contraceptive.

testes/testicles: the primary sex organ in the male.

thrombosis: clotting of blood in an artery or vein.

trimester: pregnancy is divided into three trimesters—first, second and third—each is of three months duration.

ultrasound: extremely rapid sound waves used as a diagnostic test.

urethritis: inflammation of the urethra (the tube which carries urine away from the bladder).

uterus: the womb, the muscular organ in which the foetus grows.

vagina: the passage from the uterus to the vulva.

vas deferens: the duct of the testis, which carries sperm.

vasoconstriction: a narrowing of blood vessels.

vasodilation: a widening of blood vessels.

vegan: a vegetarian who eats no dairy/fish products.

ZIFT: assisted conception procedure—Zygote Intra Fallopian Transfer.

SUGGESTED READING

The published papers, articles and books which we have used as source material number in the hundreds. To give a complete bibliography would stretch our already large book and our publisher's patience. However, we are very happy to answer any questions (which should be addressed to the authors c/- Random House) regarding specific references. What we have included here is a list of books which can add to your knowledge and understanding. For comprehensive catalogues of reading material on related issues you can also contact:

CAPERS Bookstore, Ground Floor, Spring Hill Quarter, 454 Upper Edward Street, Spring Hill, Qld, 4004; Ph: (07) 3831 5400, Fax (07) 3831 5411

Australian College of Nutritional and Environmental Medicine, 13 Hilton Street, Beaumaris, Vic., 3193; Ph: (03) 9589 6088, Fax (03) 9589 5158

Environment Centre Bookshop, 39 George Street, Sydney, NSW, 2000; Ph: (02) 9247 2228

Nutrition

Bland, J. *Nutraerobics*, Harper & Row, USA 1983.

Cheraskin, E., Ringsdorf, W. M. and Clark, J. W. *Diet and Disease*, Keats Publishing, Connecticut, USA, 1968.

Davies, S. & Stewart, A. *Nutritional Medicine*, Pan Books, London, 1987.

Davis, A. *Let's Have Healthy Children*, Allen & Unwin, London, 1968.

Hoffer, A. & Walker, M. *Orthomolecular Nutrition*, Keats Publishing, Connecticut, USA, 1978.

Hume Hall, R. *Food for Nought*, Vintage Books, Random House, USA, 1976.

Jennings, I. W. *Vitamins in Endocrine Metabolism*, Heinemann, London, 1970.

Pfeiffer, C. *Mental and Elemental Nutrients*, Keats Publishing, USA, 1975.

—*Zinc and the Other Micronutrients*, Pivot Original Health, Keats Publishing, Connecticut, USA, 1978.

Price, W.A. Dr., *Nutrition and Physical Degeneration*, Price Pottenger Nutrition Foundation, California, USA, 1945.

Werbach, M. *Nutritional Influences on Illness*, Third Line Press, California, USA, 1988.

Williams, R. *Nutrition Against Disease*, Bantam Books, USA, 1971.

Recipe books

There are lots of wholefood recipe books available; alternatively, you can adapt many of your favourite recipes to comply with our recommendations.

Brighthope, I. et al. *A Recipe for Health—Nutrient Dense Recipes*, McCullogh, Carlton, Victoria, 1989.

Buist, R. *Food Intolerance*, Angus & Robertson/HarperCollins, Sydney, 1990.

Gaté, G. *Good Food Fast*, Anne O'Donovan, Victoria, 1991.

Marsden, K. *The Food Combining Diet*, Thorsons, UK, 1993.

Sichel, G. *Relief from Candida, Allergies and Ill-health*, Sally Milner Publishing, Sydney, 1990.

Herbal and natural medicine

Airola, P. *Hypoglycemia—A Better Approach*, Health Plus Publishers, Arizona, USA, 1977.

Chapman, E. *The 12 Tissue Salts*, Thorsons, UK, 1960.

Grieve, M. *A Modern Herbal*, Penguin, UK, 1977.

Ingham, E. D. *Stories the Feet Have Told Through Reflexology*, Ingham Publishing Inc., USA, 1951.

Kaminski, P. & Katz, R. *The Flower Essence Repertory*, The Flower Essence Society, California, USA, 1994.

Llewellyn-Jones, D. *Everyman*, Oxford University Press, UK, 1981.

Mills, S. *Dictionary of Modern Herbalism*, Thorsons, UK, 1985.

— *The Essential Book of Herbal Medicine*, Arkana, UK, 1991.

Ohashi, W. *Do-It-Yourself Shiatsu*, Unwin, UK, 1979.

Segal, M. *Reflexology*, Wilshire Book Company, California, USA, 1976.

Stuart, M. *Encyclopedia of Herbs and Herbalism*, Orbis, London, 1979.

Werbach, M.R. *Botanical Influences on Illness*, Third Line Press, California, USA, 1994.

Women's health

Airola, P. *Every Woman's Book*, Health Plus Publishers, Arizona, USA, 1979.

Boston Women's Health Collective. *The New Our Bodies, Ourselves*, Penguin, UK, 1989.

Cabot, S. *Women's Health*, Pan Books, Sydney, 1987.

Curtis, S. and Fraser R. *Natural Healing for Women*, Pandora, UK, 1991.

Federation of Feminist Women's Health Centres. *How to Stay Out of the Gynaecologist's Office*, Peace Press Inc., California, USA, 1981.

Grant, E. *The Bitter Pill*, Corgi Books, UK, 1985.

Harding, M. E. *Womens Mysteries, Ancient & Modern*, Harper & Row, New York, 1976.

Howard, J. *Bach Flower Remedies for Women*, C. W. Daniel, UK, 1992.

Llewellyn-Jones, D. *Everywoman*, Faber & Faber, London, 1971.

Melville, A. *Natural Hormone Health*, Thorsons, UK, 1970.

The New Women's Health Handbook, Virago, UK, 1978.

Parvati, J. *Hygeia—A Woman's Herbal*, Freestone, USA, 1979.

Reuben, C. & Priestley, J. *Essential Supplements for Women*, Thorsons, UK, 1991.

Shreeve, C. *The Pre-menstrual Syndrome*, Thorsons, UK, 1983.

Speight, P. *Homoeopathic Remedies for Women's Ailments*, Health Science Press, UK, 1985.

Tisserand, M. *Aromatherapy for Women*, Thorsons, UK, 1985.

Natural fertility awareness

Billings, E. & Westmore, A. *The Billings Method*, Anne O'Donovan Melbourne, 1980.

Drake, K. & J. *Natural Fertility Control*, Thorsons, UK, 1984.

Flynn, A. M. & Brooks, M. *Natural Family Planning*, Unwin, London, 1984.

Kass-Annese, B. & Danzer, H. *The Fertility Awareness Workbook*, Thorsons, UK, 1984.

Naish, F. *The Lunar Cycle*, Nature & Health Books Australia and New Zealand; Prism Press, UK, 1989.

—*Natural Fertility*, Sally Milner Publishing, Sydney, 1991.

Nofziger, M. *A Cooperative Method of Natural Birth Control*, The Book Publishing Co., Tennessee, USA, 1976.

Ostrander, S. & Schroeder, L. *Astrological Birth Control*, Prentice-Hall, New Jersey, USA, 1972.

Rosenblum, A. *The Natural Birth Control Book*, Aquarian Research Foundation, Philadelphia, USA, 1976.

Lifestyle/environmental factors
Elkington, J. & Hailes J. *The Green Consumer Guide*, Penguin Books, Australia, 1989.*
Hodges, J. *Harvesting the Suburbs*, Nature & Health Books, Australia, 1985.*
Ott, J. *Health and Light*, Pocket Books, Simon & Schuster, New York, USA, 1976.
Salminen, et al. *Safeguards (Home Chemicals Guide)*, McPhee Gribble/Penguin, Melbourne, 1991.
Smith, R. & Total Environment Centre. *Chemical Risks and the Unborn: A Parents Guide*, Total Environment Centre, Sydney, 1991.
* Contains safe alternatives to use in bathroom, kitchen, laundry and garden.
Colboin, T; Peterson Myers, J; and Dumanoski, D, *Our Stolen Future*, Little, Brown & Company, USA, 1996.

Meditation and exercise
Anderson, B. *Stretching*, Shelter Publications, California, USA, 1980.
Shakti, Gawain. *Creative Visualisation*, Bantam New Age Books, USA, 1979.

Candida/allergy
Alexander, P. *It Could Be Allergy and It Can Be Cured*, Ethicare, Sydney, 1988.
Buist, R. *Food Chemical Sensitivity*, Harper & Row, Australia, 1986.
— *Food Intolerance*, Angus & Robertson/HarperCollins, Sydney, 1990.
De Ruyter, P. *Coping with Candida,* Allen & Unwin, Sydney, 1989.
Vayda, W. *Chronic Fatigue—The Silent Epidemic*, Simon & Schuster Australia, Sydney, 1991.

Infertility
Edwards, M. (editor). *Stairstep Approach to Fertility*, Well Woman Series: The Crossing Press, California, USA, 1989.
Llewellyn-Jones, D. *Getting Pregnant*, Ashwood House Medical, Melbourne, 1990.
Nofziger, M., *The Fertility Question*, The Book Publishing Co. Tennessee, USA, 1982.
Pfeffer, N. & Woollett, A. *The Experience of Infertility*, Virago, UK, 1983.
Raymond, J. G. *Women as Wombs*, Spinifex Australia, 1995.
Rowland, R. *Living Laboratories — Women and Reproductive Technologies*, Pan Macmillan, Australia, 1992.
Winston, R. *Getting Pregnant*, ANAYA Publishers, London, 1989.

INDEX

The definition of a term will be found on the page indicated by a **bold** number.

diagnostic procedures, 93, 271–87, 357
  infertility, 339–43
diaphragms, 182, 190, 356
diet improvement, 27–30
  see also nutrition
diet pyramid, 18
dietary fibre, 101–02
diets
  anti-Candida, 24, 302–03
  exclusion, 314–16
  fad, 27
digestion and absorption, 60, 196–200
digestive system, 101–03, 303
dilation and curettage, **342**
dispersing, **155**
diuretics, 37, 69, 232
  herbal, 104, 232, 235
double tuck pose, 225
douches, 242
  herbal, 237–38, 241
Down Syndrome, 37, 64, 82, 186
drugs, 61–62, 68–71, 160, 352
dysmenorrhoea, **222**–27

EFAs *see* essential fatty acids
eggs, 22
electromagnetic radiation, 90–91, 354
embryo, 31
emmenagogues, **218**, 219
endometrial biopsy, **343**
endometriosis, **251**–54, 355
endometritis, **290**
environmental pollutants, 72–91
environmentally friendly cleaning, 85–86
epsom salts, 90, 105
essential fatty acids (EFAs), 21, 23, 24,
  46–47, 50, 214, 231
  supplement, 47
essential oils, 159, 221, 235
ethics in reproductive technology, 334,
  336–37
eustress, 144
evening primrose oil, 58, 231
exclusion diets, 312–16, **314**
exercise, 112–31, 162

Fallopian tubes, blocked, 256–57
farming techniques, 50–51
FAS (Foetal Alcohol Syndrome), 64–65
fasting, 27, 102
fats, 22–23
  saturated, 24
Feingold diet, 311

female reproductive health, 201–61
ferrum phos, 39, 58
fertilisation, 321–22
fertility drugs, 151, 333–34
fertility enhancement, 7
Fertility Solution, The (Toth), 289
fibre, dietary, 101–02
fibroadenomas, **250**
fibrocystic breast disease, **250**
fibroids, uterine, **258**–59
fish, 21–22
fitness, 112–31
flexibility exercises, 120–31
flower essences, 157
fluorescent lighting, 163, 354
Foetal Alcohol Syndrome (FAS), 64–65
folic acid, 23, 42, 44, 48, 56–57, 58,
  184–85
follicle stimulating hormone (FSH), **205**,
  206, 211
food additives, 24–25, 53–54, 310–11
food combining, 26
Food Combining Diet, The (Marsden),
  26
food intolerance, 309–10
food labels, 24
food sources
  anti-oxidants, 96–98
  nutrients, 47–50
  see also nutrition
Foresight Association, 2, 12–13, 350
free radicals, **95**
free range livestock, 21, 51
fruit, 20, 26, 87

gardnerella, 236
garlic, 231, 237, 239
genital warts, **244**
genito-urinary infections, 239–43
  clearing, 288–94
  male, 270
GIFT *see* IVF
Glucose Tolerance Factor (GTF), 40
grains, 19, 22, 52
grief counselling, 153
GTF (Glucose Tolerance Factor), 40

hair trace mineral analysis, 271–78, 356
heart rate, 113–14, **114**
heavy metals *see* toxic metals
herbal diuretics, 104, 232, 235
herbal douche, 237–38, 241